The Healing Path With Children

THE HEALING PATH WITH CHILDREN

An Exploration for Parents and Professionals

by

MARK BARNES

Viktoria, Fermoyle & Berrigan Publishing House

The Healing Path With Children:
An Exploration for Parents and Professionals

ISBN: 1-896702-00-7

Library of Congress Catalog Card Number: 95-62102

VIKTORIA, FERMOYLE & BERRIGAN
PUBLISHING HOUSE

FAX: 1-613-634-0866
P.O. Box 698, Kingston ON Canada K7L 4X1
Clayton, NY in the United States

Three candles that illume every darkness:
truth, nature, knowledge.

—From the *Triads of Ireland*, a collection made toward the end of the ninth century, C.E., cited in Meyer, 1913, p. 103.

Our greatest
natural resource
is the minds
of our children.

—Walter Elias Disney

Table of Contents

Don't be bound by tradition,
be inspired by it.

—From the Inniskillen
Wine Center at Niagara-
on-the-Lake

Acknowledgements

I would like to thank a number of people who have been inspirational in my life and in some way, through their existence, have influenced the writing of this book:

The family/tribe – thanks for the genes, eh! ...and for the support over the years. Moments with family bring laughter and renewal forever. When Irish Eyes are Smiling...

Christina Ruth (Gramma), whose eyes and heart were always so full of love. I will never forget your laugh and smile. You gave so much to so many. Your soul is truly of the Goddess;

Anna Dorothy (Ma), for teaching me about gentleness, kindness, laughter and sharing;

John Leo (Dad), for teaching me about endurance, laughter, kindness, thinking of others before oneself. I miss you beyond comprehension;

Ma tante Yvonne, whose kind and generous soul has touched many, *merci*;

Viki, magic, trust, loyalty, closeness, friendship, silliness, total unconditional love and always just being there;

Erin Meadow, silent depth in an extrovert, wisdom/intuition and feelings beyond your years, for saying what one thinks, giving to one's friends. I don't think it's easy being the firstborn, but you've done so well with it;

Rory Devon, silent depth in an introvert, for being a great travel companion, always stay true to your course, for technical brilliance beyond the norm (this book may never have been completed if you, at 14 and 15, hadn't torn the computer apart, rebuilt it and made it work again);

Conor Francis, for innocence, playfulness, gentleness and a refreshing ability to make me stop the world and just play and be. Your consideration and giving to others (even at the earliest age) has always touched me deeply;

Emily Anna, your calmness, gentleness, determination and wisdom pervades all around you, your laugh and Irish/Hungarian eyes will always light up the world;

Alex, sis, integrity, playfulness, and silliness. Your honest and intense approach to the world is always refreshing. Your brash and magical existence make this world a better place in which to live;

Fred Shuh, always a shoulder, always a friend, all anyone could hope for in a friend, in so many moments of need, you have just been there;

Stuart Beck, my longest friendship in life...through the years and tens of thousands of miles, always there, always a true friend, I miss you a lot;

Tom Turner, the gift of laughter and storytelling, a loving father to your family and husband to your wife. Our time together is treasured and it is an honour to call you friend;

Shige Morita, truly a man of honour and integrity...you are like an intense but quiet fire...meaning, peace, calm, trust, encouragement, I can never thank you enough for your support and belief in my work even when there was great personal cost to yourself;

Cindy Taylor...we have given birth to so many ideas and shared so much on our life path. To you and Ken I am indebted for the friendship I treasure;

Naomi Cohn...you are a wise one, bringing gentleness and magic to all around you. May sunshine and warmth always be in your life, even in the depth of Milwaukee winters;

Mike Simpson...close to a brother, we survived undergrad together and it survived us. I learned more from you than from the courses we were supposed to be taking. You brought peace to the turmoil.

Bridget Revell...when the pieces have fallen apart, you put them back together. Thank you for the walks along the journey.

Walt Disney...Tommy Makem...Booker T. Washington...Ben Wicks... John Brunner (The Chrysalids)...Dr. Charlie Barr (would that every family physician be like you)...Dr. Cesar Guajardo (you saved my life, took me in and became a friend—without you I may not be here)...Dr. Raymond Bush (likewise, you saved my life—I can only repay your kindness by giving to others as you have done)...Danny Kaye...Francis of Assisi...Jean Seasons (a high school English teacher who had such faith in me)...Thomas Szasz (thank you for challenging my thoughts)....

The information contained in this book is not intended as medical or psychological advice. For help in these matters, consult a doctor, psychiatrist or psychologist. If you are already under medical, psychiatric or psychological care of any kind for any emotional, psychiatric or psychological condition, you are advised to consult with the physician, psychiatrist or psychologist responsible for your treatment prior to taking part in any exercise from this book.

A DISCLAIMER

REGARDING MARK BARNES

A publication released early in 1995, entitled *Victims of Memory: Incest Accusations and Shattered Lives* by Mark Pendergrast includes a section (pages 341-347) that has caused Mark Barnes, the author of *The Healing Path With Children*, great embarrassment. In the above noted pages of the first edition of *Victims of Memory*, the author, Mark Pendergrast, used the fictitious name of Mark Barnes to describe a very unethical therapist who does everything from implant memories in MPD clients to sleep with clients and lead clients into thinking he will marry them or maintain long-term relationships with them. Unfortunately, it was not until after the publication of the first edition of *Victims of Memory* that the author and publisher of that book discovered that there is a real Mark Barnes, whose reputation had suffered from rumours that he was the therapist described in the book.

The real Mark Barnes is Canadian as was the fictitious character, and, like the fictitious therapist, he also recommends relaxation training, but only for the purposes of lowering blood pressure and decreasing heart rate as part of an overall program to deal with stress, not to get at what are referred to in *Victims of Memory* as "repressed memories". Unfortunately, such similarities to the fictitiously named Mark Barnes caused suspicion with resultant further embarrassment for the real Mark Barnes.

The fictitious name was derived from "thin air" and was not based on any real person's name. Unfortunately, following publication of the book, the real Mark Barnes suffered as a result of the choice of this name by the author. As a result of the fictitious name of Mark Barnes used in the first edition of the book *Victims of Memory*, rumours about the real Mark Barnes developed in certain areas of North America concerning his work, exploits with women, and so on.

The real Mark Barnes is in no way connected to the fictitious name used in the first edition of the book, *Victims of Memory*. The real Mark Barnes is a well-respected ecopsychologist and author of the book *The Healing Path With Children* and the manual *Self Discovery Through Inner Play* co-authored with Bridget Revell. He lectures throughout North America and the Pacific.

The real Mark Barnes was a co-founder of the Canadian Association for Child and Play Therapy and in 1993 received the CACPT Annual Award for "outstanding career contributions to the field of play therapy and the community", in 1995 was elected to the International Who's Who of Professionals, and in 1996 received the Annual International Play Therapy Award for "outstanding career contributions to child psychology and play therapy".

The author of *Victims of Memory*, Mark Pendergrast, has included a clarification of this unfortunate situation in the second edition of the book. And, the fictitious name of the therapist was changed.

There is an Oriental proverb that states that "trying to stop a rumour is like trying to unring a bell" but the publishers of this text are doing their best to help silence the rumours and idle chatter about this matter.

Preface

This is a personal, as well as a philosophical and professional, exploration. I do not see these areas as mutually exclusive, although I realize that many do. If you are searching for a text written in obtuse professional jargon hidden behind a professional wall, this is not the book for you. What you will see on these pages will neither be a facade nor a professional persona.

The writing of this book has involved an enormous internal struggle. It has been rewritten at least twice. The struggle involved a challenge to integrity. At first it seemed important to create a document which would be taken seriously in the professional field. In my mind, this means being able to back up one's statements and views with scientific data when called upon to do so. I realize this is unrealistic. Moreover, in actuality most of what exists in the mental health field is nothing more than personal belief system posing as science.

Further, as I wrote and rewrote the thoughts in these pages, I felt a gnawing and nagging emptiness whenever I left out the spiritual aspects of life. The truth was being trampled on, oppressed, all in favour of being able to publish a text that would be scientifically respected. However, such scientific respect usually involves a considerable amount of collusion. First, what tends not to be acknowledged very often, if at all, is that in the mental health professions very little is known about what actually does work. The field is still in the process of being born. All of its parts are not yet working well or together.

Some colleagues who have read this book have noted that "you're not going to be Mr. Popular after this one is published. Some of this is really treading on firmly held beliefs and, at the very least, is going to be considered radical and controversial." I was informed that I would be thrust immediately into the role of radical, rebel or bad boy of the field. I'm not sure I follow the logic. The natural flow of the argument is that to remain popular I should not write what I believe in. Apparently, daring to raise issues which question the very legitimacy of the field of play therapy is considered taboo. To me, the truth, not beliefs or theories, should be sacred. I must also remember the wise words of George Bernard Shaw who noted that the truth is the one thing nobody will believe.

Besides, with regard to a solid knowledge base in the field, there isn't one. Unfortunately, if you ask typical psychologists, social workers or other mental health professionals what they do and why they do it and how they evaluate their work, you will not tend to get very coherent answers. Following such a challenge, there is usually a great deal of stumbling and fumbling around with words like self-esteem, self awareness, ego strength and the like. A usual response will include statements about various belief systems – for example, the non-directive belief system, the gestalt belief system, a structural family therapy belief system, the play therapy belief system...all masked by the word model. Many of these belief systems are very cult-like and deeply threatened by any challenge, critique, or even mere academic questioning. Two exceptions to this may be the behaviourists[1], who do have a significant body of research to substantiate much of their work, and the psychiatric use of certain medications whose known actions and effectiveness have been tested[2].

Integrity is of vital importance and consequence for the healer. It is important for the healer to commit to daily practice what he or she preaches. Integration, personal fulfilment, passion, spirituality, transcendence, spontaneity, viewing life through the eyes of a child, sharing of love...these are all vital to the healing process. It is important to model wholeness.

As you wander through the words on these pages, I ask you not to stay "up in your head". Healing does not happen from words in the head. The gut, soul and emotions must be involved for resolution to occur. Things must be felt, not just thought through. Otherwise, one is left with an empty awareness. True healing occurs below jaw level. It must be felt at our centre, in our body, in our soul. There are many exercises in these pages designed for the healer who works with children. The exercises can be adapted for different ages of children, but do keep in mind, as written, many of the exercises are designed for the adult who is reading this material.

Every one of you who has picked up this book is probably a healer or potential healer, otherwise you would have shown no interest in a text entitled *The Healing Path With Children*. A person with goodness and kindness inside them has the potential to be a healer. True emotional healing comes from loving words, thoughts, feelings and actions.

I am aware of some glaring contradictions in this text. The first is that, on one hand, in professional work, I demand that, wherever possible, a professional have empirical support for their decisions. In the same breath that I critique new age trends, I will tell you that I believe that the use of herbs, stones, Bach Flower Remedies, prayer, and other esoteric methods will one day be found to be some of the ultimate sources of healing. There is a rather strange interweaving of empirical research and mystical thought in these pages. I am aware of this and acknowledge that this can seem confusing.

Another contradiction ultimately involves my basic beliefs about "psychotherapy". In general, I believe that therapy is for people who don't have friends, or, more precisely, the good friends, faith and hope they need in life. Unmasked and stripped of its mystification, therapy, as it is largely practised today, is basically a self-indulgent form of prostitution, or "the great white whine", as I have heard some refer to it. For a fee, a professional trades intimacy, emotional closeness and attention. But it is not real intimacy, any more than sex with a prostitute is true passion or love. A major difference between therapists and prostitutes is that therapists are often sanctioned by the state through procedures known as licensing, certification and registration. In contrast, the prostitute is, at least publicly, almost always frowned upon by the state and its representatives.

On some basic level, I see therapy with children as different. Therapy with children is for kids who don't have, or who haven't had, the caregiving they need. Therapy with children should be a form of nurturing and good parenting. Thus, one goal should be helping the real caregivers to become as good at their caregiving task as possible.

However, I do believe that there is a time and a place for professional emotional support for children and adults. During, after, or in preparation for periods of severe stress, a trained professional—or a professionally designed program that a paraprofessional can conduct—can be of great assistance. After trauma or major life changes, having a professional shoulder may save one's emotional life. It is not that I see no place for professional mental health intervention. My concern is with a self-glorified profession that does not have any scientific basis for many of the beliefs of its proponents. I also think mental health professionals are severely over-used in North America and some parts of Europe.

Although I in no way condone the activity that blanketed actor Hugh Grant with controversy—i.e., a quick fling with a hooker—I did appreciate the comments of Grant as he was peppered with questions following his arrest. When questioned about why he did it, his simple response was that he was not too worried about trying to figure out why he hired a prostitute:

> I might ponder on it but, you know, there's nothing more I can say than I think it was an atrocious thing to do and disloyal, and I can't beat myself any more than that.... I'm a bit old fashioned. I've always thought that if you read enough good books you sort it out in life without having to go too self-centred and internal. [I think this] is a danger to much analysis (*Associated Press*, 1995, p. 19).

I am often asked how I got into the mental health field or why I teach on mental health topics when I have such a negative view of the field. The truth is I really do not have a negative view of helping people, I simply have a negative opinion of many people who work in the mental health field and of many of the methods and philosophical underpinnings involved in mental health. I like to quote one of my mentors on this issue:

> Colleagues often tell me that they chose to become psychiatrists because they felt they were all screwed up and thought that it would help them put their heads on straight. They ask me why, since I am "hostile" to psychiatry, I chose to become a psychiatrist. I tell them: because I felt psychiatry was all screwed up and I thought I could put its head on straight" (Szasz, 1990, p. 184).

Footnotes

[1] This is not meant to be a whole-hearted endorsement for the behaviourist approach, although I do have a great respect for many of the methods of the behaviourist. As well, the scientific basis for the behavioral approach is admirable.

[2] Nor is this meant to endorse an over-reliance on medications in the healing process. My view on medications is that we should use as little as possible, but, wisely, as much as necessary. They do have their place when cautiously monitored.

A PERSONAL NOTE

It is a dangerous and faulty assumption to believe that we can remain apart from our work. In this book I will offer a personal/ professional perspective. These pages will reflect my philosophy, spirituality, my life and lifestyle. It is foolish to pretend to do otherwise. I think it is important to lay one's perspective on the line, up front, before we even start. Given the realities of any individual's existence, each person will have a perspective unique to his or her reality. I am a white, English speaking, heterosexual male. These demographic items have significant political implications.

I come from an Irish Celtic background and I see the world through the eyes of this playful, magical and mystical culture. Although my family of origin was not at all well off financially, I never went to bed hungry a day in my life, except of my own doing. I had two parents who cared about me very much and seem to have done everything in their ability to take good care of me. I had the fortune of growing up in a family where Gramma believed that love and the giving of oneself (as well as the use of herbs and stones) are basic tools of healing.

I was a very restless child and youth. Curiosity plagued me. Exploration haunted me. I always had to see new things and try new adventures and challenges. By the age of 16 I was on the road travelling a great deal. At 17 I ended up in El Paso, Texas and other areas of the American Southwest. I became quite ill. Fortunately, I was taken in by a wonderful Mexican-American physician, Cesar Guajardo and his wife, Helen, who kept me in their own home and the home of Helen's mother. I had the fortune at this impressionable stage of my learning to experience a true holistic approach to healing which involved the use of sand, herbs, desert work, chants and traditional medicine. In other words, I was blessed very early with an ideal starting point for the exploration, study and training for the life of a healer. I welcome you to this exploration....

Mark Barnes
Spring 1996

The Healing Path
With Children

PART ONE

The Needs of Children

CHAPTER 1

Introduction

INTRODUCTION
STRESS IN THE LIVES OF CHILDREN
CHAOS THEORY (IT'S THE LITTLE THINGS THAT COUNT)

INTRODUCTION

We are at war with our children. I'm not honestly sure if we mean to be, but we are. There is an unnecessary battle of wills. It begins before the child is born. Parents are asked if they want a boy or a girl, as if one is better than the other. The very fact that one wishes for a boy or girl means there will be battles. Suppose the child is not of the sex of choice. Or suppose the child is the sex of choice but does not cling to the rigid stereotype the parents placed on that sex. Does this mean such a child is valued less?

There may be a battle with the medical practitioner whose golf game or hospital's bureaucratic commitments and procedures necessitate that the child be induced at a set time so as not to interfere with anyone's life. Shortly after birth, many unlucky children are placed on a feeding schedule. These are some of the first of many declarations of war against children, nature and life that they will have to endure in their early years.

In this text I hope to give some guidelines for creating peace and healing wounds in our relationships with children. Our own children. All children. In *Part One* of *The Healing Path With Children* I will look at children's needs and some possible results of failure to meet these needs. In *Part Two*, *The Magic of Play Therapy*, I will be exploring the healing path to deal with unmet needs and pain, the metaphoric process of emotional and spiritual healing with children. As you proceed through these pages, keep in mind that play therapy is but one piece of a total picture. It is a very important piece, but still just one part of a larger process. There are other areas and people to deal with. As a child is involved in individual therapeutic work, it is important for someone to be involved with the caregivers, the school, maybe even the cornerstore owner whose window was broken by the child or the neighbour whose garden was destroyed. These other areas are not going to be explored in this book since the focus here is play therapy. This is not meant to imply that play therapy is in any way seen as more important than any of the other pieces.

Everything I talk about in terms of the techniques used with children could just as easily be adapted for adults and their inner children. I have used most of the approaches and techniques which will be discussed with boys and girls, men and women ranging in age from three to eighty-three. Obviously there are certain adaptations made for different age groups but, in general, there are few limitations in tapping playful or creative impulses in the healing process.

As I talk about healing, therapy and mental health, remember that the entire mental health field is relatively new. It really is barely a century old and play therapy/therapy with children is so new that there is no excuse for getting locked into dogmatic beliefs about there being "one wonderful model that works." Take everything you hear in the field with a grain of salt. There are mountains of theories and philosophies concerning working with children, but relatively few facts. Models are based on theories. Unfortunately, when much of a theory has been disproved, we are sometimes still left with the models based on false beliefs. A critiquing mind is vital for a therapist.

As we explore the different techniques, I emphasize that they are largely for the benefit of the therapist in his or her role of guide, helper, or healer. A truly skilled therapist could work with only the air and emptiness. Healing comes from the heart, soul, and spirit, not from certain techniques or models. I see techniques and methods as being like tools in the tool chest of a healer. The more skills or tools one has, the better one can adapt to new situations, difficulties or problems. These tools are also resources. The more resources, inner and outer, that we have access to, the less likely we will "burn out."

Do not feel you have to have all the "right tools" before beginning. You may never have all the concrete resources you could hope for but you will always have access to your own inner voice. I am always hesitant to give opinions on the "ideal" play therapy milieu, toys, supplies, equipment, room arrangements, and so on. I have seen professionals in the most wonderfully equipped play therapy settings doing a horrible job. The toys do not make the therapy. On the other hand, I have observed therapists in what appear to be quite inadequately equipped settings doing an extremely good job. The same thing can be seen in families. How many times have we heard the joke about the best gift a child received for Christmas was the box the toy came in. Kids get bored of someone else's preconceived toy. The problem with many children's toys is that they come with such a narrow focus that children get bored with them very easily (and this is programmed into many children's toys – if kids get tired of them, parents will buy more to keep kids busy, since they don't seem to like to spend much time with them). Empty corrugated cardboard boxes, on the other hand, are invitations to creativity. Kids can play endlessly with a cardboard box. First it's a fort. Then it's a stage for some production. Now it's a hiding place in the woods. Other great creative tools for kids include blankets and tables. They can turn the underside of the table into an endless array of settings. Cover it with the blanket and it's Robin Hood's hideout. Or perhaps Peter Pan's home in a tree. Tell kids stories and give them props. These are true gifts. Skip what comes inside the boxes.

STRESS IN THE LIVES OF CHILDREN

Children today have different stresses than they did two decades ago or a century ago. It is true that we have vaccinations now that prevent many of the old childhood killers like smallpox and polio. We have antibiotics that are, at least for the present time, effective against many infections like pneumonia.

At the same time as these developments have occurred there has been an insidious deterioration in the quality of emotional and family life for children. We know that the amount of time parents spend with their children dropped 40 percent between 1965 and 1989 and divorce rates continue to climb—accompanied by a misguided modern philosophical view that a child is better off with divorced parents, each of whom love the child, than with two unhappy parents. What is ignored in this argument is that any child is better off with a loving caregiving team of two. Furthermore, the help available from the extended family continues to decline and there has been a loss of religious belief and the support of religious communities.

In response to stress adrenal glands release cortisone, and continued high levels of cortisone hamper the ability to fight off both major and minor illnesses; the thyroid secretes thyroxin which can lead to insomnia and exhaustion; cramps, nausea, bloating, and diarrhoea result from digestive tract disruptions...the list is almost endless (Sinclair, 1992, p. 5-6).

We are in a culture full of stressed kids badly in need of nurturing care.

CHAOS THEORY (IT'S THE LITTLE THINGS THAT COUNT)

Chaos theory, from aviation meteorology, was initially used to describe difficulties in weather prediction resulting from "sensitive dependence on initial conditions" (Lester, 1995, p. 16-6). The word chaos is somewhat of a misnomer. It is used to describe the apparently random or unpredictable characteristic of weather development. The truth is that weather is not random or unpredictable at all. It would be more accurate to note that it is influenced by very small undetectable factors that can be so minute as to be impossible to calculate at this time. The "Butterfly Effect" is a description used to describe chaos theory. It comes from the proposal that a butterfly flapping its wings in the Orient could influence weather development in North America several months later. Chaos theory suggests that accurate weather forecasting may ultimately be limited to about two weeks due to the fact that a huge number of tiny initial factors can have significant impact in a very short period of time.

Chaos theory, as a complete concept, grew from the work of an atmospheric scientist and mathematician, Edward Lorenz, who was studying computer generated weather forecasts in the 1960s. He knew that astronomers had been able to apply mathematical equations to understand planetary and other astronomical movements. Taking into account many components and influences of weather development, he developed a series of equations to predict future weather. Computer calculations did actually come up with accurate short term weather forecasts and this accuracy seemed to confirm the view that weather repeats itself and, over time, follows familiar patterns. Yet, in 1961, Lorenz discovered that three month forecasts diverged radically from predicted patterns. In exploring the reasons for this, Lorenz found that minute initial calculations (to the fourth decimal point, or one ten thousandth) could drastically make changes in overall outcome. It was concluded that, as a result of the "Butterfly Effect,"

> all the conditions affecting a forecast can never be completely known, and as time progresses, a forecast will diverge further and further from reality (Lester, 1995, p. 16-6).

Chaos theory has major implications for the lives of humans and human behaviour. I think there is very potent food for thought in the notion that perhaps little things I do can have very serious and important results with major implications. Perhaps the fact that I let someone who looks tired in the grocery lineup ahead of me has more than just a five second, "thanks, that's very kind of you" effect. Maybe, just maybe, that person will leave in a better mood...go home...be more friendly to a friend or partner...and maybe also end up reading a bedtime story to his or her children...who then go to bed having had their needs met...and get up the next day...and behave at school...which makes the world more pleasant for the grade 1 teacher...who has been having a rough time lately...but after this particularly good day gives her sister a call...who hasn't heard from her in three weeks...and this really cheers up this sister who.... You should be starting to see my point.

I cannot overemphasize how very important I think these little things are. In terms of influencing the world, I am convinced that doing something that we think is really big and significant is no more important than the little day to day things we do and the attitude we have in approaching life.

CHAPTER 2

What Do Children Need?

INTRODUCTION

The question of what children need has been discussed at length in the mental health field for several decades. There is much we have learned about children, their needs and development. It is accepted that there are the obvious and basic physical needs such as shelter from the elements, a nutritious diet, and clean water. Many children in the world lack these. In our so-called advanced culture many of our children are also lacking. They are fed a diet of fast food, unhealthy snacks, candy and "sit in front of the television" meals. All too often their emotional needs are met in the very same manner as their nutritional needs.

Children in our culture have taken the back seat to narcissistic parental needs. Self-absorbed mental health professionals have only served to reinforce the view of "me first." Our children come second, or worse. Time and again we hear messages like "Our relationships must come first" or "If you don't meet your own needs first then the children will suffer." I believe such views grew out of deprived mental health professionals meeting their own needs.

Children should often come first. At times, our relationships should take precedence over our individual needs. Someone other than ourselves should come first. Over a period of only a few decades we have come to believe that I/me is God. We have come to view "my needs," "me," "I" as being of paramount importance. Anyone with that view should not be a parent, therapist or healer. Children's needs must often be put above our own needs. The belief that if I do not meet all my own needs first then my children will only suffer is warped. This simply reflects the large number of narcissistic and selfish people involved in the mental health field. The history of the mental health profession is largely a story of disturbed or emotionally deprived people from pasts where their own needs were not met: S. Freud, Jung, Adler, A. Freud, Horney, Murray, E. Erikson, Watson, Maslow.... The list seems endless. It is interesting that many individuals from nurtured backgrounds and/or those who appear to have been emotionally stable themselves entered the field through developmental psychology rather than psychotherapy.

There are cultures in the world where children's needs are met but they are not to be found in the technologically advanced world.

CHILDREN'S NEEDS

IDENTITY

The very first non-physical need is a name, a place to hang one's identity. It comes as a shock to many people that there are children in this world who have not had this need met—destitute, homeless, uncared-for children of the streets who were never even named.

> A name is connected to a child's soul and gives him or her an identity.... In fact, historians surmise that it was in order to protect babies that we developed the custom of naming them as soon after birth as possible (Dunham *et al.* 1991, p. 157).

For those children fortunate enough to be honoured with a naming, there are some things to consider in choosing a child's name. It is important to understand the future impact from the naming. Remember, the name should be an honour to the child, not something to fulfil parental needs. It is important that the name be easy to spell and pronounce for a child. As well, it is prudent to look at what the initials spell. Don't give the child an acronym that would prove embarrassing as he grows up; for example, Alexander Stephen Smithers forms ASS. Unfortunately, I'm sure there are many worse acronyms than "ass." Make sure you are not giving your child one of them. Caregivers of the child need to consider potential nicknames or silly phrases that could derive from the name given to a child. It also may not be wise to name your child after living famous people. Life has an interesting habit of throwing twists at us.

Certainly, honour the past, your culture, and ancestors in the naming of a child. If you are Celtic, find Celtic names for your children. If you have come from an African background, choose an African name. If Great Gramma Christine was a very loved and influential person on the life of the family, it would be wonderful for a child to receive her name. This brings honour and respect. It helps a child take an interest in his or her own family's past.

You may have a number of names chosen prior to the birth of a child. It is wise to have several possible alternatives. As odd as this may sound, you may have a name chosen for your child, yet when he or she is born, the name just doesn't seem to fit. Have several names available that you like. Perhaps you can have a definite name that you absolutely have to give your child (such as the Gramma Christine example). Maybe that will end up as the child's middle name rather than first. The child's actual full legal name should not be given until after the umbilical cord is cut, and, some say, not until the remaining cord has fallen off (about a week or two). While children are still physically attached to the mother they are still spiritually connected to the mother. I think children should be named as soon as possible after birth on their first day on Earth so they can start hearing their name lovingly cooed and sung to them.

Some rather difficult situations may arise with an adoption, especially with adoptions involving children who are not newborns. This child most likely already has a name. The adoptive parents want a different name, impose one and legally change the child's name. I strongly advise against this. It creates a scenario where the child's basic identity is rejected. Even the six month old infant has been called by the same name for a considerable period of time. Suddenly, that being no longer exists. In an adoption, should you wish to give the child the gift of a new name, add a name, don't take one away. For example, if the child had been Claire Elizabeth Barnes, the new name could be Susan Claire Barnes or Claire Susan Barnes, or perhaps keep the three original names and make the new name Susan Claire-Elizabeth Barnes. This is a very important point and is symbolic of acceptance of the child. Suppose the adoptive parents wanted a blonde child named Susan and the adoptive baby was a red-headed child named Heather. It seems absurd to think of constantly dying this child's hair blonde simply because of parental whims. Yet that is the very thing that is done to many adopted children in terms of their names.

I have heard a counter-argument that runs along the lines of proposing that the adoptive child is older and he or she, too, wants a new name. I still don't buy the argument. Let me put it in terms of a biological child. Suppose you had a biological child of your own and at the age of 8 he said he wanted to change his name. It is highly unlikely that any healthy parent with personal boundaries and common sense is going to allow it. Perhaps a name change is considered because of a painful past. I'm afraid you cannot erase the past with a name change. We have to come to terms with pain and learn from it and deal with our futures based on the past. This is where the gift of a new name, added on to the existing name, can be a useful process and can represent a new beginning for the older child—but only if it is his request in the adoption process. It must not be imposed by the parents.

A new name can represent a new beginning, a transition, a rite of passage. The people of many cultures and religions do gain a new name at transition periods in their lives. For example, a new name is added by some Catholics at confirmation. Many aboriginal cultures give a new name upon a member reaching puberty or adulthood.

As they grow, it is so important to allow children the space to develop their own identity. We need to hear our children's opinions about issues and find out what they are thinking rather than attempting to make them repeat our own view on such things as politics and philosophy of life.

FUTURE CONSIDERATIONS

Children need legal guardians, someone to take care of them in the event of the death of parents or present legal caregivers. If you have children, you need a will to ensure the care of your children in the event of your death. Don't do this as some flippant act to simply name your best friends as godparents. Really know the person or people who will be the child's potential future parents. Do they like children? Do they share your values? Will they understand the psychological and spiritual needs of a grieving child in the event of your death? These, and many other very serious considerations, must be taken into account in choosing legal guardians for your children to be included in your will.

Perhaps you choose an aunt and uncle loved by the family to be your children's godparents. What happens if they are too old to do a good job with your children if you die when your kids are eight and ten years old? The naming of legal guardians is a vital responsibility of parents. It is one that is too often taken far too lightly for reasons of laziness, a desire to deny one's own mortality or any number of other reasons. Your children should be your first consideration. Suppose the persons you have named as your children's legal guardians never come to visit, never have any contact with your child and show no interest in your children. If this is the case, it is time – immediately – to name a new legal guardian(s). There is no law saying you have to keep the same legal guardians throughout a child's growing days. You may have several. As your children grow you may find that they develop a very strong bond with some particular friend(s) or relative(s). It may be in the child's best future interest to have such a person(s) named as the legal guardian.

There is also nothing wrong with having godparents for the child and having different legal guardians named in your will. Let your best friends be the godparents but name the best possible person for your child as legal guardian in your will. Do not delay doing this. There have been far too many legal battles and tragedies in the lives of children to ignore this parental responsibility.

BASIC LIFE NECESSITIES/ORGANIC NEEDS

FOOD, AIR, AND WATER

What we put into our bodies to nourish or fill ourselves has profound long term effects. If you live on nothing but hot dogs and hamburgers then you will live a kind of mushy and greasy life. How we nurture ourselves nutritionally can be a metaphor for the kind of energy we put out into the world. If you give thanks and bless the food you eat and ask for a transformation of the energy from the living substance to be energy for your work as a healer, then whether you eat meat or the roots of plants you grow in your own garden seems largely irrelevant. Your metaphor of how this food gets processed within your own body would seem to me to be the most important factor in how it will affect you.

Children need and have the right to nutritious food as well as clean air and water. When we foul the Earth and the air and water of our precious planet we deprive and thereby abuse children. When we feed them a constant diet of fast food we deprive them of nutritional value and the opportunity to have social and emotional needs met over a family meal.

Clinical skills are not needed to meet children's needs in these areas. Careful conservation, political planning and natural resources management are the skills needed here.

On the individual and home levels there are many steps we can each take to make the world a better place for our children. Don't water your lawn to try and make it nice and green in the summer time and you save some clean water for future generations. Don't spray deadly toxins on your lawn and garden to get rid of natural weeds and bugs. Toxins that were long ago outlawed for commercial agricultural use are still available to the neighbourhood and home gardener. There is a mountain of evidence concerning the toxic effects of all these substances, yet millions of North Americans still religiously dump an endless number of deadly substances on their lawns. It seems that many households in North America wouldn't want a beautiful yellow dandelion blossoming amidst the green carpet of death and ruining the illusion of symmetry and orderliness.

Life is not neat. Healthy gardens aren't either. It has been found that when children play in backyards treated with pesticides and herbicides, they are four times more likely to develop malignant soft-tissue sarcomas than children who play in untreated yards. How we treat our gardens, lawns and yards will eventually have an effect on our children.

If you feel you must drive a car rather than walk, rollerskate, skateboard or bike, then it is a human responsibility to have that car in perfectly tuned condition to decrease the amount of pollution entering the environment. If you can't afford the maintenance costs of the car, then you shouldn't own the car. In my ideal world, the cost of every car might double but the cost would include full maintenance and repairs for the entire life of the car. Failure to maintain such care would invalidate both the ownership of the vehicle and the driver's license of the owner.

In our recreational activities we need to return to the Earth as much as possible. We need to question whether we really need the existence of the many mechanical and powered "toys" such as Sea-Dos. They provide an adrenalin rush for the participant but at a cost to the environment in terms of noise, trampling of the Earth or fouling of water and gases released into the air through internal combustion exhaust systems.

Political action is required by anyone wishing to lead a full and responsible life. Part of that political action needs to be focused on creating a healthy planet for our children. To paraphrase the microbiologist and experimental pathologist René Dubos[1], we shall not be able to solve the ecological crisis until we recapture the spiritual relationship between humans and their environment (Dubos, 1971, p. 403).

ACTIVITY

Being active is a natural state. We have entered an unnatural state when we have children living the bulk of their lives in front of a television set or in a classroom at a desk. Whenever I consult on issues concerning classroom problems, one of the first things I want to know is how children are expected to handle pent up energy in the class or school. No healthy or normal children will sit with their hands joined and a nice smile on their faces for any extended period of time in any classroom in the world. Children need a multitude of opportunities to allow their energy to flow in both controlled and chaotic ways.

There was a time not many decades ago when all of us, both adults and children, needed to rest at the end of a long day of work. Now, in our desks with a lack of movement, at the end of a day what we need is movement and activity. This is very true for children who have spent the day cooped up in school and daycare buildings. Many families have rules such as "no tv until your homework is done." I think we also need rules or guidelines concerning activity like; "no tv[2] until you have played and become exhausted from jumping, rolling, screaming, laughing, running and having fun."

REST/SLEEP

Both rest and sleep are extremely healing. They are vital to our survival. Rest and sleep are absolutely essential for health at all ages. They are too often devalued. It is not just our mind that needs a break through sleep. In this time of sleep our body regenerates, cells mend and repair as we literally heal during this phase of the daily cycle. Sleep and rest are great healers. Glockler (1994, p. 282) notes that it is crucial "that our biological clock, this wonderful system of interweaving rhythms, is given the appropriate care at home and at school." It is also noted that this kind of consistency in a child's life will also lead to a healthy interaction of the internal organs throughout later life.

Children of different ages need different amounts of sleep. The toddler between one and two years of age needs a good 10 to 12 hours of sleep at night and a nap during the day. Two to six year olds need 10 to 12 hours of sleep at night and a rest, not necessarily sleep, during the day. The six to nine year old needs ten hours of sleep at night and some quiet times during the day.

I have had many referrals over the years for children's sleep problems. When there is difficulty getting children to bed and to sleep, one of the first things I want to know is what happens for an hour and a half prior to bedtime. All too often I have heard statements such as "well, nothing really, they just watch tv." "Just watching tv" is quite a potentially disturbing activity. With most shows, there is a tendency to promote an adrenalin rush in the viewer. It is not going to be easy to get to sleep with adrenalin flooding the body. I advise that there be no tv for at least ninety minutes prior to the time the child is expected to be asleep.

> Television is a drug. Reduce the dosage by limiting children's exposure. One hour a day weekdays and two hours a day on weekends is plenty! ...More than one TV in the house is a step in the wrong direction (Garbarino, 1995, p. 171).

Getting to sleep should be a calm, nurturing time. To create a positive transition from waking to sleeping we should encourage a pace change. This winding down time should also be predictable for kids by keeping it fairly similar every day in both time frame and kinds of activities. A lengthy, peaceful bedtime routine is the best way to allow kids to slow down from their daytime into a night of nurturing, safety, security and total, unconditional love. The period of a couple of hours before sleeptime should be filled with calming baths, water playtime, reading to children, storytelling with children, touch, backrubs, relaxing music and bedtime prayers. It is a time to begin refreshing and healing from the activity and excitement of the day. We need to heal from both positive and negative stress. Adults need this time, and so do children. I would highly recommend soothing bubble baths with lots of water and homemade bath toys available. Little empty plastic bottles, plastic bowls and spoons, plastic berry boxes, and maybe some commercial toy like a little "rubber duckie" are all the child needs. Children's bubble baths are available from many bath and scent shops like *Soapberry* and *The Body Shop.*

This time should be followed with the bedtime dressing routine involving things like "jammies," slippers, housecoat, and perhaps the inclusion of dressing the favourite teddy bear for bed as well. Before crawling into bed, there should be prayers or some kind of thanksgiving and reflection on the day. My oldest daughter, Erin, and I always did "dodays," quiet times after she got tucked into bed and we talked about "what did we do today" = "dodays." Next, quiet storytelling or story reading with the child(ren). Many children love to have stories told to their teddy bears as well as to themselves. Children of all ages love their stories and crave this time with their caregivers. When we deprive them of this, we are saying "you are not important enough for me to spend time with." Then, the all important back rubs, hand rubs, foot rubs, head rubs. Most kids love their massage time. The day should end with total loving images and feelings like a big hug and the words "I love you."

PROTECTION FROM DANGER/AVOIDANCE OF PAIN

To be in pain is a natural response to an unhealthy and unnatural condition. In an ideal world every parent would want to eliminate pain from their children's lives. Instead, many physically, sexually, emotionally and spiritually abused children grow up enduring pain inflicted by their parents.

As far as I am concerned, such parents forfeit all rights to bear further children. Anyone who abuses or neglects a child should be sterilized (castration for males and hysterectomy for females) to prevent them from any further reproduction of their own kind. This is not a popular idea in a left wing oriented culture where individual rights are given primary consideration and personal responsibility seems to come, if at all, as an afterthought. However, we have focused far too much on rights, and not enough on the welfare of our children.

Dennis Miller on the Emmy Awards took it a step further and caused an uproar in some bleeding heart social service scenes by directly stating that "the day you get to the point where you feel the need to hurt, molest or otherwise abuse a small child, well that's the day you should commit suicide." Dennis Miller made no apologies to the bleeding hearts about how the poor abusers are also victims themselves. We all make choices. Most people who are themselves victims choose to lead healthy, happy lives and contribute greatly to the world around them. Some people who are victims and some who are not past victims choose to hurt others. Some choose to hurt children. I wouldn't mind not sharing this world with the losers who choose to hurt children. I shed not a tear the day Jeffery Dalmer was found dead. I hardly considered him to be a human being. On the other hand, I was deeply saddened the day Danny Kaye died. I always thought he was more than simply human.

SHELTER/HOME

> When you know where home is you know everything.
> —Native healer

A roof, a bed, a safe place to nest—these are things that all living beings need. A child needs these. The healing process demands such a place. The healing process needs to become a shelter for the person involved.

As you read this, I would like you to take a moment to make yourself a gift of some drawings or other creative representations of a shelter. Get yourself some paper and crayons. First I would like you to draw yourself in a safe place. Take your time in this kind of exercise. There is no need or reason to move ahead quickly.

When you have finished this exercise, next create an image or picture of yourself being nurtured. This may be a drawing of a real nurturing situation or your fantasy of how you would like to be nurtured. Do this for yourself now.

Finally, draw yourself nurturing someone else. Like the previous drawing, this can be a real situation of how you like to nurture others or your fantasy of how you would like to nurture others.

Anytime there are drawing exercises recommended in this book, remember, the best kind of therapy is flexible to your needs. Healing must not be some dogmatic and externally imposed notion of how you should change and grow. You may not feel like drawing. The reasons for this are your own. Asking why rarely accomplishes anything. In my days of practise as a therapist I can rarely remember asking the question "why." To me, it is largely irrelevant. "Why" can lead to a great deal of self-indulgent meandering that accomplishes little or nothing.

If people are very self-conscious about their drawing or have a very negative opinion of their drawing skills, other options are available. It is wise to always have a huge collection of magazines available for pictures. Someone could cut out pictures and create a collage or a scene instead of drawing. Magazines like *National Geographic*, *Audubon*, *Harrowsmith*, *Canadian Geographic*, *Canadian Wildlife* and many others have a wealth of wonderful pictures that can be used.

This is an area where a tiny sandbox can be useful. People—children or adults—can express themselves with a visual scene without the need for any "drawing" abilities. Should you wish to use such a sandbox for your pictures...go for it.... Refer to *Chapter 10* on *Sandplay* for more information on this process.

Whatever method you use, it is important to have some image of shelter in your life. When we have such an image, we will be better able to help children with the concept of safety and help them in their own quest for a shelter.

A friend once gave me the gift of a poem. It was a deep, meaningful and transcendent poem, though not a long poem. It was a poem about friendship that simply read:

> Friendship is a shelter in the storm.

I think that poem could also describe home. Or, it *should* describe everyone's home. In our day to day life we need a safe place to return to, our home, a place where we can take some time away from the world. That place where the world stops. A time and space where renewal can occur. We can do it in our own privacy or with loved ones. Imagine the life of human beings where either they do not even have a home or where home is unsafe. Their home is a place to hide from. This is the life of many of those who enter therapy.

The ideal home is a shelter in the storm. Children's homes should be their shelter.

For those children who are abused sexually, physically, emotionally or spiritually, or those who exist amidst the chaos of physical violence with their mother being beaten, this shelter is lacking.

A true home is

- a shelter;
- a renewal source;
- predictable and consistent;
- playful;
- a place to laugh, have fun, be not serious;
- a place to cry, be serious;
- a place to begin our transcendence, to develop a positive spirituality and a relationship with the divine;
- somewhere that we do not have to look, appear, act in some preconceived manner;
- a place where we can be given and learn the tools for the nurturance of self and the nurturance of others;
- a place where we can learn from our mistakes rather than being chastised for them;
- a soothing calm amidst the demands of the outside world;
- a physical reality, a place.

In my own home, many things contribute to the above.... There are several canaries and other finches in our home. How we ended up with them all is another story for another time. There is also a dog, a Dalmatian named Abby, but she, too, is another story for another time. Suffice it to say that canaries are wonderful, cheerful, uplifting pets and having several of them around only serves to contribute to a pleasant environment. I remember when we were getting our first canary several years ago and we were learning all about them. We learned that, as living things, consistency is important for them. At night, it is important in their own little homes to be at a fairly constant temperature and not get a chill. Like most animals, they need their sleep and we make sure to try to let them have lights out at reasonable times. We learned how it is important, once they are asleep, not to scare or startle them by turning the light on and off or wandering in and out of the room. Even though they are in a rather large cage that would more appropriately be called an aviary, they also need to get out and stretch their wings, to fly free and play in bigger spaces than their own home. Within that freedom, boundaries are needed. When they fly free, it is important to close the curtains first. Otherwise, they may fly toward the brightest light source, the window, and injure themselves. So boundaries are imposed for their own safe-keeping.

The entire process of pet ownership can be seen as a metaphor for the nurturing that all human beings need. Pets are essentially and ideally given the home that every human being needs and deserves. I was thinking about the care I was giving our pets and I sat quietly one night thinking how this simple care is so easy to give, yet so many children do not get the consistency, boundary setting and nurturing that they need. It hardly seemed fair that many children lack what my pets get. I was sad with that thought. I was also happy that I was able to give it to my own children and our pets and that I had received it in my own life.

Many people in therapy and many therapists come from difficult and painful backgrounds and did not get what they needed as children. They may be attempting to reclaim old needs and have them met through the therapeutic situation. As well, many therapists try to meet old needs by tending to others. This is good as long as the therapists' needs do not interfere with their ability to be effective.

NURTURING TOUCH/SKIN STIMULATION

Touch is more than just a pleasant sensation. It is a biological necessity (Davis, 1991, p. 29). It is a major lack in the lives of many children and adults. This is both a basic organic need and an advanced life essential. We cannot survive with an absence of tactile stimulation.

> Touch is one of the central experiences of an infant, whether rodent, primate, or human. We readily think of stressors as consisting of various unpleasant things that can be done to an organism. Sometimes a stressor can be the *failure* to provide something for an organism, and the absence of touch is seemingly one of the most marked of developmental stressors that we can suffer (Sapolsky, 1994, p. 97).

When children cry they should be picked up and nurtured. I don't think the newborn or infant should really ever not be in arms. The child crying is crying for a reason, often only to be held. When ignored, when left to "cry it out," the wee one may sound like he or she is being tortured. "Nature does not make clear signals that someone is being tortured unless it is the case. It is precisely as serious as it sounds" (Liedloff, 1985, p. 63). Eventually, there is a decrease in the crying. The child literally gives up.

> If he is left to cry too long, if the response it is meant to elicit does not come, that feeling departs as well, giving way to utter bleakness without time or hope (Liedloff, 1985, p. 33).

The meeting of the touch need has been badly discouraged in many cultures. In our Western world the idea of ignoring the cries of children dates back many decades to the Victorians of the 1800s. In 1894 *The Care and Feeding of Children* by Dr. Luther Emmett Holt of Columbia University was published and proceeded to be republished through fifteen editions over several decades. This document influenced much North American government literature and publications right up until the 1980s. He advocated the elimination of the cradle (too much stimulation), not picking the baby up when it cries, feeding by the clock and avoidance of undue handling except for necessary cleaning and feeding (Davis, 1991, p. 33).

> Early in the nineteenth century, over half of infants died during the first year of life of a disease called marasmus, a Greek word for *wasting away* (Davis, 1991, p. 37).

These deaths may actually be attributed to a devastating lack of touch and essential physical contact. Holt foolishly "warned parents of the adverse effects of the *vicious practice* of using a cradle, picking up the child when it cried, or handling it too often" (Sapolsky, 1994, p. 91). Sadly, in orphanages, there were even more deaths.

> The majority of orphanages in the United States had close to 100 percent mortality rates.... Ironically, in the less wealthy orphanages, where the staff was often not up-to-date on the advice of this savant, mortality rates were lower than in the "better" orphanages (Sapolsky, 1994, pp. 90, 91).

Unfortunately, it has gone further than simply ignoring children's emotional needs. Culturally, we have actually been encouraged not to meet such basic human needs as touch. It is not just touch that is important. Motion is crucial to a child's development. It has been found that

> movement is essential for infants, particularly when combined with touching. The rocking or touching of a baby directs impulses to the specific part of the brain that stimulates development. This motion and subsequent beneficial development process continues until at least two years of age (Davis, 1991, p. 37).

Yet, Lisbeth Price, a well known nurse educator, stated in 1892 that the

> "baby should never be rocked nor hushed on the nurses neck". And this, of course, meant that mothers especially should desist from such practises also. The greatest influence in the campaign against the cradle was exercised by the Dr. Luther Emmett Holt...for more than a generation, Dr. Holt kept up his attack on the cradle...writing in 1916, Holt advised that the crib should be one that does not rock in order that "the unnecessary and vicious practice may not be carried on." One does not have to imagine the effect that the word vicious had upon so many mothers...the very fact that, from the earliest days of human history, mothers had rocked their babies to sleep in their arms was taken to mean that the practice was archaic (Montague, 1986, pp. 148-149).

Dr. Luther Holt himself cannot exactly be described as a full and loving human being. He is described as austere and unapproachable and not known to have even "said *good morning* to his secretary in the many years she worked for him, nor is he known ever to have praised anyone or anything" (Montague, 1986, p. 149).

Another major negative influence on modern child rearing came from John Watson, a past president of the American Psychological Association who in 1957 was awarded the APA gold medal for his contributions to psychology. Watson highly influenced the field of child care and child rearing. In 1928 his text *Psychological Care of the Infant and Child* was published. In it he paid great tribute to Holt and took Holt's work further, advocating emotional distance, lack of touch and the banning of affection. He reportedly never kissed, hugged, or held his own children, or even let them sit on his lap. At bedtimes he shook hands with them. This giant in the field of psychology influenced our world intensely in many ways from the methods of modern advertising to child rearing. Notably, his own children reportedly did not fare so well. One of his sons committed suicide and another spent extensive time in psychiatric care following a suicide attempt (Schultz & Schultz, 1992, p. 296).

Watson is hardly a mentor for the masses to emulate. He is described as having a

> penchant for violence: he often boxed with a friend until one or both were bloody, was much addicted to what he called "nigger fighting" (beating up blacks), and was arrested twice, once for racial brawling and once for firing a gun within city limits (Hunt, 1993, p. 254).

His theory of conditioned emotional responses, which did constitute brilliant academic work, was demonstrated in an experiment that can only be described as outright child abuse, perhaps even torture. The experiment, conducted with Rosalie Raynor, involved an 11 month only child who was conditioned with a fear response. Initially, the child, called Albert, was shown a white rat at the age of 9 months. There was no response. When Albert was 11 months old, the fear response was established through a number of conditioning trials that involved making a loud noise by striking a steel bar with a hammer behind Albert's head at the same time as he was shown the rat. It did not take long before the very sight of the rat would result in a fear response and the child "jumped violently, fell forward, and buried his face in the mattress...and began to whimper" (Hunt, 1993, p. 259). Watson took the experiment further to show that "this conditioned fear could be generalized to similar stimuli such as a rabbit, a white fur coat, and a set of Santa Claus whiskers" (Schultz & Schultz, 1992, p. 315). This was not a short-lived response.

> After a month's layoff, Albert was tested again, and, as Watson and Rayner reported with apparent gratification, he cried and was afraid of a rat and a number of furry stimuli shown him without any accompanying clanging of the steel bar. Shockingly – by today's ethical standards of research – Watson and Rayner made no effort to decondition Albert (Hunt, 1993, p. 259).

It seems absurd that Watson received the gold medal for outstanding contribution to psychology. Despite his outstanding contribution to baseball, Pete Rose was not allowed to be inducted into the Baseball Hall of Fame because of his gambling. I would argue strongly that, surely, the mental health professions should maintain the same minimal level of integrity as the sports world.

Fortunately, the true good that came from this evil experiment of Watson and Raynor resulted from the work of Mary Cover Jones. The abusive Watson and Rayner study led Jones (1924) to develop conditioning techniques that could be used to remove certain fears and phobia in children. Her

> study has been described as a precursor of behaviour therapy (the application of learning principles to change maladaptive behaviour), almost fifty years before the technique became popular (Schultz and Schultz, 1992, p. 315).

Empirical research has disproved the beliefs of both Holt and Watson. We now know that infant security is promoted by meeting early physiological needs immediately and consistently (Hofer, 1987; Reite, Short, Seiber, & Pauley, 1981; Pipp & Harmon, 1987). Specifically, it has been found that

> demand feeding during the first 10 days promoted earlier differentiation of day-night sleep cycles in the first days of life and greater stability in feeding behaviour and sleep-wake cycles – stability that persisted over the first 2 months of life. Infants who had rooming-in caregivers during the first 10 days had longer awake periods and longer sleep periods by the second 10 days of life. [It was] concluded that the responsiveness of the environment influences the organization of infant functioning from birth (Lyons-Ruth & Zeanah, 1993, p.20).

Tragically, both Holt and Watson have had considerable influence on our modern day child care practises. For several decades into the 1960s and 1970s their recommendations concerning letting children "just cry it out," not "overstimulating" them through loving touch and so on were actively promoted in government pamphlets given to parents. The rationale of Holt and Watson was that if you are nurturing to children, you will spoil them. This view was an extremely mechanistic one and saw children as little machines that could be controlled. Even today, many parents, physicians and mental health professionals subscribe to and encourage such cruel child rearing methods.

Touch, Touch, Touch

Children need as much touch contact as we can possibly give them. There is a mountain of consistent evidence as to the positive physical and emotional benefits of touch in the lives of children, on the physical and emotional development of the child and on their future intellectual skills and positive emotional functioning. Basically, a child cannot get too much positive touch. Emotionally healthy children will let you know when they need space and time to be alone.

One major reason that infants cry has nothing to do with being hungry or wet or in physical discomfort. It has to do with needing contact. There is a

> constant relationship between the amount and frequency of crying and the amount and frequency of nursing care: the more care, the less crying. Infants will continue to cry even when they see that they are being approached or when the mother calls to them. Such infants, however, will cease crying immediately when picked up and fondled. Affectionate tactile stimulation is clearly, then, a primary need, a need which must be satisfied if the infant is to develop as a healthy human being. And what is a healthy human being? One who is able to love, to work, to play, and to think critically and unprejudicedly (Aldridge, Sung, and Knop, 1945, p. 95, paraphrased in Montague, 1986, p. 197).

We know that in cultures where there is a great deal of physical contact, where children are carried everywhere, taken everywhere their caregivers go, there is a very low level of aggression. When children are a full part of the family and never relegated to babysitters, daycares, or electronic television babysitters, then there is a very low level of interpersonal violence. All children need to be held, cuddled, carried, swayed, rocked, touched as much as possible and taken everywhere their parents go. This is a very different view than early Europeans brought to North America. Missionaries, teachers, and others urged "Navaho mothers to give up those savage cradles and use cribs like civilized folks" (Montague, 1986, p. 369).

Research has found that sleeping with newborns and infants allows better physiological adaptation. It is theorized that the reason for this is that such an arrangement is "the best approximation to prenatal mother-infant physiological unity" (Sadeh & Anders, 1993, p. 310). However, this view may be a reflection of psychoanalytically influenced perceptions. It might simply be that babies have a crucial biological need in the present (never mind a return to the prenatal scene) that is met through touch. Even more important, it is reported that sudden infant death syndrome (SIDS) is "rare or nonexistent in cultures where cosleeping at young ages is common" (McKenna, Mosko, Dungy, & McAninch, 1990 cited in Sadeh & Anders, 1993, p. 310).

We also know that children who do not get the touch they need may tend to shy away from being touched later, even though they desperately crave it.

> They are much more likely to become violent adults than children who were given lots of physical affection.... Baby animals have been found to produce endorphins (sedative-like chemicals manufactured by the brain with a chemical structure similar to many narcotics) when in touch with their mothers. This suggests that touch deprivation and loneliness may be linked with drug abuse. According to psychologist Sidney Jourard, extensive physical contact may be a primordial sedative and tranquilizer (Sinclair, 1992, p. 3).

Liedloff[3] notes that

> in-arms deprivation expresses itself perhaps most commonly as an underlying feeling of unease in the here and now. One feels off center, as though something is missing; there is a vague sense of loss, of wanting something one cannot define. The wanting often attaches itself to an object or event in the middle distance.... [In adults there is an] unsatisfiable quality of their longing. They cannot remember its original form: their craving as infants for their place in their mothers' arms (Liedloff, 1985, pp. 110-111).

Odent (cited in Jackson, 1989) believes that separating mother and baby at birth, discouraging sleeping with babies and depriving them of physical contact lead to aggressive adults and aggressive cultures and notes that we only have to look at two of the most aggressive cultures of all—Russia and America—for proof of that. Prescott (1975), exploring modern and primitive cultures where infants have a lack of touch in infancy, notes that there is a predisposed tendency toward violence in individuals in such cultures.

Prescott (1971, 1975) takes it so far as to state that the deprivation of sensory pleasure is the principal root cause of violence. He believes that "a principal cause of human violence stems from a lack of bodily pleasure during the formative periods of life..." (cited in Montague, 1986, p. 225). It has been proposed (Jackson, 1989) that premature or abrupt weaning is the root cause of temper tantrums which emerge in many cultures somewhere between 18 and 36 months.

Pearce (1977) notes that bonding is facilitated through holding, body moulding and contact, eye contact, smiling and soothing sounds. It is strange that while in Japan it is considered pitiful and lonely for a child to sleep alone (Okabe, Takahashi & Richardson, 1990, p. 125), in North America it is considered somehow unusual to be close to and sleep with one's own children. For the benefit of our children,

> anything that blocks bonding should be avoided. Hospitals for delivery, bottles for feeding, cribs for sleeping, playpens and strollers for isolation, day-care centers for not caring, nursery schools for not nurturing, preschools—all create abandonmentand weaken the bond (Pearce, 1977, pp. 223-224).

This should not be taken to imply that if you gave birth to your child in a hospital you are a bad parent. Most good parents have had their children in hospitals. Nor does it mean that if you fed your baby with a bottle that you will not be bonded with him or her. Some of the most wonderful parents I know fed their babies with a bottle. What I am implying here is that each of these acts serves to block overall bonding. Children who are born in a rigid hospital delivery room, removed from their mother and kept in a hospital nursery—screaming for hours on end with no one paying attention to them, bottle fed on a schedule, left to cry it out in their own nursery, abandoned at a day care when old enough to go...will not have the stage set for feeling loved that children who are born in a birthing room, room in with mum, are breast fed on demand, and spend their days at home in the loving presence of a caregiver working in a garden or in the kitchen. The research is quite definitive on this matter. People's opinions and mythical beliefs may differ, but the truth about what is best for babies and children is clear.

So if your medical practitioner, or the local public health nurse, or health unit social worker, or anyone, tells you that you can spoil children by picking them up at the first sign of a coo or cry or if you carry them with you at all times and that if you sleep with them you are doing untold damage, you can safely assume they are in the wrong profession and should refrain from making any recommendations on child-rearing. It is cruel, vicious and abusive to ignore a basic biological, emotional need of children. Listen to your own heart and soul, not to some so-called professional.

None of this discussion on touch implies being indulgent with older children. Jackson (1989) notes that we "love" our children in all the wrong ways (none of which involve the early tactile contact they so desperately need).

> We love them so much that they are spoiled by the age of two. It would be better to let them be. "You don't have to go on being baby-centred," Jean Liedloff told me. If you keep saying to a baby "what would you like to do now? Would you like this, or would you rather have that?" you drive them up the wall, and their response is anger. They can't express to you that you're not supposed to be doing this (Jackson, 1989, p. 158).

Children become independent, not from being pushed out, but from having their early needs met, and then being allowed to unfold with minimal intrusion.

ADVANCED LIFE ESSENTIALS

A LOVING PRESENCE

Children need a significant day to day time commitment. I have often heard people say "I don't have much time left at the end of a day for my kids. It feels like I work all day, come home, do things around the house that have to get done and when I finally do have time left for the kids, it's time to put them to bed. So I always make sure we have real quality time at the end of a day." This is self-delusional. It is a denial of the fact that these are poor parenting skills and the children are basically neglected. It is also reflective of the fact that the amount of time parents spend with their children dropped 40 percent between 1965 and 1989 (Sinclair, 1992, p. 5). If that information alone is not frightening enough, it becomes terrifying when we consider, not just time, but quality time. It is estimated that, for working couples, the amount of quality time spent with their children each day is 3.5 minutes (Chisholm, 1996, p. 34)—yes, three and a half minutes. Many don't want to hear such words, but let's face it, if you can only swing 3.5 minutes of quality time with the children you bring into the world, you should learn reliable birth control practices or abstinence. You should not be bringing children into the world.

Children need, want and deserve *quality* **and** *quantity* of time. Quality demands quantity. I will give an analogy here. Imagine you are searching for a real quality car. You approach a dealership and see your dream car there. The salesperson tells you "Hey, I see you're interested in that car. I want you to know what a quality vehicle that is. It was made at the end of the week. There wasn't much time left for the crew to build your car. Instead of the usual number of days they only had 30 minutes left to build that car. But that didn't matter at all because the time they had was real quality time." I hope my point is clear and no more need be said about this matter.

During the Christmas season of 1993 I first heard of what I consider to be an absolutely appalling and horrendous toy. I was so personally offended by the idea, it sent shudders up my spine. Some company had designed a night lamp that doubled as a storyteller. All the parent had to do was plug in a story tape that the lamp would then tell to the child. I couldn't think of anything which we could possibly design that could better encourage emotional distance.

More recently, priming and preparing for the 1995 Christmas commercial spending frenzy in North America, I heard someone nicknamed "Dr. Toy" making her recommendations for Christmas presents for children. Although some of her rationale for choice of toys was quite solid, I was saddened that at no time did she recommend that the focus should be on the parent-child relationship rather than on the stuff we consume. One of her highest recommendations went to some toy that helps a child learn to read and spell. This kind of toy, which has recently been modernized, has been around for years. You press a button, the toy pronounces the letter displayed on that button. Well, the idea is great, but I was flabbergasted at the recommendation to buy some consumer item to say "a," "b" and so on (while sounding like a robotic computer). Why not recommend ideal books and games that parents could play with their children to help them learn to read and write? No, the consuming public was being advised to buy yet another electronic device that can essentially babysit the kids while providing a mechanical educational experience. I'm afraid what that child will learn is that Daddy and Mommy love you so much that they will spend money on you but won't spend the time of their own to teach you letters and words. Children need Mommy and Daddy, not some corporate marketed toy, to teach them these things.

With regard to spending quality time with your children, I do not believe that babysitters[4] are particularly good for children. An emotionally healthy, extended family is the ideal caregiving group for a child. Hiring a stranger or professional child watcher is a secondary choice that cannot meet the same qualities of a healthy caregiving unit and extended family. There is no way on the face of this good earth that a paid professional will be as bonded to the child as caring and healthy kin and close friends. There is, in fact, evidence that more than 70% of parents, when they get a chance to observe, through hidden surveillance equipment, how their babysitter is handling their children, find that the babysitting, at least, is neglectful and does not meet minimal standards the parents' expected and, at worst, quite often is downright emotionally or physically abusive (*American Broadcasting Corporation*, September 13, 1995). Olivia Gross Neufeld, a parent who is also a lawyer responsible for picking juries and considers herself an excellent judge of character was shocked when she and her husband had the opportunity to observe their own babysitter through hidden surveillance equipment. She and her husband discovered that their beloved sitter was abusing their children (*American Broadcasting Corporation*, September 13, 1995). This is another area where some left wing liberals have created an uproar about the individual rights of the babysitters being violated by this so-called invasion of privacy by being taped. My response to such professionals with this kind of criticism – go crawl back in your hole. The needs of children are far more important than the civil rights of the uncivil abusive babysitters. I don't hear these same civil rights people complaining about video surveillance of underground parking garages where they park their cars. Let's get our priorities straight and focus on the rights of infants and children who need to be cared for, rather than the rights of the adult babysitter.

If you are having any difficulty grasping what I am getting at here with regard to babysitters being a secondary choice to a healthy extended family, imagine this scenario. You are on a boat. The boat gets in difficulty and is going to sink. You are with your own child whom you love deeply and a child you are babysitting. You can only save *one* of the children. Which *one* do you save? Case closed.

The Quality Time of Family Playfulness

It builds strength in families when they are able to play together. The importance of sitting around a card table playing cards or some board game is the cohesion that such activity can build. Everyone sitting around playing a game means they are all facing each other. If a family really likes board games, it could be interesting if they took time together and designed one of their own. In contrast, if the family goes out to a movie, they sit in the dark, all parallel facing a theatre screen, and focused on the material on the screen, not each other. There is no opportunity to learn something about anyone else, hear anyone else's view or look into each others' eyes. When a family sits down at the kitchen table or lies around on the living room floor to play a board game or work on a puzzle, a nesting takes place. Other excellent activities for families include any arts and crafts exercises.

Many games have a number of secondary benefits. Games like "hide and seek" and charades bring a great deal of laughter and movement with them. The body gets moved around as the family gets closer. Children can only benefit and emotionally grow when such activities are promoted in their lives.

Although not necessarily playful, the serious activity of tracing one's own family history can be fun and build a sense of belonging. It also gives a sense of personal history and can mean time spent together in genealogical explorations in libraries, city registry offices, and graveyards. Life and death take on new meaning. For persons without a close biological family, they can trace their own history to the point where they chose to "adopt" meaningful persons in their lives as family members. I think I know my family very well but am regularly surprised by new information. A cousin of mine was doing some family tree work. My mother had written up a brief summary for my cousin describing my grandmother's entry into Canada. I had never known this little but very fascinating piece of our family history. Apparently, my pregnant grandmother, arriving from Ireland in the port of Montreal, had gone into labour. Concerned onlookers provided a modern day manger for her. Crates and trunks were piled around her on the docks of Montreal so she could have some privacy and there, amidst the chaos, she gave birth.

Another fun and touching way of being a family together is to seek guidance from the elders, the wise ones. I was always very close to my grandmother. A number of years ago when my grandmother was 80 years old I sat down with her over several weeks and tape recorded our conversations. I simply sat with her spellbound for many hours over many weeks and months and recorded information about her life, our family history and significant events she remembered.... the birth of my father while they lived in the rugged Algonquin Park while my grandfather worked as a telegraph operator for the railroad...the coming of the automobile, radio, television, wars, the depression, vaudeville, sneaking into burlesque houses as a teenager. Through all the talks of wars, going hungry, struggling to make a life, the death of her husband due to mustard gas in the war, his lingering deterioration until death and how Gramma felt that effected my own father.... There was only hope in her voice. She was such a positive person. I taped her when I did for I never wanted to lose a part of her. She was 80. She lived until the wonderful wise age of 92. What I remember about her most was how much she gave to others and her joyful laugh. Now, I have this tape. I listen to it every couple of years and still laugh and cry intensely when I hear her laugh. It was so life affirming. I recommend this taping activity to anyone who wants to increase closeness to another family member...a gramma, a grampa, a favourite aunt or adopted aunt or uncle, the neighbour who was always like a mother or father to you. You can do this with children. A teacher in a class can ask kids to make tapes of talks with each of the children's favourite family member, or take a picture or create a drawing with their favourite family member or favourite person in their lives.

FREEDOM AND LIMITS

These two really go hand in hand. We cannot have one without the other. Since the sixties, these concepts have been quite confused and confusing. Freedom came to be confused with license. For example, in the sixties there was a common phrase of "free love," meaning "free sex." To say "no" was seen as an indication of inhibition. This was one of the tragedies of the sixties. It resulted in an entire generation with blurred personal boundaries. What was ignored was that with freedom comes responsibilities, limits, boundaries. True freedom demands negation. In other words, it means I have to make choices, to say "yes" to one opportunity and "no" to another. Freedom does not mean saying "yes" to everything. The freedom needed in growing up is the freedom and right of the child to make increasingly independent choices. This does not mean blanket permission to do absolutely anything he or she wants. The freedom to choose exists within the boundaries of limits.

Many children of permissive sixties (and 1970s/1980s/1990s) parents are the most undisciplined, unruly, disobedient and ill-mannered brats imaginable. They think they own the world and have no sense of responsibility or respect for others because their parents did not demand this of them. This is a sad situation. These are kids who could benefit from a (metaphoric) good swift kick in the butt.

Children need the security of limits, boundaries. They need to learn that there are safe places. They are taught this when they are given limits and boundaries. Children without limits at home, at school or in the therapist's office are abused children. They are being given the message that the world is an unsafe place because there are no limits on what anyone does. Obviously, if there are no limits on the child in his or her world, then there are also no limits on adults, or what adults may do to children.

Within consistent limits, the child needs considerable freedom. Limits and boundaries will vary considerably, depending on the age and skills of the child.

A SENSE OF RESPONSIBILITY/INNER DISCIPLINE

Children in our culture are abused by being spoiled and deprived of the requirement of being responsible. When we do not require children to take an increasing responsibility for their lives and actions, we are depriving them of opportunities for developing inner discipline.

Children should have chores from the time they are old enough to walk. The early chores may be as simple as the expectation that they are capable of taking their own bottle out to the kitchen counter when they are finished with it. It is just a little task, but it says to the child that "your role in this family is important and you have responsibilities to fulfil."

As they grow, children can and should take on increasing responsibility around the family home. An early chore that most children are capable of doing is helping to clean the house. A two and a half year old is quite capable of dusting and beginning to learn how to scrub a floor and help with vacuuming. In fact, if they see you taking joy in self care for your living environment they will want to join you. If you are painting a wall they can share the fun of running the roller up and down a few times. All these things should be joyous sharing experiences that say "I care about myself and I care about my nesting environment." Pity the person who feels that taking care of one's domestic environment is drudgery rather than a metaphor for living in a well loved space.

The Issue of Discipline

On a basic level, children cherish discipline. They thrive when they know what the rules are and what the consequences of stepping over the line are. Discipline needs to be fair and consistent to be effective. It also needs to exist within an atmosphere of complete acceptance and love for the child. As James Dobson so wisely states:

> I am recommending a simple principle: when you are defiantly challenged, win decisively. When the child asks, "Who's in charge?" tell him. When he mutters, "Who loves me?" take him in your arms and surround him with affection. Treat him with respect and dignity, and expect the same from him. Then begin to enjoy the sweet benefits of competent parenthood (1992, p. 51).

Consistent discipline is a sign of stability. Children need stability. They need to know how far is too far. Without limits, children just keep racing until they are over the edge. With consistent limits, children learn that they can count on their immediate world. They know what to expect. When children have this in their life, they develop an inner security that will allow them to handle life's unexpected surprises as they enter adulthood.

One of the best forms of discipline is praise for good behaviour. There was some liberal trend that grew out of the recklessness of the sixties and into the seventies and eighties that stated that we should only encourage children, never praise them nor chastise them. Here in the real world children need praise. There will also be times when it is necessary to punish bad behaviour. It is a misguided parent who chooses to ignore all bad behaviour and recognize only the good.

Children need to be punished for wrongful acts. How are they ever to learn the difference between right and wrong if they are neither praised nor punished? I am not necessarily talking about using concrete rewards as praise, although the odd concrete reward does a child good. Nor am I in any way advocating physical punishment for wrongful acts—such should be a rare last resort. Generally, I am talking about the need for consequences for negative behaviour.

Discipline and limits should serve the purpose of helping children learn the inner discipline that will allow them to become an effective and competent adult. Thus, discipline can be overdone if the parents become too rigid. To become responsible and independent adults, children need to slowly test their independence. Parents who thrive on their own power are not acting in the child's interest. A child of such parents could easily end up as depressed or extremely rebellious.

> The child whose parents give him a balance of limits and independence learns to be secure in the knowledge that his parents will intervene when he gets too far out on a limb. These children learn that pushing forward can be harmful when it hurts you or other people. They learn that venturing ahead can be wonderful when it leads to discovery, invention, and fulfilment. Over time, they learn how to use their own judgment to decide when to push forward into unchartered territory and when not (Sanders, 1992, p. 98).

Having noted the importance of discipline, I should point out that it is no use preaching responsibility and discipline and modelling something different. Children need to have moral models. The parent must be a person of integrity who cares for others and who tries to do the right things in his or her own life. This means that parents should try not to make promises they can't keep with the child. In other words, when you say something to a child, mean it. Know what you are saying. Children not only count on our actions, they also count on our words. A child who is disappointed too often either gives up or gets angry, or both. For example, if you cannot take the child to the park later in the day, do not say to them "we'll go later."

When you are setting limits and the child asks "why?" about a specific limit, there will be times—for reasons of your own personal energy or time factors—that your only answer will be "because I'm telling you." This is not an answer that fosters inner discipline. It is more likely to lead to frustration and resentment. On the other hand, a question from little Danny like, "Why do I have to wear nice clothes to Church?" could be met with (obviously depending on the age of the child) "when you put on your nice clothes it says to people around you that *I am respecting this time with you*. It lets them hear you say *I want you to know that although I'm a kid and like to wrestle and play and romp in the mud, I also know how to take the time to make myself look really nice*. It is just another form of nice manners. And Danny, it is not right to just judge someone by what they are wearing, but the outward impression we give to others is a way of letting someone know we feel honoured to be with them. Remember how after Gramma died and lots of people came to the funeral? Everyone dressed up and Gramma wasn't even there. She had died. But people wanted to let other people around know that they really liked Gramma, and liked her enough to take the time to put on their best clothes for a special way of saying goodbye to her." That is a rather long and drawn out explanation. The younger child may not need such an elaborate use of words. But I believe that most children asking "why?" really want to know why. They may be stalling, but I think that more often they really want to understand your expectations. Take the little bit of time it takes to frame your expectations in a context that is both age appropriate for children and allows them to see a purpose behind the discipline and expectation. There is also an unspoken message in the above "nice clothes to Church" example that says "I will not let you show disrespect."

SKILLS OF TOGETHERNESS

Children need to develop the skills of togetherness. In order to succeed in the everyday world children must develop the basic social skills which allow them to get along with others. Every age needs to learn at its own level how to negotiate, how to get along with others and to work cooperatively. Social skills need to be taught by adults and learned by children. Manners are a gift that parents give their children and in turn the children give back to the world. Well mannered children can have their own opinion but they know how to express it with respect to the world.

The value of basic good manners is immeasurable. Children first learn and develop these manners and skills by watching those closest to them. Hopefully they will see these people being polite, kind and gentle with each other and being concerned about giving to others rather than taking.

It is also a good image for a child to witness two people they love disagreeing and accepting their differences in themselves and in others in the community. This is one of their earliest introductions to social skills.

In addition to basic social skills, there are also what I would call modern technology social skills—riding a bus, hailing a cab, calling for a pizza, reading directions on a map, playing on a soccer team, choosing and buying a gift for another child's birthday, making a dental appointment, sending flowers to a friend who is going through a difficult time or in need of a kind gesture, handling finances, operating a computer, obtaining information from the Internet. These are all advanced social skills which older children need to learn.

Caregiving and Caretaking Skills

Children need to learn to care for others. They need to see their own caregivers giving lovingly to each other and to those they love and their community. Just as parental and domestic violence in front of a child has a powerful effect of devastation, witnessing their caregivers holding hands or sharing a hug has a powerful effect in an opposite, positive direction.

It can only help a child to see caregivers give freely of their time in some volunteer activity in the community. "Daddy's going out this morning to help at the retirement home or the Humane Society" gives a clear message of sharing love with others.

Being able to ask for and accept being cared for is something best learned through modelling. A child seeing mum or dad or gramma being touched lovingly and giving loving looks to someone tells the child it is okay to be taken care of and to care for others.

A WRITTEN METHOD OF CONTACTING THE WORLD: EDUCATION/LITERACY

Illiteracy is a great tragedy in our culture and in the world. It need not exist. Without the ability to communicate in written form one cannot read a public transit system map, a newspaper, a menu, a death notice of a loved one, a birth announcement or thousands of other important pieces of communication.

Children in any culture need to learn and be given the skills to communicate in written, drawn or other symbolic form with other members of their own culture and the outside world.

It is my view that libraries should receive huge amounts of public funding. Much more funding should be poured into education and literacy programs. A great deal of parental effort should be directed to children's reading skills. This does not have to be time devoted specifically to teaching how to read. Better to model the joys of reading and the wonder, wisdom and pleasure that can be derived from books.

Wise parents spend a great deal of quiet time with their children reading to them as well as cuddled up side by side as each reads his or her own book. Every minute the television is on is a minute when the child is not reading, not playing, not being a child.

Ben Wicks, in his *Born To Read* (1995, pp. 19, 20, 21, 22), gives excellent pointers on helping children learn to read. They include a number of recommendations that are adapted as follows:

- Get out those football and hockey cards. Share the comics with your child (ethical comics, not just any comic).

- Show your little one that reading is fun. If you read, so will your child. There's no point in telling your son or daughter to read when you're sitting in an armchair watching tv.

◗ Scribbling and drawing are wonderful ways to enter the world of reading and writing. Have lots of paper and writing materials available.

◗ Don't forget to show how proud you are of your little one's efforts. The greatest art gallery ever invented is the fridge door.

◗ Go to the library with your child.

◗ When asked by loved ones and relatives what to give the child as a gift, recommend certain books or individual volumes from collections.

◗ It is never too early to start. Leave books around the baby's bed. Have books everywhere in the house.

◗ Have fun with storytelling. Make sounds and songs to go along with the stories.

◗ When reading with a child, no interruptions are allowed. If the phone rings, let it. The person you're with is the most important person in the world – your child.

◗ Kids love rhymes and poetry. Don't forget silly books like *Cat in the Hat* and other such playful adventures.

◗ When the child has lost interest in reading, maybe it's time for a sing-song. Make up silly songs with words that apply to the child's life.

◗ Take books on family outings. Always have them in a bag in the car or in a bag you take with you on the bus, train or plane.

◗ As the child learns to write, remember that there are many ways of writing – homework, grocery lists, birthday cards for a friend or relative.

◗ Read at least 15 minutes a day with your child.

◗ Have a daily family reading hour, where everyone reads as the tv monster sleeps.

As far as I'm concerned, the best time to start reading to children and getting books for them is sometime shortly after (well, actually, even before) they are conceived. This little human being developing inside mommy will get an early start if mommy, daddy and others read them stories even before they are born. We know that children hear before they are born. They are also aware of mommy's moods. Daddy reading to mommy will be a benefit to both mommy and the unborn baby. It is irrelevant if the 1 month old doesn't have a clue what you are saying. They feel what you are saying even if the words are irrelevant. Books like *Love You Forever* and *The Velveteen Rabbit* will surely be felt by everyone in their heart and soul.

Remember that many regular activities can encourage children to read. Cook and bake with children. Read the recipes and the ingredients in containers to them. This brings the added benefit of the fun of creating a nurturing food. There are many other reading "locations": street signs, maps, grocery store signs, comics, bills, *even* the tv guide.

The Issue of Television

It is a tragedy that

> in 1990, $1 billion was spent on children's books; eight times that was spent on children's war toys, most of which are linked to TV cartoons (Bennett & Bennett, 1994, p. 13).

By 1981, in a three year period alone, the amount of expenditures of video games increased from $200 million to over $4 billion. Basically, if you want to discourage reading and the development of both creativity and literacy skills, turn on the tv.

> "Television is one of the single greatest impediments to full literacy in society today," says Dr. Maryanne Wolf, a developmental psycholinguist and neuropsychologist at Tufts University. "It, along with video games, represents the most insidious challenge to the development of imagination among children" (Bennett & Bennett, 1994, p. 12).

Television has some secondary problems beyond the simple issue of depriving children of reading opportunities, activity and play time. Much of the programming and many of the issues arising on television deal with intense adult issues. Daily, children are confronted with murder, rape, adultery, and numerous other adult issues whenever they turn on the tv. Certainly, some very good shows are available for adults (and you don't have to worry about what kids see on these shows) such as *Avonlea*. There are also good kids shows like *Polka Dot Door*, *Tiny Tots*, *Mr. Rogers*, and certain documentaries geared toward children. I would encourage children to turn on the tv and watch them. However, these are in the minority. The predominance of airtime features the nastiness, negativity and adult orientation of *The Simpsons*, *Beavis and Butthead*, *Beverly Hills 90210*, *Baywatch* and the like. Each of these is full of conflict and bitterness. Some of these may or may not feature social commentaries full of wit and adult sarcasm; nevertheless, is this the kind of thing we want to fill a ten year old, or worse, a three year old child with? Political commentary and satire have their place in the adult world, not in the world of childhood. Realistically, would you really prefer to spend your time with a bitter, sarcastic person/environment or with a kind, funny, loving, and gentle person? If you chose the former, you are in your ideal world, for that is exactly what we have in today's tv programming. You can get your fill any time of the day or night on television.

Unfortunately,

> children lack the social resources and personal power to deal with adult issues.... [They] face a special challenge with these issues because of their relative powerlessness... (Garbarino, 1995, p. 336).

Garbarino (1995), in discussing how television teaches that violence is an acceptable means of conflict resolution, notes that

> childhood ought to be a protected space for children in the economic, political, and sexual life of the community. When we allow the erosion of this protected cultural space for childhood, we permit the creation of one important element of social toxicity—and it happens daily. It is, some observers say, like "the end of childhood" when children are exposed to and drawn into adult issues and themes well before their time. There are many signs that this is happening. For example, many children faithfully follow TV soap operas, listen to raunchy pop music, and speak in

> the cliches of adulthood. Like many features of increased social toxicity, this erosion of childhood is hard to detect most of the time because it is so widespread. I notice it most when I happen upon a child who somehow has been spared, who vividly reminds me of what childhood was before. These children are polite. They are interested in the culture of childhood – toys and games, and books that are not preoccupied with sexual violence. Meeting such a child is a bit like looking at a family photo album from the 1950s (Garbarino, 1995, pp. 35, 36).

Basing his statements on hundreds of studies on television viewing and violence,[5] Dr. Leonard Eron asserts that

> "The scientific debate is over.... All types of aggressive behaviour, including illegal behaviours and criminal violence, demonstrated highly significant effects associated with exposure to television violence".... Based on his studies dating back to the 1960s, Dr. Eron also concluded that the more frequently subjects watched television at age 8, the more serious were the crimes for which they were convicted by age 30 (Bennett & Bennett, 1994, p. 6).

My advice: every one of us who has contact with a child had better monitor that child's television viewing closely. If I ever walked into a substitute care setting and there was commercial television on, I would have to seriously consider removing my child immediately. There is nothing wrong with a child in an alternate care setting on *a rare occasion* watching a taped age-appropriate, commercial-less, video or movie. That is very different from watching commercial tv.

> A committee of the American Academy of Pediatrics found that "the main goal of children's television is to sell products to children" (Bennett & Bennett, 1994, p. 14).

The purchase of their product is their focus, not children's positive personal, spiritual and moral development. Don't turn childrearing over to the television. If you do this, don't be surprised by what emerges later. What you sow, so shall you reap.

INNER PEACE/INNER STRENGTH

Confidence/Optimism

> As a parent, perhaps the most important message you must convey to your daughter or son is: "Listen to your inner voice and trust it. Listen to and learn from others but never let them undermine your confidence in your own judgment." Of course, you won't be able to do so unless you yourself believe it, and act accordingly (Szasz, 1990, p. 4).

For children to become confident they must first learn to trust their inner world and outer world. They need to feel cared about and taken care of. Children who have been comforted when in discomfort learn that someone cares about them. They learn that by reaching out and touching the world through a cry they receive some comforting action. They learn to trust that the world is a caring place.

For confidence to develop further, children need to be allowed to become increasingly independent. They need to learn through trial and error. At the same time limits need to be imposed for their own safety. The best limits for a child do not involve a constant barrage of "don't touch," "no" and so on. The best restrictions involve an environment manipulated by the caregivers in such a way that the child can explore extensively without danger. It is in the child's best interest to be allowed to get hurt in safe ways—a scraped knee, a bruised elbow from a fall. On the other hand, children need to be protected from greater dangers—matches, the heavy lamp's cord that children could use to pull the lamp down on their head, traffic.

Confidence will develop when children have the opportunity to explore, the encouragement to explore and express themselves, and guidance to learn from their exploration and mistakes along the way. Children who are so "safe" and restricted that they never are allowed to take any chances will not be able to develop confidence. On the other hand, parents who are able to stand back (with anxiety, perhaps, but they still stand back) and watch little Billy at his first skating lesson fall down (obviously the parent has also made sure Billy has a sturdy hockey helmet on for these lessons), struggle to get back up, take two steps, fall again, look frustrated, stand up, take one step, fall again and so on, are helping their child to develop confidence.

Consistency and predictability also serve to promote confidence in a child. A child's

> trust in the world will deepen with the knowledge that certain things will be the same tomorrow as they were yesterday and today. If, for example, she knows that her father will come up and read her a story every night, she will gradually lose her anxieties and will step out into the world with confidence.... [This] lays the foundation for her to become a reliable and self-disciplined adult (Oldfield, 1994, pp. 238-239).

As our children grow, we need to ask them their views rather than tell them what they should think or believe. Even young children need to be encouraged to form opinions of their own.

A positive side effect of confidence is that "when a child is at ease with himself he can gradually feel kindness and compassion toward others" (Masheder, 1994, p. 135). Some excellent guidelines for developing self-confidence come from Masheder (1994):

- Don't try to take over your child's life – his play;
- Don't be tempted into trying to think up ideas for him;
- Don't try to "entertain" him;
- Don't feel that if he is left to his own devices he will be bored. The child knows what he wants and what is right for him.

Decision Making Skills

Part of becoming confident means learning how to make decisions. Children do not develop this skill by constantly taking orders. They learn this by being given options and being shown how to work through options to make choices. The same approach that helps children develop confidence allows them to increase their decision making skills.

They will not do this if all decisions are made for them and if the limits are so tight they never experience negative consequences from stepping beyond those limits. This process of building confidence and decision making skills in children helps them become flexible and adaptable to life's many demands. They will really become complete human beings with endless resources to deal with life's demands. Should their available resources ever prove inadequate they will also have developed coping skills.

Optimism/A Sense of Being Worthwhile

To help children develop optimism they must first feel good about themselves. They need to hear when they have done a good job. It is important to praise children when they have done something worthwhile. They deserve to be encouraged to do their best.

Children will come to feel that they are valued and worthwhile when we joyfully include them in our daily activities. If it's time to give the bedroom a new coat of paint, include your two year old. Put a hat and gloves on them, carefully guide them as they hold the roller and let them run it up and down the wall a few times. Children enjoy helping with such adult activities. Let them know you appreciate their help and you really like doing things with them. They can easily help with age appropriate activities in the kitchen (stirring), and garden and with household tasks. Teach them to enjoy caring for themselves and their living space.

Optimism develops as children learn that challenges can be faced and obstacles can be overcome. When children fail to reach some goal or don't perform a task well, instead of trying to make them feel better by denying reality, validate their disappointment and teach them active problem solving. Guide them in explaining failures optimistically and accurately (Seligman, 1995, p. 15). Help them to see what they could do differently in the next attempt. Do not take over the task for them. That only gives the message "I don't think you are capable of doing this." Instead, teach children to master the task through small, achievable steps. Teach them to solve problems rather than turning away from difficulties. Seligman gives some excellent guidelines for children. These guidelines include:

- "Don't solve every problem for your child;"
- "Once you give your child space to solve his own problems, you must not be overly critical of his attempt;"

- "Model a flexible problem-solving strategy yourself" (1995, pp. 237, 239, 240)

On the other side of the coin, pessimism in children

> is not inborn. Nor does their pessimism come directly from reality. Many people living in grim realities—unemployment, terminal illness, concentration camps, the inner city—remain optimistic. Pessimism is a *theory* of reality. Children learn this theory from parents, teachers, coaches, and the media, and they in turn recycle it to their children. It falls to us to break this cycle (Seligman, 1995, p. 51).

Self Esteem and the Value of Hard Work

Research (Felson, 1984) has shown that children who value hard work and who work hard themselves and accomplish something will tend to have high self esteem. Self esteem doesn't come from constantly being given "warm fuzzies." Self indulgence comes from such an approach. You don't tell children who can't read how wonderful they are and what nice people they are (although these are nice actions) in order to build their self-esteem. You teach them to read. This accomplishment will foster increased self-esteem.

Many of today's self-esteem programs are badly misdirected. They leave one with the impression that if you fail, it is because you have low self-esteem. And, if you have low self esteem, some kind of counselling will assist you. This kind of thinking is based on a sixties pop, feel-good philosophy, not on any scientific evidence. In reality, the relationship between self-esteem and things like academic achievement are somewhat indirect and the reverse of what many believe. The important variable is effort.

> Self-esteem [is] indeed related to achievement, but the relationship [can] be explained by the relationship between self-esteem and effort, where effort [is] the variable most predictive of success (Felson, 1984, cited in Dawes, 1994, p. 246).

Since effort is an important variable in the development of positive self esteem, we need to find ways to promote it. It is true that changing one's feelings about the importance of trying can help increase the amount of effort devoted to a task. Another major requirement is time. "Our school system does not provide time" (Dawes, 1994, p. 246). Again, due to the influence of sixties narcissistic feel good psychology, the "proportion of time in school actually spent in academic work is much smaller in this country [the United States][6] than elsewhere" (Dawes, 1994, p. 247).

Last, but far from least, is the influence of parents. It should come as no surprise that a parent's attitudes to hard work and effort have a major impact on children's attitudes in these areas. If parents do not have a strong emphasis on the value of effort schools will, therefore, need to "concentrate on these attitudes, not on enhancement of self-esteem. If the parents won't reward or discipline, the schools must" (Dawes, 1994, p. 250). A good and effective parent will be one who fosters positive self-image through compliments and encouragement and who promotes effort by simply requiring it. For example,

> wise parents may require their children to devote a half hour a day to learning a musical instrument; children who do so originally under threat of punishment may come to find that they actually enjoy it and want to pursue music on their own – a process the late psychologist Gordon Allport termed functional autonomy. Behaviour originally engaged in to seek external rewards or to avoid external punishment may become intrinsically rewarding in its own right (Dawes, 1994, p. 247).

In other words, to promote self-esteem, promote effort, hard work, and accomplishments. Parents need to set an example, as do schools. However, the primary important factor here is parental influence. Without such influence, children will need some model in their life to encourage this. It may be through the school or a hero figure they can look up to. Some excellent examples would be people like Christopher Reeves, Buffy Sainte Marie, Booker T. Washington, Tom Hanks (and Forrest Gump), Roberta Bondar, Walt Disney, and Annette Funicello. It is also good to have local heroes – people in the immediate environment that can be looked up to.

This kind of proposition will obviously not be popular in a left-wing, rights oriented, pop-psychology circuit. However, research does support this view.

ECONOMIC SKILLS

Prosperity, like self esteem, tends to come from very hard work, not from laziness or complaining about how bad one's situation in life is. You could have two people from a similar difficult background. One chooses to use it as an excuse and is always tied to his or her background and never progresses anywhere in life. The other chooses to change his or her lot in life, works hard and becomes an entrepreneur, eventually works his or her way up from scratch and becomes the owner and director of a highly successful, productive and meaningful business. This is not some fairy tale; it is the real world for many successful people who have chosen to take their painful past for what it is—a painful past—and make something new for themselves.

Children need to be taught how to handle finances, even if there is little to handle. They need to be taught how to gain prosperity from nothing. As they grow older and develop the cognitive skills to understand them, children should be introduced to books like *The Wealthy Barber* (Chilton, 1989) and *The Richest Man in Babylon*. These are real living and beneficial metaphors toward success and planning for the future.

TO BE RESPECTED AND TAKEN SERIOUSLY

Violet Oaklander (1978) notes that children singled out as needing help have one thing in common: some impairment in their contact functions. She defines the contact functions as the methods we use to contact and make connections with the world. These include: looking; talking; touching; moving; smelling; tasting.

This notion of impairment of contact functions is similar to R. D. Laing's discussions of crazymaking. By crazymaking, I mean we teach someone to become crazy. We do this by making them believe that their intuition is wrong, that their internal perceptions are in error. You can find examples of this quite readily. Simply go to a shopping mall on any Saturday afternoon and watch. You will likely see several ways of relating. You may see a very angry child tantruming and being dealt with appropriately by the caregiver. It is important to point out that we can too easily become obsessed with the negative. We need to keep in mind that the world is largely functional. On the other hand, you may hear Billy being told "Don't be angry, you have no reason to be angry." Well, internally, he does feel some reason to be angry. So a powerful authority figure telling him he has no reason to be angry will only make him angrier and at the same time makes him question his own internal perceptions. Even worse is the same child being told "You're not angry." A variation on this theme occurs with the child who is crying. He or she may be held and nurtured and listened to. On the other hand, that child may hear words like "Don't be sad, you have no reason to be sad." Or worse, "You're not sad." This tells children that their internal perception of the world is in error and that only an external source really knows how they feel. The message is "Do not believe in yourself." Children gradually stop believing in themselves and any of their own perceptions.

Children need to be respected. We need to take their ideas, words, and beliefs seriously. When my son was about two years old, his baths were a wonderful time of play and silliness. This changed when it was time to leave the tub. One of us would pull the plug. If any of his toys were left in the tub, he would become concerned. He thought they were going to go down the drain, despite the fact that they were too big. The basic laws of physics had not been part of his learning at this age and rather than try to "reason" with him, I simply put my hand over the drain hole and let him see that I was protecting his toys by preventing them from being taken away down the drain. In this way all that needed to be accomplished was. We ended the bath time, the water left the tub and he felt safe and secure about his beloved tub toys. His world view at the age of two was respected and he continued to grow in independence.

I have great trepidation about situations where parents think they need to be the ones to decide when it is time for children to "grow up." I have often heard about a parent taking all of a child's toys and throwing them out or giving them away because it was "time" to grow up and to get out of that phase. Perhaps it was all their childhood dolls, maybe the favourite "blanky," or maybe some object the adult perceived as silly, dirty or stupid like the collection of sea shells, "worthless" rocks or old leaves. These treasures of childhood must be protected, respected and cherished for their great value to the child. Explore them with your child, don't arbitrarily get rid of them to help the child "grow." All you do in getting rid of these against the child's will or without his or her knowledge is strip him or her of respect by taking away something precious.

Rather, create special places for these treasures with the child. Perhaps a giant cardboard box can be gloriously decorated and kept in their room and somewhere inside this big "cave," "fort" or "clubhouse" can be kept some smaller box containing the child's treasures. When it is time (if ever), the child should be the one to decide when these treasures should go. I am thankful to my own parents for always respecting my own childhood treasures and never disposing of any of them, despite their questionable outward appearance to adults. My mother and father put up with more bugs, snakes, leaves, and trinkets than one can imagine. The only concern I can ever remember being expressed was by my father. I was about eight years old. I had a "collection" of several snakes in my room. They had "followed me home," carried carefully in my pocket. I then kept them in my room in a wooden box with a wire mesh top on it. But the next morning I went to look at them and the wire mesh top was ajar. The snakes had escaped and were nowhere to be found. I told my father. His wise response was: "Let's not tell your mother." Until she reads this book, that secret has been kept for decades. God bless both of you for your love and respect of childhood.

The antithesis of respect was seen one day while I was visiting a friend for lunch. She is a physician with a busy practice and I was dropping in to meet her to go out to a nearby restaurant together. I let the receptionist know I was there and then sat down. In came an adult couple and a child. The child was fidgeting a bit and was quickly told "If you don't stop that you are going to get your face slapped *so* hard." I felt nauseous imagining the impact of such words on this little human being. Here I was, an adult man, and I felt like I had been kicked in the stomach upon hearing such words. What impact could it have on a young child? And, what impact or worldview does it give such a child upon hearing it day in and day out? Really, who cares what the rest of the waiting room thinks of your fidgety kid? When I see a fidgety kid I assume they have energy to burn, not that they are misbehaving.

To follow up the above story, I quickly got in to see my friend ahead of any more patients and told her of the scenario in her reception area. She could then plan some little intervention with the caregivers about parenting skills and children's needs.

Kids need to be encouraged to feel and be in touch. Their feelings must be accepted and respected. We need to be spending huge amounts of time listening to our children rather than talking at them, telling them what to do. A child who misbehaves is likely the child who has never been listened to and who has been constantly and incessantly told what to do.

CREATIVITY

A professor named Maurice Moreau who taught in graduate school and for whom I had the honour of being a teaching assistant said something that I have never forgotten: "We are only limited by our own creativity."

We need our artists. We need our authors, writers, and entertainers. They truly reflect the soul of a society. We need to offer concrete support to our artists by funding their activities. The art of a culture tells us many things about the culture. We need to support the artist in our children.

We need to pay taxes to support the arts. We spend many millions of tax dollars on the social services and even more on the military, yet far less on the arts. I think this is tragic. Given the lack of empirical support for much of what is done in the social services and many of its methods and the fact that many mental health practitioners consider their work to be an "art" and themselves to be "artists," I think much of that field should have the unpleasant opportunity of finding out what it feels like to be funded as an artist. All the money presently wasted on unfounded mental health methods and expensive but unevaluated treatment programs would free up a considerable amount of funding for the true arts. I have a sense that this would be very beneficial for our culture.

It could easily be argued that we need a high level of military defense funding. The funding we put into education and the arts should be at least equal to that given to military operations. I'm sorry that I don't know who the quote came from, but my daughter has a great t-shirt that reads "It will be a great day when schools get all the money they need and the air force has to hold a bake sale to buy a bomber."

A child's creativity and spirituality are closely aligned. "The creativity of the child is the inner driving force for spiritual realization: a seeking for wholeness" (Masheder, 1994, p. 167). There is much we can do as caregivers to promote creativity in our little ones. The first thing we can do is turn off the tv. It only fosters passive absorption and a complete lack of creativity in a child's life. Next, let your imagination run wild. Let it follow the child's lead. Turn to the child for direction: "What should the living room be today?" Maybe it will be an enchanted otherworld dwelling place of the faeries, or perhaps a pirate ship. Maybe it will even be another planet where gnomes and puppy dogs are the only inhabitants. Do not try and centre yourself in reality when in the nation of makebelieve. Pity the poor child who grows up in the home where the living room furniture is covered in plastic. Better to assume that the furniture will take a beating while the kids are young and prepare to have it reupholstered or replaced after the kids are grown.

To foster creative thinking, have as many creative tools as possible and as few prefabricated commercial popular toys as possible. Have a creativity centre in your home. A cardboard box where the crayons, paper, glue, safety scissors, assorted bits and pieces of material, pictures, and leftover construction paper are kept is ideal. Having these kind of supplies easily accessible is encouragement to create. Make puppets out of old socks, pieces of felt, glue and/or needle and thread are all you need to start. You don't need the hundred dollar plastic table and chairs that tell a child how to sit and where to create.

Make sure there are things you can use to make music: old plastic containers of different sizes for drums; little bells and jingly things to make tambourines; tools to make different percussion instruments—pieces of wood, hollow gourds, hollow logs; a guitar if you know how to play; pennywhistles, pan flutes, old soft drink bottles filled with different amounts of water, and other instruments to blow in.

Dress-up clothes can be used to create different characters. These encourage both drama and role playing. Next time you go to discard some old shirt, dress or pants, first check it out for dressup potential.

This may be unrealistic and unfair, but try to take a year where you never set foot in a toy department. Instead of always buying toys, think of how you can create them on your own, or, even better, think of ways you and your child can create them together.

Put a number of standard items on a table and ask children what they can do with each of them. Encourage them to be creative in their ideas. You could try having the following available:

a pair of drum sticks;
cotton tipped sticks;
cotton balls;
a small pot and lid;
an old jam jar filled with water;
small pieces of wood;
some rubber tubing;
glue;
various kinds of paint;
crayons;
a few tiny wheels;
some small rocks tumbled at the lakeshore or seashore;
absolutely no instruction or "how to" booklets.

See how many ideas kids can come up with based on just some small collection like this. When you do things this way you start to open up children's minds to new possibilities. You take them outside of prescribed and prefabricated modes of thinking.

To encourage your own creativity and storytelling skills, spend a month of storytimes with your child when you never look at the words printed on the page. Just make up stories to go with the pictures. Practise this on an adult partner as well. At bedtime, make a commitment to each other to tell each other stories each night for at least five minutes. Obviously my hope is that the activity will feel so rewarding to each of you that it will grow to go on longer than just a meagre five minutes.

Each of these things serves to promote creativity in both yourself and your child or children with whom you work. If nothing else, these activities can be a great deal of fun.

QUIETNESS

Children need to learn the skill of being alone and enjoying themselves without being entertained constantly. It is a treat to watch well-adjusted children playing on their own in games and fantasies of their own creation. The living room may become their domain of fantasy.

Our culture is hostile toward nature and scared of silence. Relaxation training is an important part of the therapeutic process for children, as it allows and appreciates silence and nature. It is a skill parents and therapists can easily teach children. There has been extensive research on the relaxation response and relaxation training. We know that the ability to relax leads to a number of physiological changes such as lowered pulse rate, lowered blood pressure, reduced muscle tension and increased parasympathetic nervous system activity. It is not possible physiologically to be both relaxed and anxious at the same time (Wolpe, 1958).

Relaxation is a technique which does not need extensive training to help children. It is deceptively simple and, perhaps for that reason, many mental health practitioners have missed its value. Relaxation training has been shown to be effective improving classroom attention span, academic achievement, handwriting and self-concept and to be useful in dealing with hyperactivity, behavioral disturbances, asthma, learning disability, autism, anxiety management and insomnia (Fish, 1988).

Relaxation Instruction

As already pointed out, with the skill of being able to relax comes many benefits. There is no particular age at which we should begin this training with children. It is important to assess if a child is ready and able to be involved in relaxation training, especially with younger or special needs children. I would use a modification of a simple assessment method (Cautela & Groden, 1978) to determine if children can participate in relaxation training. This technique involves some simple instructions in determining children's readiness. They have to be able to sit still, maintain eye contact, imitate movements and follow instructions.

> First the child is asked to sit still: "Gabrielle, I want you to sit on the chair while I count to five." The child is given three trials with this instruction. The goal is to sit still for five seconds.

> Next they are told: "Gabrielle, look at me." With this instruction we are assessing if they can maintain eye contact for three seconds. Once again they are given three trials at this instruction.
>
> If they are capable of following the first two instructions, they are then assessed for the ability to imitate three different kinds of movements. I want to make sure they can imitate movements involving an extension outside their body into "nothingness." To determine this, I reach up into the sky then I ask them to do what I am doing and reach their hand out as if they are trying to touch a star. The other two kinds of movements involve reaching to actually touch something concrete. I reach out and tap the table and ask them to do the same. Then I touch myself in some way. For example, I take my right hand and touch my left shoulder and ask them to copy what I do. From these three simple exercises I am able to determine if they can imitate three kinds of movements: reaching out toward the abstract, reaching out and touching something concrete outside of oneself, and also touching within one's own boundaries.
>
> If they have been able to do each of the previous steps, the final instructions involve the ability to follow instructions without demonstration. I would ask: "Gabrielle, I want you to stand up from your chair. Now sit down. Now stand up again and take some steps and walk toward the window.".

If children of any age can do each of the above, they have the basic skills for relaxation training and should be given every opportunity to learn methods of relaxation. It doesn't take a great deal of complex skills to teach such methods to children, but the results have far ranging positive implications. If you have trouble coming up with your own relaxation and visualization instructions there are a number of excellent resources on the market. Two that I would recommend would be *The Centering Book* (Hendricks & Wills, 1975) and *Spiritual Parenting in the New Age* (Carson, 1989).

The effects of relaxation training can be heightened through the use of other related methods such as breathing techniques, visualization of relaxing images, and calming music.

The setting used would be quiet, with gentle lighting. The kinds of words I would use with children in teaching them to relax would be similar to those which follow.

> Find a comfortable place to rest yourself in the room...let yourself get real comfy here...as you get comfy let your eyes slowly close and see yourself in a very safe place...no one can hurt you here...I am here with you and any sounds you hear are outside this room and I will make sure you are well taken care of as you are relaxing...first, I would like you to focus on your breathing.... As you are relaxing, let anything that doesn't feel quite right leave you now, let it go back to the earth where it is rendered harmless....
>
> Imagine that you are surrounded by a very calm, healing energy and when you breath in, you absorb this calm healing energy with every breath. As you breath out let your own goodness go out into the world...keep breathing in the calm, healing energy and let it flow through your whole body...if you don't quite feel comfortable in any way or you feel like shifting around, do that now...get real, real comfy...keep breathing in the calm, healing energy all around you....
>
> Now, as you breath in let this calm healing energy go to your head and let it fill up your head and eyes and mouth and nose and ears...let your whole head become heavy and relaxed...let yourself feel very quiet inside...as you keep breathing in this calm, healing energy...now move to your shoulders and arms and hands and let the calm healing energy flow into them as you breath...don't forget to let anything that doesn't feel quite right, leave when you breath out...now your neck and shoulders and arms and hands, right down through your fingertips are feeling all nice and warm and heavy...they are becoming very relaxed... keep breathing in the calm, healing energy...now move to your back and chest and tummy...let the calm, healing energy fill you up with wonderful feelings as your breath in...anything that didn't

> feel quite right, let it flow out of you as you breath out...move to your hips and crotch and bum and right down through your legs, knees and ankles to your feet and toes....
>
> Your whole body is becoming very relaxed as you breath in the calm healing energy...you feel very heavy and warm and safe and relaxed...let the energy fill your whole body and flow through your body and veins and cells so that inside and out you allow this very calm, healing energy to completely fill you...everything about you is quiet now....

At this point you may add some visualized scene or you may just let them experience the positive pleasure of being relaxed. The following example continues with a visualized scene.

> As you rest there very relaxed, I'd like you to think of some very soft, big and safe bubbles floating in the air...I want you to imagine that you are floating on top of one of these cloud bubbles...let yourself rest there floating...still surrounded by the calm, healing energy...filling you as you breath in...I am going to be quiet now for just a little while as you lie there relaxed and floating....

Allow a few seconds to a few minutes to pass, depending on the age of the child or children you are working with. Then continue,

> You are going to hear me talking again and as I talk I want you to keep your eyes closed. Do not open them up too suddenly, just keep letting yourself feel relaxed...let yourself begin to feel the floor underneath you and remember where you are and that you are in a room with me talking...remember how you got here today...let your eyelids start to feel lighter...start to notice the sounds outside of the room...come back to this room and try and remember walking in here today...keep letting your eyes feel lighter and lighter and slowly let them open so that you can again see the room we are in...there is no need to move or to say anything, just let yourself stay in that restful position for a few moments.

After this kind of exercise I wouldn't try to do anything else except help children see how they can use this in their daily life when feeling stressed. You have just given them a wonderful gift. Do not, under any condition, proceed from here to some painful emotional issue that remains unresolved. You've just helped them learn to relax. Don't spoil it for them.

Meditation/Entering Alpha

Children need time to quietly reflect, to "meditate." Patsy Cline sang, "If I could see the world through the eyes of a child." I love the music of Patsy Cline, but this song painted a picture of an all too rosy, zen-perceived world. Children are at the mercy of much hostility and negativity. They experience stress and depression. Many go to bed hungry, bruised, with weapons under their beds. If we can give them moments and places of peace, we have given them a great gift. The process of meditation for children means giving them an understanding of what it is to have a peaceful mind, to have a place where the world stops. This could also be quiet time, private time, perhaps just time without noise. During this time they can be looking at picture books or reading books side by side with a committed caregiver. Children who learn to meditate can improve their concentration. It can also build confidence and self-esteem. Certainly, anxiety is reduced. Being able to relax in this way fosters an independence that will be beneficial to children as they grow into adulthood.

Being in a meditative state is associated with what we call being in alpha. This refers to the state of consciousness where brain waves register at seven to fourteen cycles per second. Alpha is also associated with relaxation and dreaming. Mental alertness is associated with the faster beta state of fourteen to thirty cycles per second. This occurs when we are awake, alert, and involved in activity. This state is also associated with tension, excitement, stress and anxiety. On the other hand, deep tranquility, drowsiness and euphoria are associated with theta waves of four to seven cycles per second. The slowest activity occurs in the deep dreamless sleep state where delta waves of one to three per second dominate.

Being in the alpha state promotes and catalyses a personal healing process. In this state we become less restricted by categories, labels and daily expectations. We become open to non-ordinary realities, hope, inspiration and mystical visions.

Some people may wonder if things like meditation are congruent with their religious beliefs. I see meditation as nothing more than what many religions call prayer, "going into the silence" or quiet reflection. Even an atheist needs a spirituality in their life.

The word meditation is believed to be derived from the Sanskrit word *medha* meaning wisdom as well as the Latin and French words for measure. In other words, when we meditate we are quiet long enough to measure where we are, where we have come from and where we are going. Meditation is a time of simple reflection. I am not specifically referring to transcendental meditation here but to the simple process of stopping the world long enough to gather our bearings. It is in this place that we can begin to gain wisdom. True meditation is that reflective state similar to the silence of a Religious Society of Friends (Quaker) meeting or of prayer. It is that silent spot of the numinous, a spiritual place to gather our bearings. Going to this place should offend neither the atheist nor the highly religious person. To the atheist it could be that quiet time to transcend the rigorous demands of everyday life. To the Christian it would be that holy reflective moment of prayer. Gregorian Chants catalyze a natural entrance into such a state.

Meditation with children is a procedure whereby they focus attention, thoughts and feelings on a subject, thought or theme. They may simply look at a mandala symbol and let their thoughts flow into the image. The word *mandala* is from the Sanskrit word meaning circle. In its modern usage, the word mandala tends to imply circular images with a balanced or symmetrical feel to them. Often they have a quaternal division, appearing in some geometric form such as a cross, star, hexagon, octagon, or spiral. In some forms of meditation they are used as visual aids. They are also believed to have a calming and balancing effect psychologically. For example, Jung believed that the mandala image may be drawn by a child, traced in the sand or show up in a dream when that individual is highly stressed to the point of psychic disorientation. The orderly

> pattern imposed by a circular image of this kind compensates the disorder and confusion of the psychic state – namely, through the construction of a central point to which everything is related, or by a concentric arrangement of the disordered multiplicity and of

> contradictory and irreconcilable elements.[7] This is evidently an attempt at self-healing on the part of Nature, which does not spring from conscious reflection but from an instinctive impulse (Jung, 1972, pp. 3-4).

When we teach children to meditate we give them an understanding of what it is to have a peaceful mind. Peace of mind can also be nurtured by letting children play quietly by themselves. They can be encouraged to look at and read books rather than television. Two year olds should have library cards and make regular trips to the library with a caregiver. Instead of the television being on from 6 pm until 8 pm bedtime, they can look at the books themselves as well as being read to and told stories. They can have quiet reading time in the living room with the rest of the family, time on their own and individual, private quiet time with a parent or other caregiver.

There are many positive side effects resulting from children learning this peace. It will help them with concentration and learning. It will help to counter the destructive effects of the modern mass entertainment industry. "In the average American family home the TV is on for seven hours a day" (Carson, 1989, p. 154). The fast pace of *Sesame Street* and other "children's shows" with their rapid shifting images, monotonous music, flashing colours and other adrenalin encouraging tricks all erode children's already limited attention spans and give the impression that there is no place for silence or zen nothingness.

By helping a child feel at peace, meditation can help decrease overall anxiety. It can increase confidence when we incorporate visualized images. For example, a child can be given the image of being surrounded by a protective circle or glow that keeps out the unkind thoughts and bad energy of others. It can be a place of divine inspiration.

In using visualization with children, especially younger children, we need to keep it as simple as possible. Just use pleasant and peaceful scenes evoking peaceful sensations to promote relaxation. A caution here is not to expect too much from the 6 or 7 year old. Although research suggests that some children as young as 7 or 8 can produce and manipulate visual images, this is a fairly advanced task. Programs that build in a great deal of visualization for young children often end up with a room of hyper children. When the developmental levels of children are not taken into account, the program may not have the desired results. A room full of inattentive, confused and frustrated children is not a peaceful place.

When I do use visual images with children, I like to keep it fairly open in structure and not tell a child too much or too often what to visualize. I might give such simple instructions as:

> Imagine that you are floating in a pool of healing water. You find a message or gift in the water. Let yourself enjoy this message/gift.

> Pretend you are in a hammock tied to two very old and wonderful trees. The trunks are wrinkled and colours and shadows swirl over the tree. Let yourself float and melt into the tree.

> Imagine it is a perfect summer day and you are sitting by a tree at the edge of a softly flowing river. Watch the birds overhead. Once in a while a bird drops a twig in the water. Watch the ripples in the water after the twig enters the water.

Deep Breathing

I have often taken a few minutes to teach a child to slow down and become calm with several slow and deep breaths. Air is an immediate source of life. We literally renew ourselves with each inward breath. We cleanse ourselves with each outward breath. Under stress, a fast pace and anxiety, we tend toward shallow breathing. It is important to monitor our breathing in order to stay centred, calm and grounded.

Younger children may need very clear and metaphoric descriptions to understand this. I may ask them to let their chest and breathing be like an accordion or a slinky as a way of describing what I am talking about.

Due to some unfortunate misconceptions about these methods in the eyes of the general public, for relaxation training, meditation, deep breathing and the use of mental imagery, parental consent should be obtained. I would spend a little time with the caregivers and let them know what I do with children, what relaxation training is all about and also let them know the benefits clearly described in the research. If they are really curious, interested or concerned, I always have scientific references available for them to follow up their interest.

If you have assessed that children are ready for relaxation training or meditation but find that during the process, they are giggling or smiling a lot, they are restless or constantly moving to find a comfortable spot or position, there is a great deal of rapid movement of eyelids, yawning or uneven breathing, then you must consider that either they are not, in fact, ready or your methods need to be modified (Morris & Kratochwill, 1985).

Perhaps in such a situation, rather than viewing the relaxation training as a failure, what needs to happen is a change in the approach to quietness. Maybe at this stage you can help children learn about peace and quietness by spending a few minutes in every session telling them a story you make up or reading one. It may be appropriate to spend a few minutes at the beginning or end of a session outdoors looking at a garden or trees, bugs and worms in the ground or bees and butterflies on the plants. You could have a gardening time in every session. In one week a child could plant a seed and each week spend a couple of minutes watering it, pulling out any weeds which have popped up in the pot and thinking thoughts of growth and health to the plant with the child.

At home, the tv should be kept to a minimum and the stereo should not be on during every waking moment. Kids need to learn about the silence around them. We adults need to learn this, too. Reading every magazine that comes out may be just as destructive as a constant intake of tv images. It may be a way of keeping us from being alone and thinking our own thoughts. The art of zen mindfulness and seeing everything we see and do as if we are seeing it for the very first time with a full focus and awareness can turn all of life and even the most mundane of tasks into a wonderful adventure.

Relaxing Movement

Relaxation training through movement can be taught to even fairly young children through things like tai chi, yoga, and creative dance. Both tai chi and yoga involve wonderful exercise programs for children who are old enough to concentrate and to follow instructions and repeat the movements. One of the benefits of these approaches is the metaphoric imagery involved in movements and positions such as "stork stand," "lion pose," and "grasping bird's tail" that goes along with the movements. Tai chi movements are

> taken from nature, and they restore contact with the natural world.... By the practice of T'ai Chi Ch'uan we embody the essence of the natural world (Rainbow-Wind, 1978, p. 361).

For younger children, I would be inclined to teach them a number of the tai chi movements as exercises in isolation at first, rather than have them try and remember the whole series. Yoga exercises are perfect for any aged child able to sit still and do them.

Children of all ages like any kind of movement. Many movements can also enhance creativity and imagination. Dance can reflect the inner world and our hopes for the outer world. It expresses our full passionate spirit. Children tend to know instinctively how to move to sounds and music. When I speak of dance here, I am not necessarily referring to any predetermined set of required movements. True dance reflects the soul and is not a set of predictable moves. There is nothing wrong with ballroom dancing. It can be a horde of fun for a couple. It's just not what I am referring to here. To date, "dance movement therapy literature is scant" (Payne, 1988, p. 69). I think the use of expressive and creative dance and movement is a largely unexplored approach that holds great potential. Children are close to the rhythms of the earth. We simply need to open doors for them to enter or return to this realm.

NATURE/SPIRITUALITY

The field of mental health would be vastly improved if it focused more on heightening awareness of nature and spirituality in people's lives. Come to think of it, there would probably be no such thing as a mental health field if there were an awareness and focus on nature and spirituality in everyone's life. I believe that nature and spirituality are inseparable. Much of the mental health profession's history involves an avoidance of nature, a shying away from the spirit. One of the best—or perhaps in fact the very best—ways to avoid a natural flow—is to use words. When we use words we are up in our heads. True healing occurs below jaw level.

I am not sure if we can estimate all that we have lost in our modern, so-called advanced, corporate state, where consumption is demanded and the material world has been made into an idol to be worshipped. The following (revised and adapted from Reich, 1971, pp. 166-169) are some aspects of the natural existence of humans that are either missing altogether or are present in but a mere facade in our modern urban environment:

Nature. The experience of living in harmony with nature, on a farm, or by the sea, or near a lake or meadow, knowing, using and returning to the elements.

Physical Activity. Harvesting a crop, digging a garden from sunrise to sunset, chopping wood, walking, climbing, dancing, experiencing heat and cold, building a house, starting a fire.

Bravery. Aside from the brave souls who endure intensely dangerous environments in rescue efforts in situations like the Oklahoma bombing we have no heroes, we have no bravery. The only time we see true bravery portrayed in the media is following some kind of disaster. Professional sports figures who think bravery is going on strike to earn $4 million a year instead of $3 million are greedy, self-centred and immature, spoiled brats whose behaviour in public is often inexcusable. Unfortunately these narcissistic self-worshippers have come to serve as role models for many children.

Worship. Children need to see caregivers involved fully in a spiritual life. They need celebrations of spirituality. The joy of relating to that which is greater than oneself.

Magic and Mystery. There is a tingling child-like feeling to life that comes from believing in magic. It occurs when we don't have to know how something works. We simply know that it will when we believe we have the power to alter concrete reality.

Awe, Wonder, Reverence

Fear, Dread, Awarenes of Death

Spontaneity

Romance

Dance/Music/Rhythm. "Rhythms pervade the whole body.... Not only do rhythms permeate living organisms, they are also experienced in the relationship of the earth to the sun, moon, and stars" (Thomson, 1994, pp. 44-45).

Growth and Change. Constantly learning new things, experiencing changes of feelings and personality, continually growing in experience and consciousness.

Wholeness. Being completely present with another person, or completely given to some experience, rather than being partially withheld in a way that most modern roles and situations demand.

Sensuality. Being sensually aware of all that surrounds us. This includes the sounds, scents, amount of heat, breezes, body rhythms. Being sensually involved with all that surrounds us. Being fully sensually involved with another person.

Myth Making and Storytelling

Transcendence

Aesthetic enjoyment of life

Perceiving others non-verbally

Allowing vulnerability

Community

An Inner Life

Alterations of Time. Staying up all night, getting up before dawn, working three days straight, or being wholly oblivious to measured time. There is an incredible sensation to awakening at 4 or 5 am and being on the earth when the sun rises. There is an undescribable peace at this moment. While studying wildlife biology at university, I loved to get up before dawn, get through a shower and be outdoors and wide awake for the sunrise. This was the real morning, the one before what I call the plastic morning, that fabricated time when all the unnatural sounds of radios, alarm clocks, cars, and the unnatural scents of deodorants, makeup, hair sprays, perfumes and colognes filled the air. This is not meant to encourage a lack of sleep. Sleep is healing. It is wise to be in bed by 10 pm and sleep 8 hours.

Seasons. Observing the changes of the seasons by stopping other activities for a while and going to some place where the change is fully visible. Honouring these changes through ceremony and ritual.

Imagination

Creativity

Morality. Having a moral stand with respect to something happening to oneself, to others, or to society. Maintaining that stand, and giving it expression.

Adventure and travel. There isn't much adventure in most travel these days. Frustration perhaps, but not adventure. Plane delays and the wrong flavour of ice cream at your destination do not count as adventure.

Sex. Intense, passionate, life affirming contact.

Clothes. Clothes to celebrate moods, express the passion of the body and soul, acknowledge our harmony with nature.

Play

Passion and intensity. Today if you feel too high or too low you will quickly be offered prozac or some other "wonder" chemical rather than being allowed to feel the depths of joy and sadness. I remember feeling very sad for an extended period of time recently. I was dealing with some intensely negative issues at this point in my life and there was justifiable cause for the sadness. I remember telling someone that I felt quite depressed. They suggested I see someone (*i.e.*, a therapist) and get something (*i.e.*, a drug) for it. Hopefully, by this point, my philosophical perspective is clear and it is needless to say that I didn't "see someone" or "get something for it." I'm not so sure what's so bad about feeling depressed. What's so bad about feeling? The depth of my feelings was allowing me to come to terms with the changes in my life that I was dealing with. Medication was not going to help me and my preference was to turn to my friends and garden where I would be able to be in touch what I was feeling.

Each of the above has slowly been eroded from our day-to-day lifestyles, so much so, that when we do experience any of the above it is unusual, a high, something that really stands out rather than being a daily given.

Nature

There is much healing work we can do with children through the use of nature activities. I will discuss a number of these in following chapters. Kids can collect rocks, stones and maybe even crystals from road cuts. They can plant a seed, nurture a potted plant, plant a tiny garden. I advocate that every home and office should have plants and at least one animal, even as little as a singing canary or some fish. "According to specialists in child development, children who live in urban high-rises are in danger of becoming psychologically stunted simply because they have no easy access to the out-of-doors.... How many children have destroyed or injured plants and animal life because they have been taught, explicitly or implicitly, that anything non-human doesn't count?" (Carson, 1989, pp. 173-174).

Kids can begin to learn environmental awareness anywhere on the face of the earth. In the most urban settings, there is still night and day. There are lunar cycles to be observed. The seasons come to downtown Toronto as much as they do to rural Newfoundland. All children can watch and participate in the ebb and flow of life's cycles. Even in an ultra-urban environment, children can still grow plants in pots. They can watch and learn about weather patterns, study urban wildlife like squirrels, raccoons, pigeons, and sparrows. Children can participate in school and office recycling and compost activities. None of this has to involve field trips to rural settings. It can all be done anywhere. It is important that nature activities need to be more than naming and memorization exercises. Nature learning means watching, smelling, listening, touching, tasting.

Rachel Carson, author of the environmental masterpiece *Silent Spring* (1962), has noted that

> There is symbolic as well as actual beauty in the migration of birds, the ebb and flow of the tides, the folded bud ready for spring. There is something infinitely healing in the repeated refrains of nature – the assurance that dawn comes after night, and spring after the winters (Carson, 1965, pp. 88-89)

Things like *Winnie the Pooh*, *Wind in the Willows* and similar stories are wonderful for children. But children also need to feel nature, not just read about it or watch it on tv. Nature's feel, scents, colours, sounds....

Kids can learn to turn nature activities into a playground. With encouragement and creativity, a child can use his or her imagination "to transform the ordinary into the extraordinary. He [or she] will find endless possibilities for shells, smooth pebbles, driftwood, or autumn leaves. These *treasures* from nature will be transformed again and again by his [or her] powers of fantasy" (Oldfield, 1994, p. 253).

One of the greatest gifts we gain from contact with nature can be solitude. This time away from the madness and rush of civilization can provide deep and meaningful inner silence. It provides perspective and an opportunity to be ourselves, be with ourselves, and not fear the harsh realities that face us daily in the "civilized" world. Children need this kind of break on a regular basis.

Spirituality

By spirituality I am not necessarily relating to specific church activities in any way.

> The important question is not "Should I send my child to church?" but "What is my own attitude towards life's greatest mysteries and how do I want to communicate with my child about these things?" (Armstrong, 1985, p. 133).

I am referring to living life with reference to a greater meaning outside of oneself. This is much like the transcendent unconscious and logotherapy that Viktor Frankl has written so eloquently about. Frankl (1975) has noted that

> Human existence—at least as long as it has not been neurotically distorted—is always directed to something, or someone, other than itself—be it a meaning to fulfil or another human being to encounter lovingly. I have termed this constitutive characteristic of human existence "self-transcendence."

If we believe that a spirituality exists within all, then the exact words we use to describe our relationship with the divine are not relevant. Some wonderful words from a Lutheran pastor are of great importance here. He is referring to his

> belief [that] most Native American tribes worship the same God as Christians do...the only difference is that while Christians learn of God through the Bible, the Indians learn of him through nature and legends (Mails, 1988, pp. 16-17).

Prior to about the age of seven, children do not differentiate the day to day concrete earthly world from the world of spirituality, awe, wonder. As early as they are able to be shown and to understand, children should be taught to acknowledge the spiritual in their lives. It is estimated (Dreschler, 1976) that the average child asks about 500,000 questions by their teen years, thereby giving caregivers half a million opportunities to teach about the wonders of life.

Religion needs to happen at home as well as in the sacred institutions. Our spirituality is not separate from our day to day life. True spirituality lives daily, not just whatever some human religious guru states the Sabbath should be. Spirituality involves an awareness and contact with nature.

I think it is a parenting error to assume that when children are old enough they will decide their "religion" for themselves. Dreschler (1976) notes that many parents confuse freedom of religion with freedom from religion.

> A faith not supplied by the home is supplied by the movies, the street gang, or some other group.... More and more groups, organizations, and cults are offering destructive, enslaving, and false answers to life's problems. These people would like nothing more than to find a person who was brought up in this seemingly broad-minded way (Campbell, cited in Drescher, 1976, p. 123).

In teaching about spirituality, caregivers must model their approach. It is useless to tell a child about virtues if you are not prepared to live a fully virtuous life. "Parents must not only know the way and show the way. They must also go the way" (Dreschler, 1976, p. 119).

Prayer

A gift we can give to our children is the awareness of how to pray, to connect with the Divine, the Creator of all. Prayer seems to have taken an unfair share of criticism of late. There are many positive results from teaching children to pray. I have seen many modern books about spirituality, new age issues and so on that don't include a word about prayer. Prayer is how we relate to the Divine. It is an essential part of spirituality.

I have heard critiques of prayer that include the negative assumption that all prayer is simply a rote activity and, further, that all rote activity is bad. I find it interesting that some of this criticism comes from the same people who don't mind the rote activity of chanting the same word or mantra over and over in a meditative state.

Most children do not know how to pray. For that matter, neither do most adults. Following are some recommendations on how to pray and how to teach children to pray.

- First, prayer should not be a "gimmee" time. Requests for material things should be left out of prayer and put into the realm of hard work and effort. Neither should prayer deteriorate into a greedy time for asking Divine favours. This may be very difficult if you have a vested interest in a situation. Perhaps a loved one is very ill.

  I remember as my father lay dying over two days following heart surgery, I found my self at first praying for him to live. It was a completely blind prayer, a scream to God and the universe from a scared six year old (I was actually 35 at the time) to "let my daddy live!"

  The day before his surgery, I had driven 14 hours to surprise him and see him. We had wonderful moments together. He had checked into the hospital but was basically bored stiff in the medical environment. We left his room and explored the halls together, went to the cafeteria for a snack. He told me what he knew about the upcoming operation and what to expect. I'd brought him a stuffed toy for his hospital room and a Sherlock Holmes book I knew he'd like. If I may risk a use of the word perfect, that's what these moments together were. We had gone back to his room and as I was leaving he walked me to the elevator. The last thing I said to him as the elevator door closed was "I love you." I stood in the elevator after the door closed and tears began running down my face. I was scared beyond belief at the possibility of losing him. I did not know at that moment that I would never again see this man consciously alive.

  The next day I received the very bad news that something had not gone well. It was around suppertime when my mum called to say that the operation was over and that dad was okay but that it hadn't gone as well as expected, as there had been some complications. She told me the hospital staff would let me know how things were and that I was supposed to call them for an explanation. I called immediately and received a shock. Things had certainly not gone as expected. The nurse in cardiac intensive care told me I should get there as soon as possible and they weren't sure my father would make it through the night. It was virtually impossible to get there immediately, at least in physical form. I lay awake all night praying for my father to live. With unselfish wisdom, the prayer should probably have focused on a request for my father's present journey to be as peaceful as possible, be it to the next world or a return to his present life in this one. But I was terrified. I visualized myself going to him, I let my body go inside his and said to him "I will do the work for you now dad" and I let my heart beat for his. At some point I slept. I had a dream that two very ancient and wise people (One was my grandmother—who had died a year to the day earlier. I've come to have a serious respect for June 6 as Carl Jung, Robert F. Kennedy, my grandmother and father all left the earthly world on that day) and some other person came to his bed to take him away. In hindsight these were the angels taking him to the next world. I didn't realize it at the time.

I believe I actually kept him alive by allowing my body to cross time and space and carry him. I also think this probably wasn't fair, it was a selfish act that did not acknowledge that it was his time to leave. Fortunately, my father was a very unselfish person and probably just thought, "Oh well, kids, I'll just put up with him."

The point of this whole description is to show how our vested interests can obscure our spiritual vision. My prayers were not really for my father in that situation. They were for myself. Some sense did come to me once I reached him in concrete reality. I caught the first possible flight in the morning and went straight to the hospital. Upon seeing my father I felt dizzy. This man of strength, humble quietness and omnipresence was physically reduced to an "unconscious" body, hooked up to all kinds of tubes, machines and monitors. I knew, but consciously denied, that he was moving on to the next life. Fortunately my prayers did change. I asked for the strength to be with dad and support him however he needed. Over the next 36 hours his heart rate and blood pressure ever so slowly dropped to very dangerous, "life on a string," levels.

We were blessed with very aware medical staff. His immediate nurse told me that "I don't know and neither does anyone else here where your father is right now. But I recommend that you assume that he knows you are here now and that he can hear everything anyone says around him. So talk to him all you want and assume he is hearing you." Again, the selfish and inquisitive son, just had to know. As I held his hand I said to him, "Dad, if you can hear me let me know somehow, squeeze my hand harder or something, just let me know." Without a change in any of the monitors or life function meters or anything, he put a firm grip on my hand for a moment, then let go again. I knew I could count on him. This was the last thing I asked of him. As always, he was there for me. From that point on I tried to give my total self to him, to being at one with him.

Finally, after many hours by his side, the nursing staff took me aside and told me that he could die that night or he could hold on for weeks and there was no way of predicting when his time would come to leave. That night I flew home. I stared out the plane window, my shirt getting soaked from the tears running down my face as I watched the city disappear below knowing I would never again see my father alive on earth. I prayed "Dad, go in peace." Due to exhaustion I did have at least some sleep that night. But at 2:22 am the phone rang. A nurse was calling to tell me my father had died. Apparently he had waited and wanted to die in privacy without human company by his side.

The moral of this rather long story? In times of selfish involvement, try to remember to pray for what is best for the other person and seek guidance for yourself in handling what is best for all involved.

◗ Despite my comments in the previous discussion of prayer and "favours" there is nothing wrong with visualizing the sending of healing energy to a person who is ill, upset or in distress. The prayer component would involve words like: "Oh Divine Creator, please grant that this healing force work for the good and best interests of all involved." With that kind of wording, if it is, in fact, time for the person who is ill to leave this world, your visualization will not stand in the way of natural flow.

◗ Prayer allows a place to connect with our Divine Creator, and to listen for guidance.

◗ Prayer involves a personal responsibility. Instead of requesting peace in the world, the request should be for help in bringing peace to the world. The running of the world must not be abdicated and turned over to some outside force at a cost of ignoring our own responsibility.

Following are some simple examples of prayers I have created over the years. There is nothing earth shattering about any of them. They tend to be simple requests for guidance. Many of them are not specifically Christian or Celtic in approach and can used by a person of any faith. Also included are a couple of examples from others.

Lord, how can I help make this a kinder and gentler world? Through your Divine guidance I ask that you bring me the wisdom to find this answer.

Dear God, I come to you in humility. I ask that you help me find the path that is best for...(my career, etc.)

Oh Divine Creator I seek the strength and wisdom to handle this difficult time. May I have the dignity and endurance that my own elders would have had in this situation.

Now I lay me down to sleep, I pray the Lord my soul to keep.
In the night as you do watch, I ask you to love my family lots.

After planting a tree or seeds in the garden I always walk clockwise (this represents the rotation of the earth) around the tree or garden and simply pray: *Grow.*

God and Goddess, father and mother of all life, I request your guidance, approval, and blessing for this upcoming venture into....

Even atheists can pray. They can relate to all of life and a transcendence beyond oneself in the form of affirmation: *I am part of all nature and life. May I always walk with respect upon the Earth.*

One of my all time favourites comes from the simple writings of Francis of Assisi. I love this prayer, for it involves a participation in life and a giving rather than lazily asking God to do something for me or to give something to me:

Lord make me an instrument of your peace.
Where there is hatred, let me sow love.
Where there is injury, pardon,
Where there is doubt, faith,
Where there is despair, hope,
Where there is darkness, light
And where there is sadness, joy.
O Divine Master, grant that I may not so much seek
To be consoled, as to console;
To be understood, as to understand;
To be loved, as to love;
For it is in giving that we receive,
It is in pardoning that we are pardoned,
And it is in dying that we are born to eternal life.

Although more a visualized thought than a verbal prayer, I feel it quite beneficial for a child (or adult) to be able to envision a guardian angel or spiritual companion. About 15 years ago I had completed some very difficult medical treatment—chemotherapy and radiation—that had been used to help me rid my body of Hodgkin's Disease, a form of lymphatic cancer. This is an understatement, but my energy level was low following treatment. My whole body had been, and felt like it had been, under intense attack. I had feelings of being at my limit in terms of endurance. I didn't know what was next. I was by the shores of Lake Ontario and saying a prayer for guidance.

What came to me was a visual scene in the sky of, not one, but an entire circle of angels sitting, glowing with life energy, "chanting" what sounded like a very uplifting Gregorian chant. They stood up and I heard them say, "we will be with you. We will always be with you." Since that day they have always been there when I am at severe distress points. They give comfort, wisdom, and guidance. They are messengers from the Divine. Some may wish to dissect my previous description and read in all kinds of psychoanalytic or other psychological interpretation. No such interpretation is needed. I have angels and they guide me. Sometimes I have one. Sometimes the whole darn group comes.

Coming from the Irish Celtic background that I do, I know it is angelic and not some "complex" or "projection" or other psychological dynamic force. Likewise, children need to be given a belief in transcendence. If they can grasp a visual image of a Divine Being, an angel, whatever, all the better. Research from cognitive and developmental psychology tells me that four year olds are unlikely to cognitively be able to manipulate visual images in their heads. So if they do see an angel, and that angel is doing or saying things, I know they are not "making up" this image and they truly see an angel. This reminds me of the *Oh God* movies. In those wonderful movies we saw the reactions of people to those who actually are visited by God. We tend to think they are unstable, crazy or lying. Even United States' money says "In God We Trust" on it. So how come so many people don't seem to believe in the influence or even existence of God?

Teach children how to visualize images of an angel(s) or some other messenger of God to whom they can go for comfort and guidance. In *Resilient Adults* (1995, p. 107), O'Connell-Higgins describes an adult woman who survived horrific abuse as a child by turning to angelic spiritual companions and guides. During the abuse "she was able to envision, as a small child, a host of benevolent spiritual children with protective powers, charged with guarding her integrity in some inviolate manner." I would maintain that these "spiritual children" were gifts from God.

Some excellent times to start to teach children the value of prayer and how to pray are upon rising in the morning, at the dinner table, at bedtime, and anytime you are outdoors with a child.

- Quiet time in the morning with your child or children can include a few moments seeking guidance for the day and affirming to do the best one can over the course of the day.

- At dinner time, there can be the grace before the meal when the family is together. It should be a prayer of reflection and thanks. For example: "We thank you, Oh Lord, for this meal on the table. We thank you for helping us put our best effort into earning this meal. We thank you for the blessings of a roof over our head, the shelter that is our home, and our family we are able to share this with."

  A touching alternative from a Presbyterian background: "Dear heavenly Father, we humbly beseech thee to enjoy the presence of our fellowship, and to enable us to enjoy the presence of that Divine Unseen Guest whose coming to earth has filled all life with new meaning and beauty." I particularly like this grace before meals "We give thanks for our food, and remember those who are hungry. We give thanks for our health, and remember those who are ill. We give thanks for our family, and remember those who are alone" (Carson, 1989, p. 114).

- The bedtime routine is an ideal time to include prayer. It is a time to reflect on the day, to create peace in the home and to settle down for a night of renewal.

- In the garden, outdoors in the woods, under the night sky, by a running brook. These are all places where we can see the beautiful and natural unfolding of the Divine presence.

A Shrine

A home needs a shrine, a sacred space where one can go to in order to seek solace, quiet, say a prayer. A shrine can be a living component of a home. Without it, a certain depth and meaning is lost. The shrine is the symbolic spiritual centre. It should be simple and symbolic of your acknowledgement of the Divine in your life. It is a place of quiet peace.

The shrine may be the hearth with pictures of your elders and ancestors on the mantel above. For a Catholic it might be the mantle with the palms from Palm Sunday.

The shrine is a place to sit before and quietly reflect, meditate, or pray. During a crisis, sitting there helps one to gain peace.

It can also be the place of blessings. For example, you may put lunches for your loved ones here in the morning before they leave the house for the day. Or perhaps a little gift (not an expensive commercial doll for Sandy who fell down and cut herself) for a family member having a rough time or rough day...such as a tiny hand-made felt teddy bear with a message of love written on it.

The shrine is simply a symbol of our connection with the Divine. The shrine or the objects placed there are not worshipped. They are there only to remind us symbolically of our connections to powers greater than ourselves. I take great exception with much of the "new age" movement which takes the metaphors literally and turns the symbolic representations into actual items to be worshipped.

A SENSE OF MAGIC AND PASSION IN THEIR LIVES

If you accept the forms that be,
you are doomed to
your own ultimate blandness.

—John Lydon

Both magic and passion are sadly lacking in the lives of most people. Children learn early that most adults consider magic to be just makebelieve, that it is silly, something for little children or the very immature. Or, even worse, they consider it something evil. And passion, well, passion is just plain scary for most adults. It is too intense.

In the 1800s, Henry David Thoreau wrote that the masses lead lives of quiet desperation. It is ever so much truer today toward the end of the twentieth century than it was over a hundred years ago. Many people ooze desperation. I feel for them. I feel their pain, their frustration, their longing for meaning. We all long for meaning in life. Many fall into a rut of "is this all there is?"

In my travels, I meet and talk with a great number of people. Far too many seem so terribly sad. There is an existential emptiness and a longing that I sense from within them, a longing for a non-defined "more." They've made a life for themselves but have reached a point where they thought there was more but all they can feel is an emptiness and don't know where it comes from. I talk with them and see in their eyes an intense desire for magic and passion in their lives. They want to be loved, to have passion and adventure in their lives. They want to feel the pulse of life throbbing in their soul. But they're not even sure they have a soul anymore. They've reached a point where all they have left is a wondering if that pulse really exists anywhere outside of fantasy. They begin to wonder if, perhaps, it is an illusion and this really is all there is. I meet many women who are reaching for something that they cannot find within or from their relationships. I meet many men and I see their longing for more. They see my life and I see a longing, an envy in their eyes. So many times I have heard: "You've done it all, you have it all, is there anything you can't do or haven't done?" To me life is about fullness. It's about not letting your handicaps[8] be your limitations. It means that, yes, you were in a car accident and now you're confined to a wheelchair but you can still learn to be a pilot. Your handicaps become your weaknesses when you let them be your limitations. You cannot be a doormat until you lie down.

The longing that many feel is often assumed to be some *thing* they need to own or something they should be *doing*. It is as if only having that new house or cottage or taking the skiing lessons would make it all better. There is an increasing desperation as one gains these things, does all these things and still feels the lack, the longing. We so often lack passion that we think that by touching a lot of things (ownership) or doing a lot of things (power/control) we will then feel the passion, be the passion. But it only becomes more empty. There is an increasing desperation as one gains these things, does all these things and still feels the lack.

In reality, fullness is not about external things. It's about being in touch with spirit and nature. When you are in touch, then you feel the passion. FEEL THE PASSION. When you are in touch. TOUCH. FEEL. Passion is about being in touch, communicating with the Divine, experiencing nature. Don't get me wrong here. My idea of a good time is running amok at DisneyWorld. I like five star hotels and nice beds.

I mentioned earlier Thoreau's statement that the masses lead lives of quiet desperation. In this desperation of many lives there is an attempt to drug it away with adrenalin. An adrenalin "rush" provides a momentary respite from loneliness and emptiness. Adrenalin can also be fun but not when it is a drug used to replace fullness. When it enters the system as a result of having fullness that's a different story. Then it is a byproduct of fullness, not the quest in and of itself. Adrenalin can be psychologically very appealing when it is used to replace fullness. One who leads the life of a warrior[9] experiences fullness and does not need to replace it with a drug. Television provides most of the meaning existent in many people's lives. The very existence of soap operas is proof positive of this emptiness. Another adrenalin booster is watching sports. I can guarantee that most fans at games have almost as much, or sometimes even more, adrenalin in their systems as the players do. While watching a show on pilots and flying on TSN, a Canadian sports network, a commercial proudly extolling the joys of watching sports on TSN blared "Adrenalin can be the most addictive of life's ingredients."[10]

We hunt, we play sports, we watch television (the more intense the better, for witnessing intensity and violence triggers adrenalin), we listen to loud music,[11] we drive fast, we participate in dangerous activities (drugs, certain pastimes), we fight with our partners. All in a quest to feel and to find meaning.

Children need to learn to continue to feel throughout their lives. They need their feelings respected, intense feelings, little feelings, big feelings. We need to help them respect their inner voice, to listen to their intuition, to inspiration from our Creator, from Nature. We need to devote ourselves to always helping our children see, feel, sense the magic of life, the passion of living.

SOME BASIC REMINDERS TO THOSE CONSIDERING PARENTHOOD OR THOSE WHO ALREADY ARE PARENTS

Before becoming a parent one should be as mature as possible—at least mature enough to consider others before oneself. From studies on abusive parents, it has been found that "if such parents see a child as a rival or a playmate, they will not be able to provide their child with needed structure and control" (Fagot & Kavanagh, 1991, p. 217).

This new living being will not be a pal, a playmate, a friend. They will be a needy, totally dependent, gift from God. You will have to be open to your own need for quickly developing maturity. Someone else's needs will need to be placed before your own. Maturity will be taught to you very quickly by this little new being who enters the world helpless and needing. There can be some difficult and challenging moments as a parent. For example, that cute wee thing who was cooing and smiling at you at 7 o'clock in the evening may seem to be crying for eternity by 9 pm. Feelings of helplessness can creep into a parent's psyche. You have to remember that it is not a personal affront to you. Just keep walking. Maybe treat it as a personal meditative time. Allow the screaming to be outside of your being. Walk, move to and fro and just keep rocking and swaying with the precious little life in your arms. Because of challenging moments like this example and because it takes a lot of energy to be a good caregiver, parents owe it to themselves and to their children to be refreshed as often as possible.

This may involve a weekly (how about daily) massage,[12] a walk alone by the beach or sitting in the park for an hour digging in the earth all alone or while your children play nearby. From this time away, this stepping back, comes perspective. We gain the awareness of how trivial most of life's problems are compared to the gift of being alive that we have been given and the gift of this new life in our children.

Following are some recommended words and phrases, some to use often, some never to use. Make sure when saying the important things, to look a child in the eyes and touch them.

Things To Say Often To Your Child

I love you!

Did you ever do a good job!

What do you feel about that?

What do you think about that?

What do you sense about that?

Thank you for helping.

Thank you for trying so hard.

I really appreciate...(kids love being noticed and appreciated).

I really like being with you.

(After a child has made an apparent mistake at some task): *What did you learn?* or *Is there anything you would like to do differently?* or *Is there anything I can do to help?* (do not take over the task for the child though—help means assistance, not taking over).

When the child is challenging authority, a clear "*No*" is needed.

Never Say These Things To A Child

Never... (in unrealistic contexts). Often heard from the mouths of ineffective parents—for example, "if you don't smarten up and behave I am never taking you to a movie again"—yeah, right. Even the kid knows you're bluffing, but you sound like such an ineffectual idiot that it's embarrassing to fellow human beings, so don't say it.

Hurry up and.... Kids go at a kid pace. If you want to create anxious children then push them to hurry all the time. Unfortunately, the kind of parent who says things like this, usually says them all the time. The pattern starts to give kids messages that they should not be going at their own pace, they should not be enjoying the world around them, and so on.

Just wait until your father/mother gets home. Translated means "I'm ineffective but your father/mother isn't." Well, at least not until they get home and don't do anything either.

If you do that again, I'm going to smack you. This simply says the best way to deal with conflict or frustration is through physical abuse. Get a life and stop taking your frustrations out on your child. "Spanking" should be used rarely, if ever, and reserved only for the most severe situations and should never involve anger.

If I've told you once, I've told you a thousand times.... So why should the kid listen to you on the thousand and first time? Learn some effective parenting skills and how to use logical consequences. Stop nagging, if for no other reason than the fact that this, too, is embarrassing to fellow human beings.

Are you ever...stupid/slow/bad/etc. Nothing is accomplished by such abusive words.

If I have to tell you again.... If you have to say something like that in the first place you probably will have to tell them again, and again, and again.

Footnotes

1 René Dubos is identified as a microbiologist and experimental pathologist. In the 1940s he was the first scientific investigator to demonstrate the feasibility of obtaining germ-fighting drugs from microbes. I see him as a brilliant ecological philosopher. Some of his philosophical texts such as *A God Within* are brilliant explorations of the human relationship with nature.

2 Better yet, how about no tv, period, or not even having a television in the house.

[3] Heartfelt thanks to Elspeth Christie of the Kingston Childbirth Education Association for introducing me to the invaluable work of Jean Liedloff. The work of both of these women is helping to create a better world.

[4] I do not define someone like your best friend who is always present and is a significant part of your family life as a babysitter. Nor do I define mom or dad, gramma or grampa, uncle or aunt and so on, when they are regularly involved in the child's life, as babysitters. These people are all part of the extended family. This is the group that, ideally, should be looking after a child.

[5] Some of the most tragic effects of violent television on children, according to the National Association for the Education of Young Children, include "(1) desensitization to the pain of others, (2) increased fears of the world around them, and (3) increased aggressiveness" (Bennett & Bennett, 1994, p. 6).

[6] The comment here is in reference to the United States, but the same ridiculous situation has developed in Canada.

[7] I'm sure if there was a more complex way of making a simple description appear more knowledgeable than it actually is, Jung would have found it.

[8] Whether we like to hide from the fact or not, there are handicaps. Using politically correct phrases and calling someone developmentally challenged does not alter the fact one iota that they are retarded. It is interesting how these phrases keep changing every few years as they start to be identified with the truth. We go from moron to retarded to developmentally delayed to developmentally challenged. As the general public catches on to who we're talking about, the politically correct thought police change the phrase and, so, for another 5 to 10 years we can again deny reality and pretend everyone is equal, *i.e.*, equivalent, *i.e.*, identical.

[9] I define a warrior in a non-militaristic manner. To me a warrior is one who confronts life's challenges and seeks to master them,

rather than running from them and hiding behind one's fears. We all have fears, handicaps and difficulties in our lives. The coward hides behind them and uses them as an excuse for laziness and inactivity. The warrior does battle with the fears and the difficulties. True warriors are heroes who rise to the challenges of their particular handicaps. Cowards blame others or their own past or their own life difficulties for all future actions.

[10] From a commercial heard on *TSN*, *The Sports Network* in Canada. Commercial aired on February 8, 1996.

[11] This is not to imply that some of the things I mention like sports, loud music, or even driving fast are inherently bad. The problem arises when we become hooked on the adrenalin rushes in an attempt to avoid the emotional pain in our lives.

[12] I have a sense that there may be a reaction to the recommendation of something like a weekly massage. I am not assuming that everyone can afford the cost of going to a professional for this. Partners and friends can exchange massages. It doesn't have to be a paid professional. However, I don't think this will be the issue. In the book, *Self Discovery Through Inner Play*, written with Bridget Revell, there is one exercise we included written by Viki Takacs (1995) on nurturing your unborn child. Although I didn't hear any of it, I understand that Bridget took some flak for our inclusion of that particular exercise in our book from some people who told her that it was such a middle class viewpoint (interesting that the criticisms apparently came from middle class professionals and social workers—and since when did a middle class viewpoint become inferior?) who said it really missed the point because it didn't deal with the fears of many pregnant women. The first thing to note about this particular exercise is that it was not written by me, a male, nor by Bridget, a non-pregnant female. It was actually written by Viki Takacs who, at the time of writing it, was several months pregnant and deeply involved with and committed to her unborn child. The second point is that I feel it is important to write from the perspective of

health. The mental health field has so long been focused on dysfunction and the abnormal. I am proud to have included this healthy and positive exercise in our book. No apologies to the bleeding heart social workers who felt it didn't relate to the dysfunction of their clients (or themselves).

The previously mentioned exercise by Viki Takacs is reprinted here:

FOR AN EXPECTING MOTHER

Meditation and Celebration with Your Unborn Baby

Many women who are expecting a baby feel a wonderful awe in knowing there is a live human being growing inside them. Throughout pregnancy women can be very nurturing to themselves and to their unborn baby(ies). Being pregnant can be a time of reflection as well as preparation. Even if time is at a premium a mother should take time to talk to her baby to help him/her feel accepted. Science has shown us that babies' brains are activated at a very early stage. They think, feel, hear and see early on in the womb. They know when mommy is upset or when she is very happy. As a result, it is important for a woman to communicate to her unborn child, to share feelings of love, happiness, security and well-being (healthiness)*.

A Very Special Time

This exercise takes place in the bathtub and is healing and nurturing for a mother and her unborn baby. First, you need to choose a candle (preferably beeswax as they are non-toxic) that is a favourite colour and shape. Flowers or scented candles can be very nice. Take a thick towel, robe, some scented bath powder and your candle to the bathroom. You can find nicely scented bath powders at many bath and scent shops (*The Body Shop* has scented bath powder for moms-to-be). Run a bath and mix the bath powder with your water. You can now light the candle and turn off the bathroom lights! These lights can be very invasive and stressful. With the lights off you will become more relaxed and able to concentrate on both your body and baby.

The best part now is to get into the tub and feel the warmth of the water soaking into your body, warming up cold toes and fingers and loosening up that congestion that one always seems to get during pregnancy. While lying back in the tub (mothers at four months and on should be lying on their side so that baby is not lying on your spinal cord or major blood vessels!) start thinking about your little baby floating inside. Imagine his/her little fingers and toes, head, brain, spinal cord, etc. Really try to "see" them. Imagine a little movement (soon, you will **feel** this part), happy wriggles, and thumbsucking.

Greet your baby, "Hi baby, here's mommy," and tell him/her how much she/he is loved. Perhaps you can tell baby of future plans, about what is happening in your life, what you've planted in the garden and ways you are preparing your home for him/her. Send your baby lots of warm feelings and think really happy and safe thoughts. Remember that this is a very special time for both the baby and you.

You will find that as the baby grows she/he will react with movement when you are in the tub doing this exercise. One thing babies particularly like is having water swept up over a mom's belly in a somewhat swishing/rhythmic motion. It is comforting to the baby and it feels neat for mom! Add a lullaby that you can sing every time you are in the tub. If you don't enjoy singing then use tape-recorded classical music. It has been noted that after birth babies will calm down when they hear the same lullaby/taped music*.

You can finish by telling baby about the love and joy that will be part of their life and how excited people are waiting for the birth. Then, send the baby a warm, calming feeling before letting him/her know that it is time to get out of the tub.

Try and let this become a habit—to talk to your baby every time you are in the bath. It only requires a few minutes of acknowledgement and, as the pregnancy "increases," it gets easier to do whether in the tub, car, or in the office chair.

You can help your baby come to feel loved and secure before she/he is even born. Perhaps this extra stimulation will have other benefits to the baby. It is a peaceful celebration any woman and her unborn child can enjoy.

* For further information in this area please refer to Tom Verny's (1981) *The Secret Life of the Unborn Child* (Takacs, 1995, pp. 87-88).

PART TWO

Transitions

• • • •

The Magic of Play Therapy

Food for Thought

I personally feel that, and I feel this about very few things—as you know I have libertarian feelings, I don't like the State to get involved in these things. But I would think the State ought to ban child therapy for the same reasons it has banned child labour. Child labour is not a bad idea if you think about it. Educationally, economically, it wouldn't be bad necessarily for a child to work for a few hours. It would be good for a lot of children. But the possibilities of abusing child labour are so much greater than the benefits which can be gotten, that all modern Western States have made child labour illegal. Now I think for the same reason, all child psychiatry, psychology and therapy should be made illegal.

—Dr. Thomas Szasz

(In conversation with Mark Barnes)

Nature is my teacher.

—Ludwig von Beethoven

The magic is never ending.

—C. S. Lewis

CHAPTER 3

Play Therapy

INTRODUCTION

In this section I will be looking at methods of working positively and productively with children. These methods may be used with children who have emotional problems or they may be used with your own children as they spend precious special time with you. You do not have to be a skilled child psychotherapist or play therapist. In fact, the research on psychotherapy in general notes that the level of training of therapists, the amount of experience they have, as well as their professional credentials are all irrelevant when compared to a client's outcome in therapy. This speaks well for the possibility of paraprofessionals being therapeutic agents and for parents themselves being agents of healing with their children. This is not meant to imply that you should be your own child's therapist. It means that parents can spend quality time with their children in ways that have been proven to be quite beneficial emotionally. Parents who do this will be less likely to have children who need professional help.

Play that is known as play therapy—actually all play—is truly a magical process. Through this contact between child and adult, the child's world can be transformed. Reality can change for a child and this is true magic.

Children may need some special help after a stressful or traumatic event or during life changes. As we leave a familiar spot, no matter how confident and secure we are, there is an anxiety that goes with change and new situations. In transition from point A to point B, a safe place is needed. To emphasize the point, by help I don't necessarily mean the child will need a therapist. A wise parent with therapeutic skills would be ideal. The notion that to help children heal and grow, we must separate them from caregivers and put them with professional therapists is a bizarre thought!

HISTORICAL BACKGROUND OF PLAY THERAPY

In giving a brief background on play therapy, it does not necessarily mean that all or any of the methods mentioned are still in use or that they necessarily work. I will be examining what works in the final section of this chapter. What is being explored here is our beginning, the "roots" of therapy with children. Many of the methods would definitely not be used today for reasons that will be discussed. They are only mentioned to indicate the growing process of our understanding of work with children.

There are already a number of histories of the field of play therapy available in the literature. Almost every play therapy text seems to have one. Only the briefest of outlines will be provided here.

The earliest organized psychological work with children began in 1896 with Lightner Witmer's child guidance clinic at the University of Pennsylvania (Reisman & Ribordy, 1993, p. 6). Here, learning principles were applied in the treatment of such troubles as autism, anxiety, and conditioned fears. The success of some of these treatment procedures brought considerable scepticism toward traditional, and largely unsuccessful, psychoanalytic methods. It also "heightened the receptivity of a new generation of professionals to conditioning and behavior modification" (Reisman & Ribordy, 1993, p. 6).

Unfortunately, play therapy has historically been dominated by psychoanalytic viewpoints. One of the earliest pioneers in using play directly in the therapy of children was H. Hug-Helmuth (1919). Given her outcome, it is surprising that play therapy ever got off the ground. Hug-Helmuth was murdered by a client while she was using psychoanalytic methods to treat him for emotional problems. This particular client was a nephew raised by Hug-Helmuth as a son (Reisman & Ribordy, 1993, p. 4). Obviously, personal boundary issues need to be considered here as well.

Anna Freud and Melanie Klein, both psychoanalytically oriented, incorporated play into their sessions with children. Anna Freud maintained that she used play to help build a relationship. Klein took this a step further and used play as a substitute for verbal communication. Freud founded a psychoanalytically based school in Vienna in the 1920s. Her work was characterized by a "mixture of naivete and arrogance" (Szasz, 1994, p. 75).

> Ostensibly, the students in this Freudian parody of education had mental problems "treated" at the school; actually, they were the pampered rejects of rich parents. Typically, the children were denominated as sick because they were upset by the parents' extramarital affairs. For a fee, Anna Freud took the troubled and troubling children off their parents' hands (Szasz, 1994, p. 75).

The idea of considering children to be disturbed in their emotional lives first appeared when "the term *emotionally disturbed* was applied to children, apparently for the first time, in an article that appeared in 1932 (Despert, 1970)" (Reisman & Ribordy, 1993, p. 4).

In the 1930s there was the beginning of a movement known as structured play therapy. This approach was in no way associated with the Minuchin systemic family therapy model known as "structural family therapy." The structured play therapies grew from a psychoanalytic framework and still believed "in the cathartic properties of play" (Knell, 1993, p. 10). The therapist in this approach was highly active in determining the course and focus of therapy. Three of the key authors were Levy (1938), Soloman (1938) and Hambridge (1955). Levy developed an approach known as "release therapy" in which materials were made available to re-enact a specific trauma. It is my view that all sorts of materials should be available to the child, not just those which would precipitate the re-enactment of trauma. Priority should be given to creating a nurturing sense of protection for the child rather than pushing him or her into what could be an intensifying of the traumatic experience.

Soloman (1938) developed a technique called "active play therapy" which was used with impulsive, acting out children (Schaefer & O'Connor, 1983, p. 6). Today, we know that the best methods for use with impulsive, acting out children are behavioral. There are highly structured impulse control group and social skills group formats available for work with this population.

Hambridge (1955) set up play much like Levy but was even more directive. The traumatic event was directly recreated in play in order to aid the child's "release" of psychic pain (Gil, 1991, p. 30). I consider such an approach to be completely out of the question. It is far too directive and can possibly lead to two very negative outcomes. The child may completely shut out the therapist or the child may lose his or her grasp on reality.

Also in the 1930s there was another approach known as relationship therapies. This developed out of the thinking and views of Otto Rank (1936), who stressed the importance of the so-called "birth trauma" in human development. It was Rank's view that "the stress of birth led the individual to cling to the past and to fear individuation" (Knell, 1993, p. 12). This notion that birth is traumatic is quite a bizarre thought from a biological and ecopsychological[1] standpoint. Birth, life, and death are natural processes. To assume that birth, by its very existence, is traumatic runs counter to biological knowledge. Living organisms are designed in species-specific ways to give birth to other members of their own species. If birth were truly traumatic, our species would no longer exist. This view indicates the influence of the highly negative and bizarre psychoanalytic viewpoint.

Jessie Taft (1933), Frederick Allen (1942) and Clark Moustakas (1959) all adapted Rank's line of thinking to work with children in play therapy. Through therapy, the child is given the opportunity to establish a deep, concerned relationship with a therapist in a safe setting. This approach tended to emphasize the child-therapist relationship and de-emphasize the significance of past events. However, there was still a strong tie to psychanalytic theory.

Allen (1942) was largely responsible for our present view that the relationship between therapist and child is therapeutic. Gaining insight and awareness were not seen as being significant therapeutic issues or goals.

> Allen's system of psychotherapy stressed the importance of creating a special kind of human relationship between the therapist and child. It was held that this relationship was what was therapeutic, rather than the bringing of unconscious conflicts into awareness and the communication of insight. Since Allen's time it has become appreciated by therapists of almost every orientation that the relationship between themselves and their clients is of great significance (Reisman & Ribordy, 1993, p. 5).

In 1949 there was an influence from Bixler which began a movement where the development and enforcement of limits was to be considered the primary vehicle of change in therapy sessions. The therapist sets limits with which he or she is personally comfortable (Schaefer & O'Connor, 1983, p. 8). Bixler suggested that limits include: the child not being allowed to destroy toys or property in the play room other than designated items; the child not being allowed to physically attack the therapist; the time limit of the session being enforced; the child not being allowed to take toys from the playroom, and; the child not being allowed to throw anything out of the window (Bixler, 1949, p 2). Bixler's material indicated a meaningful new direction in child therapy. No longer would "catharsis" be a primary focus for many therapists. The concept of boundaries, limits, and an orientation towards the reality of daily life was beginning to take hold. There was agreement by Ginott (1959, 1961) on the value and significant reality orientation that limits offered in allowing the child a feeling of protection by adults.

It should be stating the obvious to note that setting and enforcing limits is an important part of parenting. As mentioned earlier in the section on children's needs, I truly believe that a child without limits is an abused child. Without limits there is no sense of safety, boundaries or protection in the world. Children without limits cannot trust adults to act in a consistent manner.

We owe children limits. This is not to imply rigidity or inflexibility. The limits I am talking about stem from loving concern for the child, not from a desire for power over the child. A child should have as few limits as possible but as many as necessary.

Therapy does not mean "anything goes." Therapy should be a lovingly and carefully guided process. There is a time for many different pieces to the process. It must not deteriorate into what I call "cupcakism" where the adult does only what pleases the child and does nothing that would make the child dislike him or her.

Parallel to the humanistic psychology movement was an approach to working with children developed by Virginia Axline (1947). Based on the client-centred, non-directive approach of Carl Rogers, Axline developed a client-centred play therapy method for working with children.

Axline stated a number of principles underlying her play therapy approach. These principles include:

> the therapist developing a warm, friendly relationship with the child; the therapist accepting the child exactly as he or she is; the establishment of a feeling of permissiveness in the relationship in order for the child to feel completely free to express his or her feelings; recognizing the feelings the child is expressing and reflecting those feelings back to the child in such a manner that he or she gains insight into his or her behaviour; maintaining a deep respect for the child's ability to solve his or her own problems if given an opportunity to do so – the child maintains responsibility to make choices; there is no attempt to direct the child's actions or conversations in any manner; there is no attempt to determine the pace of therapy; the only limits imposed on the child are those needed to orient the therapy to reality and daily life (Axline, 1969, pp. 73-74).

The 1950s and 1960s saw the development of behaviour therapy techniques applied to children. These have been very useful in treating anxiety, impulse control, deficient social skills, and certain acting out behaviours. However, there is a certain concern that we should not rely too heavily on these techniques to simply modify all children's behaviour at a cost of masking underlying issues. We know that children, lacking adult verbal and cognitive skills, may indicate their underlying distress through their behaviour. If we eliminate children's behaviour that is causing difficulty for the adult world around them, do we then run the risk of creating even greater problems later? This is an important area worthy of considerable research efforts.

Some more recent influences have included the wonderful work of Violet Oaklander (1978), who put together a great toolchest for working with children in her text *Windows To Our Children*. In this text she describes hundreds of techniques for working with children. It has been inspirational and a highly influential adapted gestalt approach with children that can be used by parents, teachers, and counsellors in a number of settings. Another modern contributor of significance has been Dora Kalff who was responsible for the popular use of what is known today as sandplay therapy.

Over the past three decades there has been a landslide of theoretical and philosophical literature on play therapy, but little or no research. It has been proposed that the

> current renaissance in play therapy can be attributed to the following sociocultural developments: (1) high divorce rates, (2) blended families, (3) socioeconomic pressures requiring both parents to work, and (4) greater pressures for children to show academic proficiencies at younger ages. These events have been consistently shown to place children "at risk" for the development of emotional difficulties and adjustment problems (Kissel, 1990, p. 5).

In 1986 the Canadian Association for Child and Play Therapy (CACPT), a recognized non-profit and registered (by the Government of Canada) charitable organization, instituted the first standards in the world for those wishing certification as a child psychotherapist and play therapist. The Canadian Play Therapy Institute (CPTI), accredited by the Canadian Association for Child and Play Therapy, began training programs in play therapy and many other mental health issues. CPTI became the very first organization in the world dealing with child psychology and play therapy to go on the Internet and World Wide Web, thus opening the door for a mushrooming in the growth of play therapy throughout the world. By the 1990s, an international play therapy association, Play Therapy International (PTI), had formed and become active through intensive Canadian and international efforts. Through Play Therapy International, the formation of the International Board of Examiners of Certified Play Therapists (IBECPT) has allowed professionals from different countries to become certified in child and play therapy. It has also allowed the development of international standards for certification in play therapy. Not the least of their efforts has been the establishment of bursaries and scholarships for those in need to receive training in play therapy. Professionals who will be able to take their acquired knowledge and apply it in their own settings are eligible to apply for these bursaries to further the growth of play therapy worldwide.

The greatest present need in the field of play therapy is research to determine what works and what doesn't. Without an understanding of research and empirical methods one can quickly deteriorate into a dogma of unproven beliefs rather than facts. This will be highlighted in a later section of this chapter.

THEORETICAL BACKGROUND OF PLAY THERAPY

It is a gift of life to be watching a child play. This can bring a wealth of information. Play can be used to gain a diagnostic[2] understanding of a child, but only if great care and caution are taken not to read too much into the child's inner world. Perhaps little Susie has been playing with dinosaurs for several months and doing little else in her play scenarios. This may mean only that she is playing with dinosaurs, not some deep intrapsychic message. Freud did give at least one worthwhile thought to the mental health field when he noted that "sometimes a cigar is just a cigar," meaning that we do not have to read deep meaning into everything. Such a search is the realm of self-centred narcissists and anal retentives. The less indulgent inner exploration we need to do, the healthier we probably are. Some of the most maladjusted people I have met in my life and career are those who are constantly trying to be in touch with themselves, analyzing everything in their lives, always trying to analyze their family and past, looking for meaning in everything *ad nauseam*. There is a whole wonderful world out there to explore without constantly and obsessively looking for meaning in everything.

In attempting to gain an understanding of a child, we need to watch for themes and trends over time. Do not take any one piece of information as *the* diagnostic picture. We must fit all pieces into an overall context.

Play can be used to establish a relationship with a child. The younger the child, the less likely that words will be of any use anyway. When children are anxious, allowing them to play can help to break through that anxiety. Play allows children to put feelings into "words," the words of play. Children may have unresolved issues that, if put into verbal form, could be overwhelming. However, when children play out different issues through toys, it can help them relieve an inner tension.

All children need to play. Play is a learning place for all animals. Play processes are ways of learning that are carried into daily activities and give children greater strength and potential abilities.

The Personality

In the healing process in play therapy, it is important to watch for indications of change and improvement. To do this we need a working model. Let's first examine a hypothetical construct of the personality.

Our psyche[3] or personality consists of a number of different aspects. At our very centre is the elusive concept called the self. We constantly use terms like self, self-esteem, self-control, self-image and so on. It is difficult to define this ambiguous concept. As a rather simplified explanation, I think one could easily substitute words and phrases like soul, inner divinity and guiding light to describe the concept of the self. It is that innermost centering part of us. Truly, this is the inner guide, the wholeness of being for which we strive. The self is often symbolized in dreams, in art, in sand and other play and creative processes as a divine image and on a deeper, more primitive level of the unconscious as the circular or mandala form (Kalff, 1980). Objects like the sun or star may symbolize the self, for they are a representation of wholeness and completeness. However, please keep in mind that an individual's interpretation of his or her own symbols must take priority over any guidelines or suggestions I am giving here.

An example of self-symbolism comes from a session with a ten year old girl. A mandala-like scene was created by this young girl who appeared quite disturbed in her daily life. In one particular session about ninety minutes following a severe tantrum at home, including much physical destruction in her household, she walked into my office, sat down and without speaking did a beautiful and symmetric mandala sand scene. She appeared very relieved after making this scene and was significantly calmed. I felt great relief, realizing that the self was solid enough to make a symbolic appearance.

As Dora Kalff notes,

> The manifestation of the Self, this inner order, this pattern for wholeness, is the most important moment in the development of the personality. Psychotherapeutic work has proven that a healthy development of the ego can take place only as a result of the successful manifestation of the Self, whether as a dream symbol or as a depiction in the sandbox. Such a manifestation of the Self seems to guarantee the development and consolidation of the personality (Kalff, 1980, p. 29).

Despite the previous rather obtuse description of the concept known as the self (and the Jungian glorification of this concept, even capitalizing it to read "Self"), what is really important about this description is the basic idea that when one is centred and grounded, the personality can unfold naturally.

Another important component of the personality is the ego. The ego is the centre of consciousness, the organizer and gatekeeper of consciousness. The ego allows us an identity. Our ego must make the decisions that allow us to be human. A healthy ego has strong, clear, flexible boundaries. Symbolically, it, too, may be represented by numerous symbols such as an automobile, a baby or some animal with which the person identifies. The actual item is irrelevant. What is important is the fact that the person is clearly identified as the symbol. Cars are often used. If you think about it, they do make an ideal ego representative. In our modern world, cars are our tools for moving from place to place, meandering here and there along the way. Similarly, the ego gets us from psychological and emotional place to place.

Concepts

There are certain concepts relevant to the therapeutic process. These specifically are those which relate to certain personality aspects and their functions, as well as assumptions upon which I base therapy:

1) *The self is the directing centre of the personality* (Weinrib, 1983, p. 20).

2) *The psyche and self, like the physiological aspects of humans, can metaphorically be wounded and can heal metaphorically.* There can be both little hurts and big wounds along life's path. Under proper conditions, we heal ourselves. Like the setting of a broken arm, there is nothing particularly mystical (except how and why those cells and tissues mend) about the arm repairing itself. Remember, the physician does not mend the broken arm. He or she simply promotes as opportune an environment as possible for healing to take place. Likewise, the psychological healer also sets the stage for the ideal healing environment.

3) *There is an inner trend toward health.* Only under certain pressures and stresses do we end up unwell or dis-eased. This seems like an obvious fact, but over the course of their careers many mental health and medical professionals come to assume that we tend toward sickness, unwellness and neurosis and that life is a struggle to conquer pathology. I think it shows the considerable influence S. Freud has had on the ideas in modern psychology and medicine. I do not believe this is the case.

4) *The metaphor of psychological healing occurs on many levels, both within and outside of our awareness.* Conscious awareness can be quite important because the person, with proper knowledge, can set the stage for his or her own emotional growth and metaphoric healing. I equate this kind of abstract idea with the scientific use of antibiotics. You don't have to know how they work for them to have their effect. However, with proper information and knowledge about dosage and type of antibiotic, you can speed up the healing process.

5) *Healing occurs below jaw level.* Getting stuck *up in our heads* only serves to stop or delay the process. Many therapists I have worked with and supervised over the years have said things like: "I've been working with her for so long, so many months we've been dealing with the depression yet still she is still stuck there feeling depressed." I will watch or listen to a tape of their work and the depression, the pain, is not being dealt with. Both are simply talking about dealing with it.

Therapist and client are prancing all around it with words. The pain is not felt. They both fear the pain, the healing crisis.

6) *Play and creativity tend to operate on impulses from outside our awareness, from what some refer to as the unconscious.* As such, they can be vehicles for the healing process to emerge and promote itself. "The making of a sand picture [or any creative image] is, in itself, a symbolic and creative act" (Weinrib, 1983, p. 23). Keep in mind that many natural folk healers already act on this awareness.

Goals

The primary goals of therapy include a growth in ego strength, an increased ability to meet one's needs directly, increased decision making skills and coping skills, accessing inner and outer resources, personal empowerment and an increase in self esteem, and an ability to act independently and assume full (as full as is realistically possible, depending on the age of the child) responsibility for one's own actions. People can accomplish this by facing themselves, learning about their feelings, experiencing respect and acceptance, and learning to make decisions by accessing power from within. Self esteem increases through hard work, not by sitting back making wishes to feel better about oneself and not by receiving an endless stream of compliments from a therapist.

In therapy children are given the chance to acknowledge and express feelings, conflicts, joys. They are given some breathing space, an opportunity to let their inner world come to the surface, to integrate feelings or to work them through to resolution. They explore their own inner world and learn alternate, perhaps more constructive ways to experience/express their inner feelings and processes. They not only work through conflicts and difficulties—they also discover hidden strengths.

Therapy involves helping children gain inner power, exploring their resources that come from within, accessing needed resources from the outside and helping children learn to make decisions and feel a mastery of their own life while accepting what cannot be immediately changed about their own environment and family.

THE ENVIRONMENT OF PLAY THERAPY

In working with living beings, I am making the assumption that there is a purpose to my work. It is not just some haphazard occurrence where someone—a powerless "client," "case," "patient"—comes to see me, a powerful therapist, in my office where he or she is somehow, by contact with me, "fixed" or "cured."

I believe that each child (or adult or animal or plant) I work with tends toward optimum functioning, toward wellness, not disease/pathology. I find it a curious situation where many in the mental health field focus on dysfunction and pathology and work as if they assume that the human race tends toward pathology.

Each living thing has within a tendency to function as well as it can, toward healthy emotional growth. There is an urgent force inside compelling us toward being well. When that force is disrupted or blocked—through a harsh environment, difficult family relationships, painful or frightening experiences—children can become blocked on their growth path.

Ideally, all therapies and play therapy are interventions to move children forward on their path of growth by providing an opportunity for their own natural force toward health to emerge and be nurtured.

As a healer/therapist, I do not come in and fix people or cure them. I do not assume there is anything "wrong" or "broken" about them. All I can do is set the stage for their own inner healing trend to occur. Therapy can thus be seen as stage setting rather than some mysterious event where the "client/patient" has no power or resources of his or her own.

In the therapeutic process there are certain elements which create a safe, optimum environment for the child's healing processes to emerge. These include:

1) *A safe space*. This includes privacy, no interruptions. A place where children can be free to express themselves and be listened to. This is not necessarily a highly equipped play therapy office. I have worked in the corner of a school auditorium. But remember, privacy is very important. I have seen some very talented adult therapists treat children in a negative manner that they would never have considered appropriate in their work with adults. For example, the phone rings

in the middle of a session and they answer it when they are with a child. Or they allow other kinds of interruptions that would have been considered completely taboo when working with adults.

You may find yourself working in an agency where clinical work with children is not fully understood. You may find that, although you understand the need for confidentiality and privacy with children, others around you don't. You may be in the middle of a session with a child and someone knocks on the door. You may wish to ignore it, and this is the best choice if the person on the other side is not particularly persistent. If the knocking continues despite you ignoring it, it could become a distraction of its own. I would advise opening the door and relaying some message to the person who has been interrupting you that says something similar to: "I am in the middle of a meeting with Johnny. Please, don't interrupt us again when we are in the middle of our appointment." I would not wait for a response and would immediately close the door upon making this statement. You may not be very popular in the agency after such an incident, but you will maintain your integrity in your work with children.

2) *A mode of expression.* Given that play is the primary and natural medium of expression for children (Axline, 1969, p. 9), it makes sense that toys be available to foster an environment that is conducive to self-expression and the sharing of feelings. How many of us can remember at some point in our school years going into the "guidance office," a mysterious spot with no toys, art supplies, creative outlets. Having these kinds of supplies in your office gives a clear message that you like having kids in there and you know what kids like to do. A lack of kid tools will only stop a child from being expressive.

3) *An accepting therapist who offers a trusting relationship to children.* A therapist is one who encourages children to face themselves, to express their feelings, to make choices and decisions. By acceptance, I mean that children are accepted with whatever they bring to the session—sadness, anger, joy—their stuff. I have found that therapists who begin working with children often have their preference of issues they find easy to deal with. Some will say: "I find it easy to deal with the aggressive, acting out child, but don't know what to do with the

withdrawn, depressed child." Others may say the reverse. Over their early training, they usually develop a competence in dealing with both kinds of issues. However, an area of lack in mental health training is what to do with the child who brings in joy. Now, I'm not talking about children who are avoiding an issue or denying. I'm referring to children who honestly come in "up." Our tendency, from a mental health perspective, is to bring them down to some negative agenda we feel they should be focused on. I think it is much more appropriate to find out what has been happening over the past few hours, the past day and the past week—what preceded this "up" phase. Since one of our goals in play therapy is to help children with resources and coping skills, when children come in "up," they have obviously tapped some resource or inner strength. We should be helping them gain access to strengths and resources for similar situations in the future.

4) *Freedom, and* 5) *Boundaries.* These two really go hand in hand. You cannot have one without the other. Since the sixties these concepts have been quite confused. Freedom has often been confused with license. True freedom demands negation; it means I have to make choices, to say yes to one opportunity and no to another. Freedom does not mean saying yes to everything. With freedom comes responsibilities, limits, boundaries. The freedom involved in therapy is the right of the child to make increasingly independent choices. This does not mean blanket permission to do absolutely anything he or she wants. The freedom to choose exists within the boundaries of limits.

6) *Confidentiality.* I include this as a separate category although, in reality, it really is philosophically related within the concept of boundaries. However, I believe it is important enough to merit its own discussion. I believe that every child I see has the right to confidentiality. I realize that this does not fit with certain systemic family therapy models. I don't concern myself with them though, for followers of such models sometimes seem like they are inhumanly discussing the arrangement of pieces of a machine rather than human beings with lives, hearts, and souls of their own.

I like to explore the concept of confidentiality with children. It sets the tone of how we work together. It says "I respect you." I use the word "confidentiality" with children and ask if they know what it means. What I like to tell children is something along the lines of "Everything you and I talk about is private. That means I won't go blabbing on you or talking behind your back about the things you say with me. *You* can tell anybody you want all about our time together and the things we talk about and do in here." Notice that I never use the word "secret" with the child. I do not like to use that word. In a way, using the concept of "secrets" sets the child up for abuse—sexual, physical, emotional. When there are secrets there are things that must be hidden and there is nothing that the child should have to hide about the therapeutic process. There is another important part to this discussion of privacy and confidentiality with the child. The child also has the right to be protected. The notion that the child can have total and unquestioned confidentiality is a denial of reality. I, as a therapist and adult, also have the responsibility of protecting that child. So, in our discussion, the child is also told that "I will break that rule (confidentiality) if I think you need to be taken care of or be protected or made safe. Then I will tell whatever I feel necessary to whoever I need to in order to make sure you are taken care of. I will not ask your permission before doing this, but, if possible, I will talk with you about it before I do it." Obviously, the words you choose to explore the concept of confidentiality must fit the age and cognitive abilities of the child you are working with but, in some way, the above messages are conveyed to the child.

This process of discussion with the child builds in a number of things to the therapeutic process. There is a great deal of respect given to the child. There is also nurturing, love and concern conveyed. I believe that relaying everything and anything from the child's session to the parents is incredibly degrading to the child. It is unnecessary and serves no purpose except to reinforce the power of the therapist and parent over the child.

This is not meant to imply that the parents are left totally uninformed. There is a delicate path that must be followed in this process. The parents/caregivers, although not necessarily involved in the child's individual sessions, must very much be part of the process. You can help them feel included by regularly meeting with them and recommending home activities with the children as well as instructing them in parenting skills that will be beneficial for their development as good parents.

WHAT MAKES AN EFFECTIVE THERAPIST?

It may seem like a severe case of stating the obvious, but to be an effective professional who works with children, you must like kids. I had hoped that such a statement need never be issued, but I have seen far too many professionals who work with children who don't seem to like them. They don't respect them, enjoy them or appreciate or understand them for what they are. Such persons can be found in any profession but, unfortunately, there appear to be an overabundance of them in certain professions such as teaching—every level, from preschool and nursery school to high school, and child care work. If you don't like children, don't work with them.

It highlights and catalyses our work with children when we have a sense of humour. This allows our own playful child to emerge. Humour is healing. It allows perspective and relief from stress.

An important aspect of our work is openness and honesty. We shouldn't lie to children or make up excuses for their situation or behaviour or the behaviour of others in their life. This honesty facilitates the development of two way acceptance and trust. The child who knows you can be trusted to be honest and consistent will come to trust you.

Children need to be treated with kindness, gentleness and respect. Generally, when I hear a caregiver saying that their child has no respect for them, I can almost guarantee that this person has rarely, if ever, shown respect for and to the child.

HOW TO EQUIP A PLAY THERAPY SETTING

There are no "musts" or "shoulds" with regard to how to equip a play therapy setting. Perhaps there are some ideals to strive for. However, the only real ideal is an open mind and warm and caring heart. True healing comes from the heart and soul, not from a well-equipped office with all the right equipment and toys. So the following are really only guidelines and possibilities. There are no musts.

Boxes

Simple, plain old cardboard boxes. They are easily obtained and infinitely catalytic of creativity. You can build with little ones, put things inside them, hide things in them, protect things in them. You can crawl inside bigger ones. They might be a bedroom, a kitchen, a house, or a fort or tree house or cave. That old discarded cardboard box is also a puppet theatre. You can decorate them, colour them, glue things on them, cut them, rearrange them. And, when they are finally no longer able to stand the wear, they are recyclable. They might, in fact, be one of the few mandatory supply requirements. And they are free!

Crayons and Paper

Crayons and paper open up many doors. Perhaps no better play therapy tool was ever created. The presence of crayons says "it's okay to be a kid" and make colours and have fun. Crayons are colourful. They are also sensuous with that waxy feel as you move the crayon across a piece of paper. Kids can colour for the sake of colouring or you may suggest some specific technique. Some are outlined in *Chapter 9, Art and Drawings*.

Creative Arts Supplies

The above mentioned crayons, paper, construction paper, non-toxic glue, safety scissors, string, pipe cleaners, egg cartons, empty paper towel rolls, empty plastic berry boxes, material, thread and all kinds of household leftovers, old clothes, discarded cardboard boxes (great puppet stages, caves, hideouts, forts, tunnels), and whatever else you can collect that could be used in the creation of new artsy items in your work with children and adults.

Sunglasses

Make sure to have a pair of sunglasses in your play room for kids to wear. I learned this one from a state trooper in a conversation about fifteen years ago. He was telling me about investigations he had to do involving children and how children were much more open and disclosed far more extensive and intimate details when he let them put on his own sunglasses for the interview. I immediately tried this and found how helpful this could be. It makes sense though. When we put sunglasses on a few things happen. First, we feel a bit tougher, in the sense of being a "cool," "hip" person. Second, we build in some safety, a slight amount of distance and anonymity.

Puppets

Puppets—as many puppets as you can afford. I always have at least one cute little teddy bear in red overalls (the trade name of this little beastie is "Penny Bear" and used to be made by the Dakin company). I also have quite a preference for the use of a full body puppet (by the trade name of "Wiki Tut Bunny" also by Dakin. Unfortunately, I am told that each of these is now extinct as the company has discontinued these wonderful little creatures). Suppose your agency has limited funding and you operate on a minimal budget and there simply is no money around to purchase such supplies as puppets. Don't give up hope. Your agency most likely still has enough money to buy legal size business envelopes and, if so, you have the potential for puppets. Just put an envelope over your hand and then bend it in the middle. Now you have a talking puppet. This can become a very personalized puppet. The child can colour it, make the face and eyes, maybe glue on some felt or cotton balls. It becomes a very individualized puppet. Or how about all those old socks with holes in them just sitting around on the floor beside the washing machine, or all the "singles" you have—you know, the socks with no matching mate. These are all potential puppets. For those of you in climates warranting them, mittens serve the same purpose. What a great way to recycle such items. Turn them into tools for working with children!

Sandbox and Numerous Figurines

Those that are "needed" (read, those that can be useful) are described in *Chapter 10, Sandplay.*

Plants and Animals

I think it is imperative to have a number of representatives of nature in your working environment. I would recommend some plants, an animal like a dog or cat or a singing canary, some rocks and, in some ideal world, maybe a fountain with running water. A miniature fountain with water bubbling over stones and marbles was one of the nicest additions I ever made to an office. Please refer to *Chapter 11, Working With The Earth: Plants/Rocks/Animals in the Healing Process.*

PRINCIPLES TO APPLY IN THERAPEUTIC WORK: How to Play With Children (and Adults) in a Way That is Healing

1) *Do not interpret or analyze for another person.* It may be appropriate to say nothing. If talk does seem to be in order, explore the artwork, stories or sandbox scenes with the person who has made them. Ask questions like: "Do you ever feel the way that animal does?" or "What do you think that person feels (or needs)?"

I like to simply ask the person, child or adult, without pressing or imposing an analysis or interpretations, to tell a story or to talk about specific components of his or her drawing, sandbox scene or other creative product.

I was "working with" ten year old Rebecca in play therapy. One week she made a very complex jungle scene in the sand tray. She threw in two plastic snakes very quickly because she did not want to touch them. I asked her what the snakes meant and she got a repulsed look on her face. I suggested we talk to the snakes and see if we could learn anything from them. At first she was very "grossed out" (her words) by this idea so I suggested that I could hold one of the snakes and we could ask it questions. Upon holding it, I told her, I just couldn't seem to hear it well enough to figure out what it wanted. I told Rebecca I heard the words "I want to be closer to Rebecca." Upon hearing this Rebecca said maybe she could hold it. This was within seconds of having displayed repulsion toward the snake. I gently handed it over to Rebecca and then I started to ask the snake questions about what it wanted to tell Rebecca and what it thought she needed and Rebecca then started to respond for the snake. One of the very important things we learned from this little plastic snake was that Rebecca should be "doing music." Rebecca was not a child who was reported to be particularly musical, but she was telling us quite clearly that music certainly seemed to be important to her.

From that session on, we often included music in our work. Sometimes she just wanted to play music on the synthesizer that would describe her feelings and other times she would dance to the sounds I would make on the synthesizer. In general, music became a way for this little girl to express her emotions. And the clues for this new path came from a little plastic snake that seemed so offensive to her when she first added it to her sand tray scene. Truly, it was an unacknowledged part of herself.

2) *Let the client discover and choose to work with whatever toy or method he or she wishes.* I would recommend you rarely even suggest using any method. Let the client discover the possibilities.

3) *The child in therapy, especially a younger child, may try and tempt you into his or her play.* Should a child be particularly insistent that you take an active part, you could get into a power struggle with the child and say "No, this is your sandbox, I want you to do it." The child then says "No, you do it" and so on....

I would suggest you take the approach in the following example. A child says "You put the trees in" the therapist responds: "Where do you think this one should go?" or "Tell me where you want them to go." In this way the child maintains directorship and production control and responsibility.

4) *Sit close but don't smother.* I think it is important to symbolically be in touch to say "I am here with you." This may be as simple as having one's knee or toe touching the sandbox in which the child is telling stories. I definitely think you should be on the floor near the child with whom you are working. There are some therapists who believe that they practice a very non-directive approach and sit on a chair the whole time and think they never actively participate. The truth is that there is no such thing as non-participation. Sitting in your chair, watching, simply gives the message that adults are aloof, don't play or get close to you. Interestingly, when the child does something, the therapist interpretively says, "You're feeling angry today Johnny." There are a couple of issues here. For one thing, it presumes the therapist has perfect vision into the child's life and knows exactly what the behaviour of the child means. This is very dangerous. Further, I find it much more intrusive and directive to sit on a chair telling children what they feel than to be on the floor exploring their work with them.

5) *Don't lie to children.* They get enough of that from the outside world. I was particularly challenged some years ago during my last appointment on a Friday afternoon. At one point during my session with nine year old Billy, I was very tired and glancing out the window at the falling snow. Billy looked up at me and said "Are you paying attention to me?" I felt caught in the dilemma of whether to tell the truth or to lie in order to avoid making him feel rejected or angry. I sat silently for a moment as I looked at Billy. I smiled rather sheepishly and said "No, I'm sorry, I wasn't, but I'm back now." I went with the decision that, no matter what I said, Billy knew the truth. I felt it was more important to acknowledge what he already knew and in that way maintain Billy's trust in both his own perception and my willingness to be honest with him. As it was, he was quite satisfied with my answer and we immediately got back to the work at hand.

6) *Do whatever you need to do to facilitate a safe, healing environment.* This applies to all work with children, play therapy and therapy in general. This may mean playing soft, relaxing or meditative music in the background, a candle burning, or incense. The options are numerous. However, it should always be geared to the client's framework. If the client is threatened by certain music, then it is not going to create the desired ambience to play that music. Or the client who was sexually abused by a priest or minister as a child may find the burning incense a trigger to all kinds of negatives. The guidelines should be to create a protective and safe ambience for each individual client.

7) *A client's resistance to participating in any particular method such as the sandbox, fingerpainting or whatever, should be respected.* There may be good reasons for a person to abstain from the process.

8) *Parents as healers.* A parent cannot be a child's therapist any more than your professional supervisor can be your therapist. Neither should try. But the parent who consistently responds therapeutically to their children will not likely have children who need therapy.

THE THERAPEUTIC JOURNEY

Beginnings

The initial meetings with a child set the tone for the therapeutic process. I like to discuss issues like confidentiality and privacy in our early meetings. I also like to ask children why they think they are present and I like to let them know what I know or what I've been told.

Over the years I found that with many children, the early phase of our work together involved a great deal of tactile exploring around the room. They reach into all kinds of boxes and toys to see what's inside, lift up blankets and boxes to see what's underneath, open doors to find out what is inside. They are exploring their physical terrain in the office to become comfortable by making this setting familiar. You may find that children do this over the first two or three sessions or they may do it for the first five to ten minutes of every session. I see this exploring resembling dust settling.

Also in the early sessions there may be a general getting acquainted. You need to know ahead of time how open you choose to be in disclosing certain aspects about your own life that children may be curious about. I do think it is an unfair arrangement if children are expected to bare their heart and soul to you, yet you are unwilling to share anything about yourself. This is an unrealistic expectation.

Trust develops in the therapeutic process slowly over time. If you are working with a child who has been abused, trust can easily take six months to begin to develop.

Boundaries/Limits

At some point in the therapy sessions, the limits may well be tested. Children are seeking guidance and direction and are pushing the limits to find out what is safe. Will you still like them after the limit testing? Will you continue to have sessions with them? These are things many children need to find out by pushing the limits. How you handle the conflict in session can model healthy options for handling conflict outside.

A child pushing you and triggering you and trying to go

beyond what is acceptable will quickly need to hear that what he or she is doing is not permissable in session. There are many issues regarding limits. The clearer you are in your own mind about what the limits are and what consequences exist for the child who steps beyond the limit, the easier a time you will have in your sessions.

Some typical difficult areas for therapists might include children who become quite aggressive in their play, children who keep stepping over the line of a recognized limit by doing something like breaking toys or throwing sand, or a number of sexual issues such as children who masturbate or who want to take off their clothes. You need to know what you will allow in your therapy space. For example, children who take off their clothes—well, for a start I would wonder how they got their clothes completely off before being stopped. These children need the safety of hearing that their clothes are not to be removed unless they are in a private place at home. Children who begin to masturbate need to know that this is a private act that should be reserved for a time when they are in private, not in the office. Children who insist on breaking toys need to hear that "the toys are not for breaking." Should they continue, the therapist would then appropriately state that "if you keep trying to break that toy I will see that you are telling me you are not willing to play with it in a safe way right now." Obviously, some toys in the room need to be ones that can be taken apart, wrecked (perhaps old egg cartons), or somehow literally or symbolically destroyed. If your room is too neat and has too many rules you may as well do it in the living room with all the furniture covered with plastic. Play therapy turns into just another oppressive event. Play, like life, has an underlying natural rhythm and beautiful pattern, but on the surface can be quite messy.

Impulse Control/Social Skills

Children with impulse control issues or lacking in social skills may not be prime candidates for much of the inner world exploration of play therapy. A group and/or cognitive-behavioral approach involving limits, behavioral reinforcement, the learning of day to day survival skills and social skills are likely much more in their best interest. They need to learn to survive the system and exist within social expectations.

Moving Along

Over time you will see both subtle and glaringly obvious changes in the child. Initially, or any time you deal with "hot" issues, you may see regression. By regression, I mean a returning to an earlier developmental phase. Regression is a very valuable tool for dealing with stress. We go backwards to a more familiar time and place when there were less demands on us. Everyone regresses. Everyone needs to at times. There is nothing wrong with regression in and of itself. The problems arise when individuals don't know they've regressed or when they become trapped in the regressed state. As mentioned, we all tend to regress when under stress, when tired, or sick and in greater need than usual. For example, in all my travels on the road presenting training programs, I can become very tired. I tend to put 110% into my presentations, so that at the end of a day, I am sometimes exhausted. I feel quite "wussyish" and will actively regress. I allow myself to feel like a six year old. I may call room service in whatever hotel I am staying in and ask for hot lemon and honey (despite this being an unusual request, most hotels can come up with it). Why hot lemon and honey? Well, when I was a kid, that's what my mum or dad would often give me when I was not feeling well or was just out of sorts in some way. So, to me, it is also symbolic of nurturing. I allow myself to be pampered that way in a regressed position. Having taken that step backwards I am refreshed and renewed and able to do my best again the next day.

Children under stress who regress are not going to be aware that "oh, I'm under stress, I guess I'm just regressing." Nevertheless, they can be taught to ask for a hug when feeling "under the weather" or sad. They can learn to go curl up in a blanket and understand the metaphor of a cocoon. Upon leaving the cocoon, a butterfly emerges.

Therapy is about empowerment for children. They learn to tap their own inner resources and how to access external resources. Children also gradually become aware of their own needs. For the six year old, it may be knowing when to ask for a hug or a snuggle or when to play a game of kick the ball. For the twelve year old, it may be knowing how to turn to mum or dad or aunt or uncle for a hug or a shoulder that will listen to his or her concerns about nobody liking him or her at school. Therapy also involves learning how to put forth effort to make changes and succeed at tasks. With effort and hard work come an improvement in self esteem. Therapy may involve referrals for help in learning to read or write or do math (unless you are a skilled teacher yourself, as some therapists are). If a child has been referred to you who has low self esteem because he or she keeps failing at math, no amount of cutesy work you do will increase his or her self esteem until someone deals with the underlying issue of failing at math. You had better make sure that someone teaches the child math skills.

A haunting aspect of therapy and a very painful aspect for anyone who has chosen to work with children is that therapy is also always about saying goodbye. Your work is, or should be, constantly geared toward the child not needing time with you anymore. You are forever trying to work yourself out of a job. Thus, at the end of your work with any individual child, that child may feel grief over the loss of you and time with you. However, therapists will experience a constant grief as they continually leave children behind. For this reason, your own support network outside of work is vital so you do not become consumed by your work. I mention more about this in other sections of this book.

Toward the end of your work with a child, it will really start to feel more like fun and less like hard work.

Endings[4]

Without the colourful dying leaves of autumn there would be no spring buds. Rotting organic matter brings life to new seeds. Through death comes rebirth. Without endings there can be no new beginnings. Without a goodbye we cannot appreciate the past. When we are trapped by the past we come to be controlled by it and resent it. When we are able to let go we are able to appreciate and learn from our roots. On the other hand, many live deep in the earth's "belly" in a self imposed death-like misery, clinging to the pains of the past which they choose to dwell on and blame for all life's difficulties.

Many of the children we work with come from environments which do not teach them to say goodbyes. They do not develop clear boundaries. Many will spend their lives clinging to the past and attempting to escape responsibility by blaming a harsh background or emotional/physical/sexual abuse and so on for all of their own present problems, wrongdoings, and difficulties.

I see it as a clinical responsibility and necessity to create clear goodbyes with symbolic elements to emphasize the process. There are many ways of doing this. Simply mentioning the process of goodbye on a regular basis can set the stage for its unfolding. For example, when running a children's (or adult's) group, make a point of mentioning each week something to the effect of: "This is our second week and we have six more weeks before we say goodbye." In the second last session, make a point of noting that "next week is our last week. Is there anything you would like to do as a way of saying goodbye?" This may involve a drawing that portrays the goodbye process, it may involve a "goodbye party" (especially in group) or it could involve a fun outing.

One little fellow with whom I had worked for many months chose that we would go bowling as the final piece of our goodbye process. We went bowling, had soft drinks and popcorn and a very good time. However, the purpose was not to produce a "good time" and avoid the pain of parting. The purpose was to highlight the ending of our time together. After this young fellow and I had been out bowling and we were driving home, I felt sad and was silent. I was lost for words. I knew it was our final session and our bowling outing had been planned as the final part of the goodbye process. In the car driving home, young Robbie put it all together: "I will never forget this day. I didn't think you'd take me seriously when I picked bowling for our goodbye. You really listened to me. I'll never forget this." At that point the goodbye was real. We had finished. Robbie had much to take with him, but one thing that would no longer be there would be the weekly therapy sessions. He had grown beyond that need. Had we not had this goodbye built in, the boundary between then and now would not be clear and Robbie would not have been able to have had a clear new beginning.

As often as not, the person we are working with may say: "I don't say goodbyes." There is a tendency to avoid the process of ending. This is natural, for who wants to let go of something they perceive as beneficial and helpful. But there comes a time when to maintain the therapeutic relationship would start to work against the client since it would foster dependency rather than independence. It is therefore the responsibility of the therapist to guide the way through ending.

I have so far focused my comments on the client, but we must remember and be wary of our own responses to the transition away from any and all of our clients. To avoid our own feelings and avoid the issue of goodbye is only modelling similar behaviour for the person with whom we are working. We have a clinical responsibility to be aware of our own inner processes. It is perfectly natural for anyone going through some kind of ending or any separation process to grieve, to feel sad, confused, angry. If you do not stay on top of this, the chances of you putting your own inner process onto the client become heightened. Through chats with colleagues and friends, supervision and such inner processes as active imagination you can deal with your own "stuff" so it doesn't impinge on the client's "stuff."

In terms of modelling, I see no problem in sharing feelings with a client as long as it doesn't become a dump session or result in the client offering support to you. For example, in children's groups, in the last session, I always let kids know exactly what I am feeling (It is vitally important here not to ask for any support whatsoever from such a group. You still have the adult responsibilities of caring for children, not leaning on them). A good way to start off a goodbye session is to say something along the lines of "I am feeling a whole bunch of feelings today. I'm very happy to have gotten to know all of you. I'm also very sad to be saying goodbye. I know that next week at this time when it would have been time for group I am going to feel a little empty. I will realize that we no longer have this group and will probably feel an emptiness right in the middle of my tummy. I will miss all of you." You may wish to say something special to or about each child in the group. Then it is their turn. The tone has already been set not to take this session lightly.

It is important for the therapist to model a clear goodbye. This may be difficult. Keep in mind that ending with one particular child who is doing quite well and who may be a real joy to be around in favour of taking on the next intense referral, little Jake, who may come into your office next week very sullen or extremely belligerent is not an easy task. We are all human. Therapists need to remember why they are there. We may wish to hold on to the child who no longer needs sessions with us. We may do so by having an unclear goodbye. Perhaps, in meeting our own needs, instead of saying goodbye, we say, "Well Billy, maybe we'll see each other downtown/at the movies/at the mall sometime." This is not a clear goodbye and pieces are still dangling. Now Billy can fantasize, with your permission and outright encouragement, about continuing to see you.

The saddest fact is that as long as we avoid goodbyes, we deprive ourselves of a full joyous life. Through denial and avoidance grow bitterness and resentment. Through grief, by working with it rather than against it, comes joy and rebirth. We owe it to ourselves and to those we work with on the healing path to come to terms with the goodbye and grieving processes.

Hand in hand at any of these stages go a number of interwoven processes such as special education, parents' marital therapy, family therapy, parenting skills programs, specific skills/issues programs (e.g. separation and divorce, social skills groups, streetproofing, etc.).

Play therapy must not be done in exclusion to the outside world and other processes. It may be a private time for that child, but the context of a much wider environment in which the child lives must always be considered.

SUBPLOTS WITHIN THE PROCESS

◗ Self

Initially a little human being perceives him or herself as totally part of the caregiver. Gradually, the infant begins to gain a sense of his or her own being in relation to others. Finally, a wholeness and independence develops. With this psychological wholeness come representations and symbols of wholeness. Such representations may include circles drawn, mandala symbolism obvious in art, the sand, or movement, the development of towns in stories where previously there had only been chaos.

◗ Ego

Our egos develop, gradually increasing in strength and stability. Initially we all function at a primitive level, which some from the Jungian movement have best described as the "animal vegetative" stage because what is seen in creative output is a great deal of animals and vegetation. Next comes the conflict stage when fighting predominates. Finally, there is what the Jungian movement calls "adaptation to the collective." It is a time of balance and cooperative skills.

ROADBLOCKS AND HOW TO WORK WITH THEM

Over the course of therapy with children, they should gradually start to come to sessions looking more hopeful and relaxed with an apparent increase in confidence. Over time, they become better able to reflect on what has been happening in their sessions and what they have learned along the way.

You should see changes from the original baseline as your work progresses. For example, if the child was, at first, never able to concentrate and sit still in a session, as you proceed, the child may come to sit quietly in play with you. Or, you may have had a child who always "froze" upon entering the play room. Now he or she enters and gets right down to business. There may be changes in the child's patterns of play, the kinds of toys and tools preferred, and in the involvement of and with the therapist.

Sometimes it may appear that there is not any progress. Roadblocks in therapy do not mean that there is no way through and it is time to end the journey. They simply mean we are likely going to have to slow down; the road may not be as smooth for a while and we are going to have to find some alternate way around from our preconceived original pathway. There are a number of reasons that the healing process may come to a temporary standstill. The biggest reason is our own impatience. On the other hand, we may think the process is stuck simply because we don't recognize the true healing process occurring.

Some signs of roadblocks or of being "stuck" on the healing path include:

- Not knowing what the child's play and symbols refer to for an extended period of time, or being unable to abandon oneself to the process and just wait for things to be revealed. This may only be a sign of the therapist's impatience. Things may be unfolding, but the therapist is unaware of the process in front of them.

- Regretting seeing some particular child. It's Thursday at 3 pm and you start to get uneasy feelings in the depth of your tummy thinking about the child you are about to see in your next appointment. You know the thoughts of "Oh God, no, my next appointment is with Johnny." A variation on this would be feeling like shortening or cancelling sessions or going to bi-weekly instead of weekly sessions with some particular child for no relevant reason other than your own discomfort. No one likes to admit to having these kinds of feelings. We are all supposed to like everyone and to be able to work with anyone. This is simply not the case. Some kids are harder to work with than others. The kind of child who is difficult to work with will vary between therapists. It is important to admit negative, ambivalent or confused feelings if you have them. It will help to uncover what is triggering these feelings and, in so doing, you will be better able to help the child with whom you are working. The important point when experiencing these kinds of feelings is to have supervision or consultation of your work.

- An apparent deterioration over a period of time. Initially, when a child enters the therapy process it is not at all unusual to see an apparent deterioration over a brief period of time as all kinds of issues are uncovered. However, if this continues for more than 3 or 4 weeks, I would be very concerned that you are doing something wrong or are missing something. Again, immediate supervision and consultation are critical.

- Finding yourself feeling overwhelmed by your own personal feelings. These may be anger, sadness, or even a sense of inadequacy. In this situation, you obviously have some unresolved issues of your own that are interfering with your work. Deal with them.

- Discovering that you have a model child on your hands. There is no such thing as a model child; when one acts that way for an extended period of time, I would be concerned that he or she is trying to please me.

In terms of getting "unstuck" in therapy with children, and adults as well, it is important to have fun, to be loose enough to not take everything too seriously. If you subscribe to a rigid school of thought or model, you may quickly find that your beliefs will not work with all children. They may not even be effective with many children. In fact, no one technique or method works with all children. The more methods and approaches you have in your "toolchest," the more you will be able to fit methods to an individual child rather than vice versa.

A most effective route to becoming "unstuck" and finding your way along the path again is to have highly competent supervision or consultation. What I have found over the years in my own work and in supervising many others is that one of the prime reasons for becoming stuck in the therapeutic process is moving too quickly with a child, forcing issues, dealing with what you think is important rather than going at the child's pace. Pushing your pace, your preconceived ideas of what the issues should be, or even what toys to play with or how to play with them can cause the child to put up personal barriers that will eliminate progress. This whole thing is called "play therapy" and sometimes we forget the play part. It is important to make it playful, to have fun and generally create a low- or no-anxiety environment. Always try and think of the metaphor of *following*. Try and see children ahead of you on a path through the fields and woods. *They* are leading. *You* are following. *They* decide how fast or slow to go, which twists and turns to take, which trees and plants to stop and look at and which to ignore, what fences to climb over, go under, what gates to open and what to look at once proceeding through. Going at the child's pace is the greatest way to become "unstuck." You are there as a support when children turn to you for help. You are not there to drag them through the mud that they might not be able to handle simply because your theory says they must deal with the mud before being "cured."

DIRECTIVE VERSUS NON-DIRECTIVE APPROACHES

There is an on-going debate in the play therapy field over which approach is "better"—non-directive or directive. There are two issues of concern here. First, there is not one right way to proceed in our work with children. Many approaches work with children. Be wary of those with dogmatic views about there being only one way that works in the mental health field. Second, I do not believe there really is any such thing as non-directive therapy. There is a continuum of directiveness versus non-directiveness that varies between sessions and children. The term "non-directive" is a misnomer.

There are different levels and areas of directiveness, but no non-directive approach. There are three main areas of directiveness: 1) the therapeutic process itself; 2) the content of sessions, and; 3) the interpretation of material that emerges within the process.

I recommend being fairly non-directive in the therapeutic process, often quite directive with regard to the methods of a session, and as non-directive as possible with regard to the interpretation of material which arises in a session, and quite directive in issues in the safety and best interests of the child. What I find in some professionals who call themselves non-directive is that they are only non-directive in the process and methods used in a session. They can suddenly become extremely directive in interpreting and analyzing the child's inner world and feeding back to the child what they happen to think they are seeing and what they think the child is feeling. This is taking a god-like approach. It is saying to the person in therapy that "I know more about your inner world than you do." This is very disempowering for the person in therapy. Therapy should be about empowering clients, not disempowering them. Therapists should not be in there interpreting clients' art, dreams, play or behaviour for them. To analyze for someone else is degrading to that person. It is a form of psychic rape.

Keeping in mind that I do not think there exists such a thing as a non-directive approach, imagine a scene in a therapy room where such an approach is used rigidly. In some client-centred or non-directive approaches, it is believed that the therapist should in no way "interfere" with the play of the child. This view is sometimes interpreted as meaning therapists should always remain outside the play, often sitting in a chair watching and reflecting their personal opinions on what children are doing. This seems like an odd Freudian-like image that only gives children the message that adults are aloof and don't like to interact with children. This is a **non-involved** rather than non-directive approach. It does give a very clear direction by providing an image of an aloof adult unwilling to have fun with children. This resembles an image of some rigid school teacher from decades ago who was both distant and aloof, and who at no time became involved or playful with children or, heaven forbid, had fun. The passion and intensity of playfulness were definitely lacking in such a person. This gives children a discouraging image of the world of adults. Beware of play therapists who don't play with children. They resemble voyeurs who would rather watch a nature program on television than dig in the garden.

Now despite this critique of some so-called "non-directive" or "client-centred" methods, I know of therapists using such an approach who care deeply about the children with whom they work and who seem to be doing a very good job with those children. Research on the non-directive methods also points to positive outcome results. So take my critique with a grain of salt. Perhaps I'm all wrong on this philosophical point. However, I do not believe the research that supports a so-called "non-directive" approach was with therapists who never became involved in play. Rather, it involved therapists who followed the children's lead, going at the children's pace, and imposing no direction on the course of therapy.

In work with others I like to give little or no direction with regard to the process or what the issues are that need work. Keep my metaphor of following a path in mind. Do not tell the path where to go. Follow the path and see what emerges. This is what the therapy process should be. Once an issue arises, then I am directive with regard to methods and techniques for dealing with the issue.

Finally, with regard to interpreting the creative output of a child or adult with whom I am working, I would not give interpretations or analyses. I would simply explore clients' material with them to find out what it means from their perspective.

THE PRESENT STATE OF THE FIELD: RESEARCH

Psychotherapy in General

In the 1940s, 1950s, and 1960s, early work on efficacy of psychotherapy was not particularly complimentary. Some studies found that those in control groups involving no treatment actually did better than those in treatment. A number of studies found that with both controls and treatment groups a small percentage improved, the bulk remained largely unchanged, and a certain percentage deteriorated. A frightening finding of some studies has involved the deterioration of the same amount or more of those in treatment compared to those receiving no treatment. Fischer (1976) reached the same conclusions with regard to a number of varied social casework approaches. Fischer went so far as to state that:

> Despite the lack of clarity over what exactly causes deterioration – indeed, the causes are probably multifactorial – the evidence on the presence of deterioration among clients of professional caseworkers is strong enough to justify the warning that professional casework may be hazardous to our clients' well-being (1976, p. 109).

Over the next few decades, there were numerous less-than-rigorous studies that showed that psychotherapy can be effective. Many of these studies had major flaws with regard to their experimental design. Many studies indicated that, following treatment, with a certain type of therapy or level of therapist, there was improvement. Unfortunately, such general studies tell us almost nothing, since there was no control group built in. Two other major flaws of many studies looking at therapeutic outcome are: 1) extremely low numbers of subjects, and; 2) poor methods of measurement. For example, many studies in the marriage and family therapy field have used therapist impression of improvement as an indicator of improvement. This is not exactly what one could call an independent and highly reliable instrument. Due to an inherent conflict of interest, therapist impressions are some of the least reliable measurements available. Some thorough reviews and research through the 1970s "concluded that there was still no solid empirical evidence for the effectiveness of psychotherapy" (Russ, 1995, p. 377).

More recently, there have emerged some major empirical studies that have concluded that at least some forms of psychotherapy, in general, are effective (Smith & Glass, 1977; Smith, Glass & Miller, 1980; Dawes, 1994). However, contrary to firmly held popular beliefs, the level of qualification of therapist, methods used by the therapist and length of therapy do not seem to be factors in successful outcome.

The work of Strup and Hadley (1979) has shown that there is no better therapeutic outcome for clients of professionally trained therapists than there is for paraprofessionals. Stein and Lambert (1984) as well as Smith and Sechrest (1991) have proven that the level of experience of professional therapists and length of treatment is unrelated to success in treatment. Smith and Glass (1977) have shown that neither type of therapy[5] nor length of therapy are related to its success.

A summary of the emerging studies (Berman & Norton, 1985) indicates that there has failed to be any definitive indication that there is any difference between paraprofessional and professionally trained therapists in terms of efficacy of treatment. Nor does research indicate any difference when types of problems and treatments are analyzed. In an analysis of psychotherapy, treatment types were broken down into the categories of behavioral, cognitive-behavioral, humanistic, crisis intervention, and undifferentiated counselling. No significant differences between paraprofessionals and professionals were found between experimental and control groups when a number of sources of outcome were used—patient, therapist, independent observer, behavioral indicators. We now know that "training, credentials, and experience of psychotherapists are irrelevant, or at least that is what all the evidence indicates" (Dawes, 1994, p. 62).

There may be personal and emotional reasons for a professional to believe that training, credentials and experience make a difference in outcome, but there is no scientific evidence. Again, from the work of Dawes:

> All mental health practitioners are susceptible to an overinflated belief in their own position, and they should constantly subject themselves to the discipline of testing their ideas empirically or reading about others' tests of them (Dawes,1994).

This begs the question, "so why bother going to a highly trained—and costly—professional at all?" I'm not sure that with our present knowledge this question has a justifiable positive answer. This is not to imply that advanced training and skill do not have a special role to play. Someone with advanced scientific training, a high level of skills and empirical knowledge still has to design, evaluate and recommend interventions to use. That does not necessarily mean they need to be the same ones carrying out the work. There is also the further question of who should pay for services.

> While therapy generally is effective, and while it would be nice to provide therapy to everyone who wishes it on the basis of their own judgment of need or desire, society as a whole should not pay (Dawes, 1994, p. 198).

Therapy is a luxury, not a right. Often it is only a by-product of a self indulgence, not need.

If you are actually looking for a therapist for yourself or a child, I would recommend certain criteria for your choice of a professional: 1) find someone certified in the specialty you think would be most beneficial—for example, an IBECPT Certified Child Psychotherapist and Play Therapist, neuropsychologist or cognitive-behavioral therapist; 2) I would want a referral to someone who reads several professional scientific journals and periodicals such as the American Psychological Association *Monitor*. You need someone who is on the cutting edge of recognizing innovative methods, who also realizes the importance of up to date research, and; 3) find someone you sense is empathic, someone with whom you feel you can connect.

Therapy with Children

Historically, children have been a largely ignored group within the mental health field, despite a large number of them presenting with problems. There would appear to have been an assumption that, whatever their problems, children will grow out of them. Although children have received mental health and psychological treatment for several decades, the aspects of therapy which are beneficial have only just begun to be analyzed. In the past three decades there have been three major influences on child therapy: psychoanalytic, client-centred, and cognitive-behavioral.

The family therapy field, which grew out of the needs of schizophrenic adolescents and their families, has not had much, if anything, to offer children. This is a peculiar development when one considers that most traditional families and even many modern alternate family forms include children. Since problems with children and their behaviour cause a great many concerns for parents and caregivers, it seems prudent for mental health professionals to focus attention on this population.

Therapeutic endeavours with children are a relatively new phenomenon that can be traced to the development of psychoanalysis. It has been stated that the profession's own resistance to evaluating itself stemmed partly from its psychoanalytic origins (Dawes, 1994). One of the first recorded case histories in the literature was that of "little Hans." Freud recorded, at length, his child guidance recommendations to "little Hans'" parents. Prior to this time, children's behaviour was perceived as resulting from being wicked, ill-bred, ill-mannered or similarly socially distempered (Reisman & Ribordy, 1993, p. 3).

> The prevalent view among professionals, meanwhile, was that the disorders of childhood were indicative of deficiencies in the child's education and training. Therefore, in treatment the emphasis had been on the teaching of proper habits and on persuading the child to overcome immorality and to behave correctly (Reisman & Ribordy, 1993, p.3).

The first known empirical research in child psychology was conducted in the late 1700s by Dietrich Tiederman. A century later, Stanley Hall administered a mass of questionnaires to young children and served as a key catalyst for the field of developmental psychology. Hall was one of the most significant figures in modern psychology. He founded the *American Journal of Psychology*. The American Psychological Association was founded in 1892, "largely through Hall's efforts" (Schultz & Schultz, 1992, p. 219). Hall was also responsible for the opening of the Child Study Institute at Clark University. His child study movement reached its height in the 1920s with the opening of a research laboratory for the study of child welfare at the University of Iowa.

Theoretically, at least, we believe

> that play helps children deal with fears and reduce anxiety and that something about play itself is important and serves as a vehicle for change (Russ, 1995, p. 382).

It is not yet clear if, or why, play used in therapy is beneficial. The earliest research on children's psychotherapeutic methodologies reported grim results. Indications were that children who benefited from child psychotherapy were not significantly different from the numbers who improved without therapy. This may have been due to the fact that early approaches were largely psychoanalytic. Fischer (1976) has concluded that

> to date, not a single piece of controlled evidence is available to clearly demonstrate the effectiveness of any form of psychodynamically-based approach in casework, counseling or psychotherapy (p. 324).

Increasing research over the 1970s and 1980s started to find that there were greater improvements with treatment than with no treatment. Some studies have shown that children respond better to treatment than adolescents do (Reisman & Ribordy, 1993).

Newer research to date has given us the information that therapy with children seems to be effective. The research does not yet definitively make clear which techniques are best. Given this rather glaring lack in our knowledge base, I believe we should be very careful about what we scoff at and what we consider true clinical knowledge. The truth is we do not yet have the knowledge. Kazdin (1990) offers "evidence that psychotherapy is more effective than no treatment with children" (Russ, 1995, p. 378). However,

> Weisz and Weisz (1993) cautioned that the evidence for the effectiveness of psychotherapy is based on studies that are not typical of conventional clinical practice (Russ, 1995, p. 378).

In the successful outcomes, the therapy focused on a target problem or issue. Typical clinical work is more vague. Phillips (1985)

> concluded that the play therapy research that found positive results were those studies of a cognitive-behavioral nature that were carefully designed (Russ, 1995, p. 379).

Some of the more important and extensive studies of children have been developmentally oriented. Piaget posed a cognitive model of child development in which human beings are considered to be "little thinkers" and his theory is framed around that view. Following extensive and painstaking research, Piaget concluded that cognitive development requires both experience and maturation and is the result of an interaction between the individual and environment. Although offering considerable insight into the lives of children, there are certain flaws with the Piaget approach, primarily in the generalizability of Piaget's findings. The cognitive development of children from different cultures does not proceed at the pace predicted by Piaget. Further, Vigotsky challenged Piaget's findings on mental development and speech. Vigotsky proposed that there exist two speech systems, inner speech and socialized speech.

Research studies need to examine the needs of children, the results of ignoring the needs of children, treatment methods which have been used with children and those methods which have been shown to be beneficial in treating children. Studies also need to raise questions concerning the direction of the specialty of child therapy.

Several years ago I realized that an important question is whether therapists who work with children have adequate evaluation methods to determine the efficacy of their work. Ongoing data obtained on this question will have practical value in promoting an increased credibility in the field. Initial research dealing with this issue has begun to examine such concerns (Barnes, in press).

To date, scientific research on the treatment of children is sporadic and limited. Most of the material classified as research is little more than philosophical discussion and extrapolation of belief systems. There has been little promotion or encouragement in the area of research or evaluation. Even the CACPT periodical, *Playground* (published since 1987), and the APT Inc. periodical, *The International Journal of Play Therapy* (published since 1992), both of which contain interesting articles fostering the development of the profession of child and play therapy, clearly lack any focus whatsoever on the process of evaluation and research methods. Any "research" articles published in these periodicals indicate a significant lack of scientific research understanding and tend to be philosophical and/or theoretical discussions rather than empirical research.

For example, in the *APT Inc. Journal*, there is one study entitled "The Evaluation of Process and Outcome in Individual Child Psychotherapy" in which an "objective method for the evaluation of therapy process and outcome in cases of individual child psychotherapy" (Rosen, Faust, & Burns, 1994, pp. 33-43) is described. It is a description, a fairly good description at that, of how 14 children were seen by therapists and sessions were videotaped. Two "judges" viewed the tapes and used a rating scale to assess the process. Their evaluations of the videotapes revealed an agreement ranging from 89% to 100%. Psychodynamic and client-centred treatment groups were compared and no difference was found between the two.

Positive changes were seen in the children over an eight week period. However, in this study, there was no control or placebo group, nor was there even a mention of control and placebo groups or the reason for the absence of control and placebo groups. To its credit, the study does indicate that the rating scale used may be sensitive enough to discover changes. Thus, based on this minuscule sample, we can say that the observation instrument being used may be useful in the evaluation of process. However, the title of the article is "The Evaluation of Process and Outcome in Individual Child Psychotherapy." There is, in fact, absolutely nothing in this article related to evaluation of outcome. This is fairly common in play therapy "research".

The journal in which this article appeared contained no other article which included a control group and placebo group in the research methodology. There can be no evaluation of outcome without a control group and placebo group.

Thus, we are left with what are essentially a large number of theories with no true empirical basis to determine efficacy. One might wonder whether control and placebo groups are not included in studies because we have "educated" a generation of psychologists and other mental health professionals who do not understand the scientific method.

Reisman & Ribordy (1993) believe that treatment with children has been found to be effective. Such treatment has been found to

> reduce the severity of symptoms, speed the process of healing or recovery, and help people acquire new techniques for coping with their personal problems (Reisman & Ribordy, 1993, p. 11).

The studies examined by Reisman & Ribordy were not all particularly rigorous nor empirical. As in other forms of mental health therapy, to date, there is little indication of the superiority of any particular treatment approach. An examination of research (Reisman & Ribordy, 1993; Dawes, 1994) suggests that we currently do not know what treatment methods work with children.

While offering a fairly thorough review of client-centred play therapy research, Guerney notes that

> compared to many therapeutic approaches, there has been a considerable amount of outcome research in client-centred play therapy. It has consistently demonstrated positive treatment results (1983, p. 53).

However, she then outlines "research that has employed some sort of control condition" (p. 53). We are presented with a sum total of seven studies over four decades, with five of the studies conducted prior to the end of the 1950s (Fleming & Snyder, 1947; Cox, 1953; Bills, 1950a, 1950b; Dorfman, 1958; Seeman, Barry, & Ellinwood, 1964; Schmidtchen & Hobrucker, 1978). I would hardly classify an average of one study every 5 years as "a considerable amount of research." To Guerney's credit, she does note that the "considerable amount of research" relates to outcome research. However, the limited control studies that are available do indicate that children in treatment seem to enjoy improvements in a number of areas including increased social skills, intellectual ability, and self-concept, and decreased anxiety and behaviour problems.

> Positive changes consistently take place in therapy for children between the ages of three and ten, even when inexperienced, nonprofessional therapists are providing the treatment (Guerney, 1983, p. 57).

Recent Developments

...basically, there aren't any. I have already mentioned the historical inadequacy of so-called research. In the past few years we have not been faring much better with respect to research in the field of play therapy.

Reams and Friedrich (1994), in a population specific review on therapy with maltreated children, found that

> only two group-comparison outcome studies of therapy...with maltreated children have been published.... No published controlled outcome study on individual psychotherapy with maltreated children is available, although the treatment needs of maltreated children appear obvious (p. 889).

Reams and Friedrich (1994) conducted a study on individual play therapy treatment with maladjusted preschoolers.

> No consistent support was found for the hypothesis that time-limited [15 sessions] play therapy would improve the adjustment of maltreated preschoolers who already were attending a therapeutic preschool. This lack of support was evident at both post-test and follow-up.... Little success was found in this first controlled outcome study of any form of individual therapy with maltreated children. Yet play therapy is a popular approach with abused children despite this lack of empirical support. Certainly, this one finding with regard to the efficacy of a particular form of play therapy does not necessitate conclusions about the usefulness of play therapy in general. It does, however, raise larger questions about why there has been so little research on the treatment of abused children and the possibility that practitioners may not be using the most efficient means to treat abused children (Reams & Friedrich, 1994, pp. 897, 898).

The authors raise the issue that "perhaps time-limited play therapy has little or no effectiveness with abused preschoolers" (Reams & Friendrich, 1994, p. 897). The authors also suggest that the time involved, 15 weeks, may have been inadequate for abused children. Significantly, it is suggested that perhaps only so much can change in any given period of time. In other words, the children were already in a therapeutic preschool milieu and perhaps there was "no room for individual therapy to have an effect" (p. 897).

In the 1994 study (Hellendoorn, van der Kooij & Sutton-Smith) with mostly European contributors, *Play and Intervention*, chapter one by Jerome Singer, who teaches psychology and child study at Yale University, is called "The Scientific Foundations of Play Therapy." Although it is quite interesting, there is not a single empirical study on play therapy in the chapter. It is a typical play therapy philosophy chapter. Such explorations are important and valuable to the development of the field, but we gradually erode scientific credibility by interweaving and confusing philosophical beliefs with science.

In another chapter there is a section entitled an "empirical study of the structural learning process in play therapy." In this section we are presented with what is basically a single case transcript. I realize that such studies can provide useful information, but, if this is the best research we can do, we can pack it in now. Fortunately, there is considerable reason in this text with some wonderful and significant material presented on "play training". As well, in the epilogue by Hellendoorn, van der Kooij and Sutton-Smith (1994), it is noted that "as a serious scientific enterprise, play therapy is still in poor shape." **That is a mild understatement.** In 1953, Lebo described the state of play therapy research as

> "still meager, unsound, and frequently of a cheerful persuasive nature." Twenty five years later Barrett, Hampe and Miller (1978) contributed a modest paper to the authoritative handbook of Garfield and Bergin, in which they had to admit that this unsatisfactory situation was essentially unchanged. And in the third edition (1986), the editors decided that there was insufficient new material in the field of psychotherapy with children to warrant a chapter of its own. (Hellendoorn, van der Kooij & Sutton-Smith, 1994, p. 217).

Sadly, in 1996, the emphasis in therapeutic literature remains on beliefs, theory and philosophy, often confusing these with scientific facts.

I think child and play therapy may have much to offer but theorists had better get off their obtuse, multisyllabic mumbo jumbo bandwagons. It is time for them to get down to serious scientific examination of the field to discover what, if anything, works so these methods can be used to children's advantage, as well as what doesn't work so that we can get rid of these ineffective methods.

A study by Russ (1995) on play psychotherapy research shows the field in the early stages of becoming scientific. As Russ notes,

> The road map for therapeutic change has come mainly from the clinical and theoretical literature. There is little direct empirical support for these intervention strategies and the use of play in psychotherapy. However, there is a strong empirical base in the children's play literature about the role of play in child development (Russ, 1995, p. 371).

Fortunately, the field of play therapy has neighbours in developmental psychology, anthropology, and ethology. From these fields we gain considerable evidence developmentally, cross culturally and cross-species on the positive effects of play and the negative effects resulting from a lack of play in an individual's life.

There is also substantial evidence suggesting that there are considerable benefits to children from play training. For example, it has been found that if parents engaged in physical play with their children in sensitive, responsive ways, their children were more likely to be popular with peers. With conventional research designs, a number of researchers have reported that children who experienced play tutoring showed gains in areas of social, linguistic and cognitive competence (Hellendoorn *et al.*, 1994, p. 190).

MAJOR FLAWS IN OUR PRESENT WORK

Four areas that should raise real concern in mental health work with children are the use of projective tests, the use of anatomically detailed dolls and general child abuse investigations, self-esteem work, and, finally, psychiatric hospitalization.

Projective Tests

> Projective Tests: Hocus-pocus used by psychologists to prove that they are smart and their clients stupid. The general acceptance of these tests suggests that this claim may not be without foundation (Szasz, 1990, p. 195).

A projective test involves asking a client to draw, tell a story, or in some way respond to questions asked or pictures shown by the therapist. It is thought that the client's response is a "projection" of unconscious material in his or her personality. The validity of such tests has never been proved. Their lack of validity has, in many cases, been proved beyond a doubt. Yet, their use is rampant in the mental health field, especially in play therapy and other creative arts therapies.

Dawes (1994) examined the reasons for the popularity of projective tests and notes that they are great fun but they are only interpretive of the interpreter. It is noted that as compelling as the theory underlying the projective tests may be, as fun and compelling as the interpretations are, as fun at they are to give, they do not actually provide the insight about the subject that users allege they provide. The only reason there is any controversy or unresolved debate regarding projective techniques is that professionals who still employ them do not accept the compelling evidence that they don't work. Despite thousands of publications about projective tests, the large majority, including the Rorschach, have never been validated empirically.

> Worse yet, licensed psychologists and others in allied fields are permitted to use techniques that the research has shown unambiguously not to work – and they do so. Most commonly used are the "projective techniques" (Dawes, 1994, p. 145).

The Ethics Committee of the Philadelphia Society of Clinical Psychologists warn against the use of such tests in a court setting:

> "any psychologist who chooses to use instruments whose validity has not been demonstrated as predictive of desirable arrangements (for example, projective tests), should be prepared to be challenged on ethical grounds." I ask, however: If the use of an instrument (a projective test or any other) can be challenged on ethical grounds in a court of law, how can its use be ethically justified in any context at all? My answer is that it can't (Dawes, 1994, p. 152).

Despite the lack of empirical evidence for the use of projective techniques, they are used pervasively in the field of play therapy. Play therapy training programs and texts are full of such projective and interpretive methods. There are even those who foolishly believe that projective techniques actually enable an outsider to determine the state of children's psychological functioning, right down to past trauma and conflicts. Loosely interpreted, this means that we should use techniques that are not based on empirical evidence but consistent with theories that have never been proved and which, in fact, have been definitively shown to be erroneous. Lighten up, for heaven's sake. With such an approach, it is no wonder that many courts and the legal system don't take play therapy assessments at all seriously!

Anatomically Detailed Dolls and Child Abuse Investigations

These dolls have often been referred to as "anatomically correct" and this description is still often used today. However, the phrase "anatomically detailed dolls" is somewhat more accurate. I don't know about you, but I certainly don't resemble any of those dolls. They are all caricatures of human anatomy, but the only thing funny about them is the outright stupidity of the beliefs concerning their use.

Here is an instrument used to assess children which has neither any standardized measurement method for assessing or normative data, nor has there been found any validity to the use of such dolls. They are an item of superstitious belief. In research studies into the efficacy of the assessment potential in such dolls,

> there is no scientific evidence that doll play has any validity in determining whether a child has been sexually abused. This lack of validity, however, does not prevent professionals from using the technique...perfectly normal children often play with the dolls in ways that the "experts" believe are diagnostic of abuse, as a number of studies have indicated (Dawes, 1994, pp. 159-160).

Dawes (1994) maintains that it is "blatantly unethical" to use such techniques as anatomically detailed dolls or projective techniques. Yet such methods are often used in the most serious of assessments in very important settings such as court proceedings.

It is estimated that "for every person correctly identified as a child sexual abuser through such techniques, four to nine are incorrectly identified" (Moss, 1988). This technique for the assessment of sexual abuse belongs in the same category as the use of spectral evidence in the Salem Witch trials three centuries ago.

In their study (1994) on the treatment of sexually abused children, Reams and Friedrich wisely note that the lack of results in their study on treatment "does have significant implications for the continued unexamined use of play therapy with abused children" (p. 897). If anything, this is an understatement. The treatment of abused children is practically a religion in North America with almost as many zealous beliefs about the approach to take as there are practitioners. Notably, there is no empirical evidence supporting what works. I hardly think that it is a matter of nothing working. I think it is more that a situation has developed where there are so many beliefs and vested interests that no one has stopped the hysteria long enough to say, "Hey, we have a very serious issue here. Children have been badly hurt through adult exploitation. Let's end our ranting and find out what children need and how to really best provide it."

In fact, an abundance of authors compare modern child abuse investigations to the Salem Witch Trials and other Inquisition style persecutions. Award winning author and journalist Debbie Nathan, from El Paso, Texas has outlined the process of witch-hunting mentality in child abuse investigations (Nathan, 1991, 1995). In two chapters of her book *Women and Other Aliens* (1991), "The Making of a Modern Witch Trial" and "The Ritual Sex Abuse Hoax," she outlines the incompetence of many social workers and child protection workers involved in such investigations. As well, she details the bizarre thinking and processes involved in a number of investigations in which totally innocent people were persecuted, prosecuted, convicted and then had decisions overturned when the rationality of appeals took place. However, many lives (child and adult alike) have been ruined by zealous child abuse fanatics. As Nathan notes,

> kids involved in this hysteria have indeed suffered, but not at the hands of their teachers. And the abuses perpetrated against them by a child-protection movement gone mad are every bit as awful as the tyranny of incest (Nathan, 1991, p. 167).

Self-Esteem Work

There are a large number of popular myths concerning self-esteem. Modern culture, influenced by sixties' narcissism and pop psychology, has come to believe that self-esteem results from constantly saying nice things to kids. It is a simple equation in the minds of many mental health professionals and educators. It is also an erroneous equation. Self esteem does not come from a constant barrage of "warm fuzzies." Self esteem comes from hard work followed by accomplishments. It is recently being discovered that constantly giving "compliments" to young people, with no basis in fact, may result in their overinflated self perception which, if challenged, results in violence directed towards anyone who would dare challenge their value or worth.

> There is no evidence that for the majority of people a change in internal state and feeling is necessary prior to behaving in a beneficial way. There is, in contrast, good evidence that changing our behavior will change our internal state and feelings. Just do it (Dawes, 1994, p. 293).

To foster self-esteem, we should be promoting programs that involve children in learning new skills, achieving, and participating in activities that lead to pride. These programs should involve external incentives.

> For example, Albert Shanker, the president of the American Federation of Teachers, suggested on National Public Radio on November 9, 1991, that establishments such as McDonald's might select its teenaged employees on the basis of their academic accomplishments. Another way is to instill a sense that working hard is the "right thing" to do. Still another way, very much discouraged by New Age psychology, is simply to require it.... Wise parents may require their children to devote a half hour a day to learning a musical instrument; children who do so under the threat of punishment may come to find that they actually enjoy it and want to pursue music on their own – a process the late psychologist Gordon Allport termed functional autonomy. Behavior originally engaged in to seek external rewards or to avoid external punishments may become intrinsically rewarding in its own right (Dawes, 1994, p. 247).

You do not improve the self esteem of an individual who cannot read or write by extolling their virtues. You improve their self esteem by teaching them to read. Our modern self esteem programs have completely missed the boat on this one. I would say the major problem with our modern

> obsession with self-esteem (aside from the absence of evidence for its validity) is that it discourages action.... A second and pernicious problem is that the obsession discourages *trying* to change one's behavior or life course. Instead, it encourages shoring up self-esteem first by running to a therapist or group (Dawes, 1994, p. 243).

In an interview in my own home area the education director of the Leeds and Grenville Board of Education noted that

> "The critical component of learning is self-esteem. If I feel OK and I feel I have a gift, I normally will excel. But if I feel I'm a loser [then I won't]." Once the student feels self-esteem, Kinsella proposes, the next step in education is to expand that self-esteem to encompass the world. (Mills, 1995).

Again, the grandiose vision of the importance of self esteem is put into public mind through the apparent authority of a representative of the educational system—who unfortunately has bought into the narcissistic pop psychology myths about self esteem. The public has been and is being seriously mislead with regard to self-esteem.

Hospitalization

Psychological "care" of children often results in jailing (hospitalizing) them. Like most forms of therapeutic treatment of children, even child psychiatrists acknowledge that there is no evidence that hospitalizing children for psychiatric treatment helps them. "Supposedly successfully treated children *fared poorly at follow-up according to objective measures used to assess outcome*" (Szasz, 1994, p. 78). In situations where hospitalization is considered by many to be justified to deter suicide,

> even the most ardent supporters of psychiatric coercions admit that the confinement of allegedly suicidal adolescents does not help to prevent their suicide (Szasz, 1994, p. 81).

Szasz' frighteningly accurate criticisms of the field proceed to outright condemnation of children's mental health programs:

> The United States loves to dispose of its unwanted children by means of psychiatric storage.... Out of sight are the countless catastrophic consequences of child psychiatry, such as the wholesale pathologizing of child misbehavior and the mass poisoning of "hyperactive" children with Ritalin and other neuroleptic drugs (1994, p. 84).

Once again, extensive human resources and financial resources are wasted, locking children away in psychiatric settings that are essentially prisons. The crime: misbehaviour. The cause: poor parenting. The punished: the child. These mental health prisons—psychiatric facilities and residential treatment programs—exist despite a complete lack of evidence that they meet their stated goals.

Conclusion

We need to scientifically study the treatment of children's emotional difficulties. Perhaps we will find that treatment makes no difference compared to simple child guidance techniques or a child's involvement in a social group or club. Maybe we'll find some of the methods are contraindicated, while others are highly beneficial. At the moment we have only belief systems with no indication of efficacy.

I fear that the present system is only meeting the emotional and economic needs of mental health professionals. They get paid particularly well and get to feel good about themselves by "helping people," *i.e.*, being involved with people who perceive themselves as suffering. Professionals feel good being with others that are classified as dysfunctional, disturbed, and so on. There is a sense of power in being a "therapist" for many seem to translate this as "the wise one."

The greatest tragedy inherent in our present milieu is that billions of dollars have been wasted, yet the children we are supposed to be helping remain at risk, in pain. The child welfare system is a farce and in shambles, psychotherapy is a modern exercise in science fiction, and a great deal of our educational services and schools do not have programs based on existing empirically tested and solid educational methods.

The fact that, in general, we do not currently know what works in the mental health field supports my view that there should be no long term and *carte blanche* public funding for any clinical programs that have not been supported by solid and extensive empirical evidence—obviously this includes most programs. Long term funding should remain withdrawn until such time as evidence is produced. It is quite likely that we are wasting millions or even billions of dollars of public funds in programs that are not actually effective. We know some things work (many early intervention, prevention and literacy programs). Let's start funneling some of this mental health and social service money into programs that do work and fund only pilot projects for treatment that are willing to be empirically examined. Failure to do this will only result in continued hocus-pocus and dabbling with no scientific basis.

Although funding cuts can be painful, if all funding were immediately withdrawn for any programs that were not using empirically tested methods, or were not willing to be evaluated, we would finally and immediately get down to serious study and examination of our present system. This would probably cause some short term chaos. What **do** we do with all the unemployed mental health professionals? If they really want to "help people" as stated, let's retrain them to help others learn to read and write. Let's increase our programs and research in the area of vocational rehabilitation. Let them become involved in Meals on Wheels deliveries and pushing trays around with cookies and books in hospitals. This is the realm of true help.

In the long term, I think we would be living in a better world. For example, if we can get the same results from therapeutic preschool programs working with groups of children as we could with much more expensive programs with individual children, why fund the more expensive individual programs—providing the programs are of equal quality. If this were the case, then we could be running several preschool group programs with the same amount of funding presently used for individual work. My suspicion is that what would be of greatest benefit would be an ongoing and intensive program of training for those with the most contact with children—parents, caregivers, teachers, child care workers. This is the group with which we need to work. They need training much like the filial therapy programs designed by Guerney. We may find that these more "simple," direct and socially oriented programs would have a better effect than most of our present treatment programs. But the sad fact at the moment is that we don't know what methods, if any, work.[6]

For this reason, I encourage every professional to take those research courses that give us the ability to determine efficacy. Bring on those dreaded, experimental design courses that make the artist in us sweat. This improved scientific knowledge and ability to know what works and to prove that what we are doing does work will benefit prospects for future support and funding of programs we hold so dear to our hearts.

Footnotes

[1] I use the term ecopsychology to describe the relationship between the natural environment and humans. It refers to the influences of naturally occurring ecosystems and biological processes on the body, mind, and spirit. It is a separate, and very different specialty from biopsychology which is a "study of the biological principles underlying behavior" (Kalat, 1995, p. 22). Further, my use of the term *ecopsychology* has no relation whatsoever to the psychological model that is described as ecosystemic.

[2] I use this word with the utmost concern and caution. I use it in a metaphoric sense only. Diagnosis has a certain implication of an underlying illness. I am not talking about illness here, nor do I accept the medical model of the mental health field.

[3] The term psyche is used here to refer to the personality as a concept. It takes into account all mental and emotional aspects of an individual (Hunt, 1993, p. 184): in other words, the mind and its workings. Aristotle called "the part of the soul where thinking takes place the psyche, although sometimes he uses that term to mean the entire soul" (Hunt, 1993, p. 31). No offense to the original Psyche, a soul filled with passion, a human who was Cupid's lover and would eventually become immortal. The word psyche has been translated from Greek as soul or butterfly.

[4] This section on *Endings* was previously published in *Playground* (Barnes, 1991).

[5] With regard to the type of therapy being unrelated to effectiveness, there is one possible exception of behavioral techniques, which seem superior for well-circumscribed behavioral problems (Lazarus, 1990).

[6] As stated previously, with the exception of certain cognitive-behavioral approaches.

CHAPTER 4

The Holistic Approach

THE HOLISTIC APPROACH

The following exploration on the magic of play therapy will be a holistic approach to working with children. Such an approach includes a focus on mind, body, spirit, culture, and politics. I will talk about some of the tools I have used in working with children. Please keep in mind that they are only tools, not answers. Tools need to be adapted in many different situations. Do not take these tools as unchangeable. Any technique I describe in these pages is a starting point. There is no one right way to work with children. There certainly are some wrong ways, but that should not imply that there is one dogmatic and definitive method.

When I am working in the realm of the holistic, I am taking into account a potentially infinite number of influences on a person's life. Wholeness implies a completeness, a completion. Yet, we are never complete. Wholeness is always just beyond our reach. It is that essence of the Divine that we strive to touch and be part of. The wholeness of this approach means that there is an understanding of the interweaving and interlocking aspects of our lives. The mind, the body, the spirit, our culture and the politics of our society all are part of the same whole. How and what we think can influence our bodies. What we eat can influence our minds. A positive relation to the sacred can give us meaning in life and protect us from depression. Being able to understand the subtle energy fields of the human being can allow a whole new focus of healing. No one can "see" energy meridians. Yet, Japanese shiatsu (pressure point massage) therapy can calm the hyperactive child, soothe the stressed executive, eliminate tension headaches and a long list of other physical and psychological complaints.

Some recent trends in the healing fields have included a blending of psychology and medicine. The work of physicians like Deepak Chopra and Stanislov Grof represent the cutting edge of bodymind medicine. Over the past three decades there has also been a return of interest in older knowledge of such methods as acupuncture, shiatsu, herbalism, and therapeutic touch. We are seeing the development of the use of combinations of psycho-physical methods such as reflexology, yoga, tai chi, aerobics, nutrition, exercise, shiatsu, biofeedback, gestalt therapy and Bach Flower Remedies. We have seen many innovations in psychiatry and psychology and owe a great debt to Laing, Verny, Szasz, Grof and Reich.

THE CONCEPT OF MAGIC

In the Introduction section of *Chapter 3* on play therapy, I note that play is truly a magical process. I am not implying anything mystical in this use of the word magic. Following are some examples of magic:

- *Electricity.* There was once a man by the name of Benjamin Franklin. He was ridiculed, harassed and tormented by others who thought he was a little in left field. He was a magician who harnessed electricity. First, he believed in electricity. Then he chose to explore it, to find out how to work with it.

◗ *Flight.* In the world today, we have massive oblong objects with a long flat oar protruding from each side. These objects weigh thousands of kilograms yet manage to float from the earth carrying hundreds of people to destinations many thousands of miles away. Cessna, Boeing, and McDonnell Douglas are agents of magic. They take elements of the earth and combine them to form implements of transportation called aeroplanes. These vehicles are so safe that your likelihood of being injured or killed by entering one of these objects is less likely than if you live in many American cities and walk or drive to the store.

◗ *Computers.* By pushing buttons on a keyboard in my home in North America I can be communicating instantly with someone in Japan or Peru, Iran or Morocco, Ireland or Sweden.

In the last century our magical skills have increased at an unfathomable pace. Radio was an amazing achievement of magical skills. Then came television. Now we have the Internet and, to date, the ultimate information exchange method. Through the use of radar, we can determine the speed of cars on a highway, and locate aeroplanes in the sky all over the world. The Boeing 767, a wonderful tool of technology, is a comfortable and safe aeroplane. It is a huge creation. This big whale in the sky even has not just autopilot, but even autoland capabilities. With only the pilot's monitoring of essential data, it can actually land itself centred and safely on a runway.

These are all examples of magic. The concept of magic, to me, implies nothing supernatural.[1] The word is derived from Persian and Greek sources meaning wise. Wisdom involves the use of information, turning it into knowledge and adapting it appropriately to the benefit of the world. To be able to work true magic, one must be in tune with nature and the natural world. For example, the computer would never have been designed without knowledge of electricity and electromagnetism. Everything about computers is based on an understanding of natural processes.

Magic is a word and concept that enchants, scares.... What is it about this concept that is so powerful? Is it a fear of taking full responsibility for changes in one's own life? When we touch magic we take responsibility for ourselves and take charge of our own destiny.

Magic means having the ability to change concrete reality. It means we are in tune with nature and natural forces and are able to apply them for some desired result. To work magic implies nothing at all supernatural. It simply means being in touch with nature and natural energies and forces. Magic means not working against yourself or nature. When one taps the true source of healing, magic occurs. Being in touch with nature means going back to a primitive knowledge base and tapping what is valuable there as well as claiming what is valuable from the present. When we truly touch natural healing forces, then we perform magic.[2] To heighten our process of change, a consistently holistic approach needs to be applied.

THE CREATION OF A HEALING ENVIRONMENT

What is meant by "healing?" Healing refers to a restoration to health, to wholeness. It means an undesirable condition is overcome and a situation or being is restored to original "purity" or integrity. When I speak of healing in these writings I am referring to a restoration of integrity of mind, body, soul and culture. Of note, even *Webster's Dictionary* refers to health as "the condition of being sound in body, mind or spirit." It is interesting that we so often leave out everything but the body in considerations of healing. In many seemingly holistic approaches, spirit and culture are ignored and so is the political realm. Only recently, in the last few centuries and especially this century, have we separated the body, mind and spirit. Healing is a sacred task. The parent who comforts his or her emotionally wounded child or the physician who operates on the person with a ruptured appendix is each participating in sacred roles that connect the realms of nature and the Divine.

No one from outside a person can heal them. At best, an outsider can help set the stage for that person to heal him/herself. We delude ourselves as healers if we start pretending or actually thinking or maintaining that we are responsible for the healing process in others. All any healer can do is set the stage for healing processes to unfold.

Every culture has healing methods. It is remarkable how the healing processes of cultures separated by both time and space can be so similar. To use but a few examples I will draw from Celtic, African, Huna, First Nations (Native North American), and Oriental cultures. The healing processes of each of these tend to involve an activation of the parasympathetic nervous system. When such activation occurs, the heart rate and pulse are lowered, breathing slows down, pupils constrict, and, indirectly, blood pressure is lowered. In some of the more intense healing processes and ceremonies, a person enters an alpha state. I am referring here to a state of relaxation wherein EEG measurements would reveal alpha brain waves as discussed in a previous section of this text on relaxation and meditation.

The value of many Native American/First Nations[3] healing methods is only beginning to be recognized outside of Native cultures. Native culture and Native healing methods are highly spiritual and deeply intense. Healing methods are synchronous with nature and natural cycles. Many natural substances are used in healing processes. I had the fortune to become very ill when I was seventeen years old and wandering around the American Southwest. I was taken in by a wonderful Mexican-American physician who had a very holistic approach (many years ahead of when this was popular and trendy). In addition to surgery and antibiotics, there were also healing rituals in the desert at night under the moon and stars that involved the sand, herbs and chants.

Celtic Culture, Afro Culture, and the Hawaiian Huna are all highly spiritual. Their methods are in tune with nature, natural cycles and rhythms. There are seasonal celebrations that honour the natural flow. Herbs are used as part of healing ceremonies. Music and dance often play a big role. The Huna healing techniques come from the Kahuna, ancient Hawaiian and South Pacific healers who believed that "anything which is out of balance, disharmonious or distorted in any way can be brought into harmonious function" (Hoffman, 1981, p. 167). This view is synonymous with the Celtic and Black NTU healing perspective.

Oriental cultures have provided the western world with alternate views on "energy" and healing approaches. We have recently discovered the value of working with energy meridians through acupuncture and shiatsu. The healing process of this system has evolved from the theory that there is an energy system circulating through the body in channels called meridians—when an energy imbalance develops in the meridians, physical and psychological difficulties follow. Like other cultures, natural substances like herbs and the return to a natural balance is a focus of healing.

IMPORTANT PARTS OF THE HEALING PROCESS FOR THE HEALER

- Destressing;
- Creating metaphoric sacred space;
- Completion and wholeness;
- Thanksgiving.

Destressing:

One who walks the healing path is always on the edge. There are fine lines and judgment calls with regard to the healing process. In working with those who have been wounded either literally or metaphorically, we work within stressful situations. Thus, for the healer, a process of destressing is constantly required.

Creating Metaphoric Sacred Space:

Our working environment must be considered a sacred environment. It is here that we touch life most intimately. Here we reach the Divine and learn to set the stage where others can heal.

Completion and Wholeness:

The healing process is not an endless path. There are beginnings and endings which need to be acknowledged. As part of our endings with each person we work with, it is important to acknowledge when our work is done and to see the present circle as complete.

Thanksgiving:

When completion occurs, there is a thanksgiving to be processed. We need to give thanks for being a part of life and having been able to work with this person and touch a part of his or her life. There is a thanksgiving for the precious gift we have for relating to others and helping them along on their path. Ceremonial thanksgiving is in order at the point of any completion of a cycle. I sense the celebration of Thanksgiving Day in North America is one of our most important festivals.

CREATING SACRED SPACE

The healer needs to work within a defined sacred space. This concept of sacred is a word which is used a great deal but has not been adequately defined. I have read stacks of books relating to the sacred that never define the concept sacred. When I am referring to the sacred I mean something that is sanctified, blessed, consecrated and considered hallowed, holy, and touching the Divine. These are its numinous qualities. But there are concrete ways of making an area of work sacred. We can use a place that is specifically dedicated to one service or use—that being healing. That does not necessarily mean that we always use the same place. Sacred space is about what we create with what we've got, wherever we may be. Sacred space means a place where we are taking an active role in life processes while at the same time abandoning ourselves completely to the flow of life.

Perhaps there is something you do to make a sacred place. You may imagine there is a circular area in a high school auditorium that is to be used for a counselling session today. You envision this space being dedicated to the healing process before you begin the session. The place which is sacred is also a place that is blessed. It is held in reverence. Honour and respect are shown and felt there. In this sacred space we devote ourselves to the work of the Divine.

For example, a metaphor of sacred space for the healing process in terms of searching for wholeness is the ancient focus on

Earth, Air, Fire and Water in connection with the Divine. This is also the "Way" of Native and Celtic healing. Connecting with nature is a vital part of healing. The following are two practical exercises for being in touch with the sacred. The first, *Your Sacred Space*, is a practical example of creating sacred space. The second, *The Wise One Within.... Your Inner Healer*, is a method for touching our own inner wisdom.

Your Sacred Place

There is a place for everyone to go to where life, time, space and all beings are sacred. It is a place where reverence is shown, where the Divine can be touched and contacted and where honour and respect are felt and shown.

Each living thing has such a place. It is also the healing place. A world between the worlds...the Otherworld as the Irish Celts knew it...that place where the world stops for a moment and infinitely... time loses its relevance here.... Everyone must find their own sacred place.... It comes from within and may be projected onto the outside world. As well, there are some places on the Earth which demand sacred status. You may have had the fortune to have come upon one of these places....

You can create your own sacred place at any time and in many places.... You simply, through your mind, enter a place that is not a place in a time that is not a time in a world between the worlds.... Your own healing powers create the scenario in your mind and then symbolically create an external representation.

> To create your sacred place, pick a time and location where you are not likely to be disturbed. If it is in your own living space do not allow yourself to be interrupted. If you feel uncomfortable letting a phone ring unanswered, disconnect the phone cord before you begin any exercise like this. If you have an answering machine, turn down the volume before you enter your sacred area. Loosen your clothes. Remove your watch and any distracting jewelry. If you can, wear all cotton or some other cloth symbolic of the Earth.

Choose a location where you will keep special items which you use in your healing processes and where you will work. This may be a little table in front of a window in your living room, a window ledge where the sun or moon can shine light on these special things or a drawer with some scented herbs or cedar chips. Your equipment may be as simple as a plant, some string (you will find an upcoming exercise called "The Making of a Lei" that requires string), a candle or a few rocks. You don't need a complex collection of symbolic items to create a sacred space. For example, the simplicity of a Japanese stone garden or the Japanese tea ceremony heightens the beauty and sense of awe and captures the essence of the creation of the sacred.

When you are in your chosen location, imagine that you are surrounded by all of creation. You are connected with your divine source, with all of humanity and nature. This is the place of prayer, of meditation, of inner peace. Know that this image is your sacred place.

See yourself surrounded by a calm healing energy. When you breathe in, take deep breaths and breathe in this calm healing energy. As you breathe out, allow any negativity inside to leave your being and return to the Earth, where it is transformed back into harmless neutral energy.

Reverence is shown in your sacred place. You can use your time in this place for whatever purpose you wish. You can be here before you begin your day. Here you can quietly reflect on the day's journey you have completed.

In the middle of the rush and business of the day you can quietly slip away and take a few moments in your sacred space to renew. It is always there for you.

Once you are able to reach your sacred place, the next exercise can be used to contact your own inner wisdom.

The Wise One Within....Your Inner Healer

We each have a wise one within...the part of ourselves which can heal...the psychic one...the one who transcends and connects with the Divine. It is important to be in touch with the wise one....

To meet this inner healer sit quietly and relax...go to your sacred place within...breathe deeply...watch your breathing... breathe in the calm, healing energy that surrounds you....

When you are ready...imagine yourself outdoors...the sun is shining...your sacred place beckons...imagine that you are in a natural amphitheatre formed by huge boulders...you have a sense that this place is ancient...it has been used by many others throughout the ages...there are towering and majestic evergreens around the circumference of the boulder amphitheatre.... Sit softly and quietly amidst the boulders in this place that has become yours...a safe and protected place.... You cannot be seen by the outside world while you are here.... As you stare at the megalithic trees all around, you start to see movement among them.... There is a person there...this person appears to be emerging from within one of the trees...there is an almost overwhelming gentleness, kindness and wisdom within this person.... He or she has come to be with you on your healing journey.... This is the wise one from within....

The wise one has brought a gift for you.... It is a healing object, image or message...gracefully and with great care the gift is handed to you.... Put your hand forth and receive the gift.... Your entire being and body tingle with the sensations emerging from the hand and touch of the wise one....

Focus on the gift...come to know the gift and the meaning and power within it.... Stay in this place for a few minutes....

The time has come for your healer to return to his or her world...time to say goodbye for now...you each must return to your respective worlds...thank your inner healer for the gift he or she brought you...ask for his or her blessing as he or she departs....watch the wise one return to the woods as he or she begins to blend into the trees...into a tree....

Now it is time for you to slowly return.... Begin to let yourself become aware of your present surroundings...gently and slowly allow your eyes to open...when you are back in the room where you began your journey describe, draw or write the healing image or message you were given by your inner healer... keep this in a special place.... Any time you feel the need for the gift you can return to it...you always have this precious gift with you...you can always return to the sacred place of this journey...to the natural amphitheatre and call upon your inner healer, the wise one....

As you return to the day to day world, try to be the healer to others...give them gifts of gentleness and kindness...help them know what it means to have a sacred place...to know the peace of inner and outer wisdom and kindness.

PRACTICAL APPLICATION OF THE HOLISTIC APPROACH

Here are two examples of taking a holistic approach in specialized practise:

- An oncologist tells her patient, Sandy, that she wants her to try something in addition to the chemotherapy that is being used to treat the lymphatic cancer in the Sandy's body. She recommends that Sandy try daily to take some time to herself, perhaps in a bathtub alone at dusk. In a relaxed situation Sandy is to visualize herself floating and healing. She is to imagine the cancer cells being defeated in her body and to see herself in the future—thriving, happy, and healed. The doctor suggests that Sandy alter her diet, return to her spiritual roots and seek guidance from the Creator. Finally, the Doctor recommends that Sandy learn about the Bach Flower Remedies and to use these as an adjunct to her ongoing chemotherapy.

Sandy follows these recommendations and finds that, although the chemotherapy is close to unbearable, she does not suffer many of the longer term side effects that were expected. The chemotherapy also seems to have its effect much faster than expected. Quickly, Sandy is in complete remission. She continues under her physician's care and heeds most recommendations. The modern scientific approach, when combined with new holistic and traditional healing methods, seems to become even more effective.

◗ My own dentist in no way defines herself as a holistic practitioner. She is fully qualified in Canada as a dental surgeon and practises as such. Yet, her work typifies an increasingly holistic approach in the medical fields.

I had an appointment to have two fillings in my front teeth. This is a particularly sensitive area and the average human being is more than slightly discomforted by dental work in this area, or at least by the application of anaesthetic via hypodermic syringe. At this dental visit the doctor was talking with me and kept making sure there was not discomfort. She asked me if I felt anything as she examined my mouth. I had seen her holding the hypodermic syringe (I was sure it was the size of a baseball bat at the time) and wondered why she had not applied it yet.

Then she announced "okay, you're ready." "Okay, go ahead" I responded. "You're ready" she repeated. Ready, what was she talking about? Ready for what? I was still waiting for the nasty discomfort of the syringe. I then realized she had already completed this task and I had felt nothing. I couldn't believe this, yet my mouth was already becoming numb. I was dumbfounded. I have no fear of dental treatment but I had at least expected a certain sudden and piercing discomfort from the syringe entering the gums around my front teeth.

As she knows my professional background we talked for a while and she told me her approach to dentistry. Without defining it as such, she was practising a holistic method. First, she explained that she tries to put herself in the position of the patient and understand what he or she might be experiencing. This, in itself, is a wonderful alternative to viewing the person as a patient without feelings, anxieties, hopes, and so on. She explained three areas of her approach which aid in the elimination of pain.

After empathically trying to understand the patient from his or her position, she warms the anaesthetic to body temperature so there is not a shock to the system from a substance of much lower temperature entering the body. She had found that this helps to lessen any discomfort involved in the application of the anaesthetic.

She uses the dynamics of the mind to help control the perception of pain by distracting the patient. As she had examined my mouth I had felt her rigorously grasping a fold of skin on my lips and in my mouth and shaking it. I couldn't figure out what on earth she was doing when she did this but, in hindsight, I understood this was her distraction method.

Next, with a slight hesitation or sheepishness, she explained that she had studied Oriental approaches to medicine and the management of pain. Her studies had included a focus on acupuncture and the energy meridians. Prior to inserting the syringe, she had applied pressure to the appropriate pressure points so no pain would be felt. Given the effectiveness of her approach, I certainly do not feel any critique or recommendations for improvement are required in her method. Well, perhaps one minor suggestion. The only thing I would recommend to improve her approach might be the addition of fish in her waiting room, as this has been shown to promote relaxation in a dentist's office.

There are many wonderful exercises you can design for use with children. You can create little meditative tools. I like to have children sit quietly and do some work with each of the "elements".... Even the most hyperactive of children seems to be able to participate in this kind of fun activity.

The Earth

> I'd like you to sit quietly and think about the Earth. Imagine all the different forms the Earth takes...big boulders, little pebbles on the beach, sand for building sand castles, dirt in your garden, forests, deserts.... See all the wonderful gifts which we are given through the Earth.

Exercises involving getting and being in touch with the Earth can be adapted for different ages of children and may include centering, grounding, growing some of our own healing substances, and rock collecting.

Centering: Being centred means to metaphorically be in a position of balance. Our mind, soul, heart, and thoughts are not teetering all over the place and pulling us flat on our face when we are balanced. We can withstand stresses and continue to grow when we are in touch with our own centre. When we are centred

> there is a feeling of balance, a feeling of inner strength that we feel when we are centred. To feel centred is to experience one's psychological centre of gravity—a solid integration of body and mind (Hendricks & Wills, 1975, p. xi).
>
> One of the most meaningful skills we can teach children is the process of psychological integration that we call centering. Centering helps people develop a pool of inner stillness that facilitates appropriate action. To be centred is to have the intellect and the intuition working in harmony. As we begin to integrate our bodies and minds, we feel balanced and more responsive to our environment. Schools should help people become more responsive to their environment (Hendricks & Wills, 1975, p. 5).

There are numerous wonderful exercises to promote a feeling

of being centred in *The Centering Book* (Hendricks & Wills, 1975).

Grounding: To help children feel grounded, we can get them in touch with the Earth, literally and symbolically. It may mean you sit on the Earth with a child. On the other hand, you may be on the 9th floor of an office or apartment building. In your office you may find that a sandbox or pile of sand that children can run their hands through helps with this. When people are grounded they have a sense of roots and stability. They can be psychically pushed, yet able to maintain the symbolic strength to remain standing.

Each of us can feel ourselves become a part of the Earth, connected to Nature fully in the here and now of life. The next exercise can help with this.

The Life of Trees

> Allow yourself to relax fully. Sit in a chair or on the floor. Feel your bottom in touch with the spot upon which it is sitting. Take deep, healing breaths, inhaling the precious air around you.... Start to feel a connection with the Earth below you.... Feel little roots begin to form from your body to the Earth.... You feel something stirring inside your being, something wants to grow and stretch. Let your fingers begin to grow as branches. they need to reach out.... You realize that you are a tree, or at least a tiny seedling beginning its growth...let those branches reach out to the sky...if you feel the need to stand at any point, do so....
>
> Allow yourself to take deep breaths, enjoying the quiet, natural sounds all around you. Let yourself be very still, a part of the natural flow. You are comfortable and relaxed. Be aware of your shoulders, back, legs and entire body. Move around as you need in order to become more comfortable.
>
> Your friends are fellow trees, plants, animals, birds who land on you and build nests in you.

Your branches are becoming much bigger and stronger... reaching to the sky and sun. Leaves have formed on your branches, bringing you the nourishment of the sun. Your trunk has become very strong, sturdy and flexible. Feel your roots connected to all of the Earth, deeply embedded through your feet in the soil around you. You are connected to the mountains, streams, oceans, rivers, forests and lakes on the Earth.

The sun feeds you, nourishes you, brings you life renewing energy. Feel this energy flowing from your leaves at your fingertips, into your branches down into your body and trunk and finally to your roots, deep in the Earth.

From your roots, feel soothing and nurturing water moving into you, up to your trunk and out to your branches and leaves. There is a constant interflow. Energy from the sun, nutrients from the soil.

Watch and feel the seasons moving by. The summer's warmth and rains fill you with life.... Autumn arrives, your leaves change colour, fall to the ground, nurture you and form a protective blanket over the soil around you. You have made your own quilt to sleep under as winter approaches.... All is quiet and still over the winter. You are groggy and sleep much of the time. Occasionally you peak an eye open to see what is going on outside during the winter days...a restlessness starts to fill you as spring arrives. Little buds on your branches turn to beautiful spring leaves. You are refreshed and beginning life anew.... Allow everything to appear new and fresh in your life....

You can use this feeling of being part of the Earth whenever you want to feel solid and connected, whenever you want to feel yourself part of the flow of energy through the Earth. On those chaotic days when you are feeling disconnected from the Earth or generally disoriented, you may want to take a moment and do this exercise.... Feel your connection to the Earth now...begin to feel the chair or floor beneath you....slowly come back to the room at your own speed.

Air/Sky

I'd like you to focus on all the different forms the air takes...feel a gentle breeze on your face and hands...a strong gusty wind blowing your hair...musical sounds carried in vibrations through the air...the oxygen which fills our lungs and keeps us alive.

To get in touch with the "element" of air, you can use breathing exercises, stretching with deep breaths, flying a kite, and meditation processes. The following is an exercise that can be used to help turn breathing into a healing process.

Healing From The Heavens

Allow yourself to become very comfortable.... See all the stars up in the sky. One glows slightly brighter than all the others. Your focus goes to this star. Amidst the darkness of the night sky glows this beautiful creature. You feel that it is almost alive. It is full of a Divine energy, almost angelic. There is a healing force contained in this star. It glows, it fades, then returns to an even greater glow. It is throbbing. It wants to open and blossom.

You see one tiny spot on the glowing star that is much brighter than the rest of the star. The spot gets larger and you realize that the star is slowing bursting open. As it opens, millions of multicolored tiny stars emerge. They fill the sky above you and rain down on you. Each of these little stars is filled with a calm, kind, gentle, healing energy. Each twinkles and sparkles with its own special colour. They are dropping in your hair, on your face, into your eyes and ears, in your mouth and nose, down your shirt and pants, even into your socks.

Every time you breathe or swallow, the tiny stars with their healing energy enter your body.... They flow to every cell in your body, they fill your skin, hair, and heart. Even your fingernails, eyes and toes glow with healing energy.

As you breathe out, this goodness returns to the world around you and starts to bring peace to the community.

Allow these little angels, the tiny stars to fill you all night long. When you waken in the morning you arise and enter the world with a renewed desire to bring peace and wellness to all around you.

Fire

Imagine the many forms fire can take...the warmth of a fireplace...the glow of a candle...the radiance of the sun...the physically warm loving sensations of a hug....

To experience fire in a safe way, you can sit in front of a fireplace or campfire, watch a candle burning, feel the sun, or bring your hands so close together you can feel physical warmth.

Water

Imagine the forms water can take...the sound of waves at the ocean...raindrops as they are falling on the roof...a soothing bath...a calming cup of herbal tea....

Feeling the "element" water can be done through baths, walking in the rain, drinking tea, or even sitting running hands through a container of water, or sitting by a lake, river or ocean.

Nature's Healing Arms

I have designed the following ceremonial exercise, based on Irish Celtic beliefs, to acknowledge our place in nature through the metaphor of Earth, Air, Fire and Water. The exercise is based on some of the ancient healing practices used by the Irish Celts over the centuries.

This is a visualization which initially needs to be acted out. After you have participated in it once, you may simply visualize the enactment of the experience in the future. Or, you may find it so rewarding that you like to do it rather than visualize it. In Celtic healing and spiritual ceremonies, many of the symbolic practices and metaphors used are very similar or even identical to Native American healing ceremonies. It is interesting how such similarities cross time and space boundaries.

The purpose of this exercise is to acknowledge our place as humans in the natural world in much the same manner as Francis of Assisi. When we feel we are an important part of the natural world, we come to feel grounded and centred and we are kinder and more respectful of nature, other people and ourselves. Another purpose to this experience is to symbolically give yourself an emotional place of shelter when you need it. You may wish to choose a friend or friends with whom to do this exercise.

For the exercise you will need a plant or a little bowl of sand to represent earth, some fragrance to represent air (such as a scented oil, an appealing plant, or incense like sandalwood, cedar, copal, or frankincense), a beeswax candle to represent fire, a little bowl of water, and some meaningful symbol of life such as another plant that will function as your centrepiece. You may wish to have other items honouring nature and the Divine, but the above are basic to the ceremony.

The metaphor used in this exercise is the vision of the circle, symbolic of wholeness. Imagine there are four directions within the circle. Four is a very stable number in the world of physics and chemistry. Perhaps psychological stability reveals itself through the same number.

> The four "elements" of Earth, Air, Fire, and Water are used in this visualization. Imagine you are in a peaceful place of protection...a safe, nurturing space that no negativity can penetrate. At the centre of the circle, place some meaningful symbol of life such as a plant. Determine which direction is North and face that way. On your right side at

the edge of the circle in the East, place the scented and fragrant object (Air). Behind you at the South, place the candle (Fire). To your left in the West, place the bowl of water. In front of you, at the upper edge of the circle in the North, place the bowl of sand or another plant (Earth).

Walk fully around your circle, beginning in the East. See a flow of energy surrounding you so that when you have completed your walk there is actually a glowing sphere protecting you. See the energy flowing upwards to create a teepee-like enclosure.

Say the words: "May this be a meeting place of love and joy, peace and truth, a space protected against any evil and negativity." Go and sit on the floor facing the East and focus on the fragrance. Imagine the many forms that Air can take. Take a deep breath and imagine a gentle breeze soothing you, a strong wind, the refreshing feel of a deep breath of fresh air in the sunshine after being cooped up indoors for several hours, the sensations of air on a humid day in the tropics, a chilly day in the autumn in Canada...sit with these sensations...then proceed to the South and face the candle. Sense all the forms that fire can take. Let your eyes watch the flickering of the flame. Take a deep breath and imagine the warmth of the sun, the warm feelings from the hug of a loved one, the glow of a fireplace, the heat of a raging campfire...sit with these sensations.... Move to the West and face the bowl of water. Imagine the many forms water can take. See a cool glass of refreshing water, a rain shower, ocean waves crashing on a seashore, a stream trickling by, a pool of water with birds bathing in it, snow falling on your head and shoulders, the gentle drizzle of a morning fog...sit with these sensations.... Finally, approach the North and focus on your plant or bowl of Earth. Imagine the many forms that Earth can take. Rocks, sandy beaches, gardens, trees...sit with these sensations.

Move back to the centre of this space, sitting just in front of your plant. See yourself as a part of all creation. Think "I am thankful for my existence. I am thankful for the gifts I have been given." Think of all the things you are thankful for...aspects of your being and your personality that you treasure and wouldn't ever want to change...some special relationships in your life...some particular skills or talent....

Sense how safe you are within this shelter....Within this place you may wish to meditate or go through some of the other exercises in this manual alone or with a friend.

Be at peace.

To leave your shelter, first approach the East and the fragrance and give the message, "I am thankful for the air that I breathe. It is healing. It sustains me."...move to the South and the flame. Give the message, "I am thankful for the warmth I receive and am able to receive. I am thankful for the heat of the fire." ...next, on to the West. Give the message,"I am thankful for soothing water. May I be always able to care for myself and others." ...to the North and the Earth. Give the message, "I am thankful for my place on the Earth. May I give back to the Earth the care and living support I have received. May I always walk on the Earth with respect for Nature and the creatures of the Earth."

Once more, walk around the shelter of the circle and, this time, see it fade and disappear as you say goodbye to the images within.

You can go back to this circle anytime you wish by simply imagining it. Or, you may actually recreate the scene using a respectful ceremony like the one just described. Anytime you return to this place, remember the Navajo prayer, "In a sacred manner I return."

In some of the professional training programs in which I am involved, I have been asked by a few therapists, especially those who have described themselves as Christian focused therapists, to help them understand how to reconcile the Native and Celtic metaphor of Earth, Air, Fire and Water with their own beliefs. I would like to offer some of the writings of St. Francis of Assisi (born, 1182 - died, 1226) and allow you to extrapolate from this how there is not really any conflict to be perceived between spiritual belief systems, as so eloquently phrased in *The Canticle of Brother Sun*:

> Be praised, my Lord, through Sister Water,
> who is very useful and humble and precious and pure.
>
> Be praised, my Lord, through Sister Moon and the Stars,
> in the heavens you formed them clear and precious and beautiful.
>
> Be praised, my Lord, through Brother Wind
> and through Air and Cloud and fair and all Weather,
> by which you nourish all that you have made.
>
> Be praised, my Lord, through Brother Fire,
> by whom you light up the night;
> he is beautiful and merry and vigorous and strong.
>
> Be praised, my Lord, with all your creatures,
> especially Sir Brother Sun,
> who is day and by him you shed light upon us.
> He is beautiful and radiant with great splendour,
> of you, Most High, he bears the likeness
>
> —(cited in Skolimowski, 1993, p. 110).

I would highly recommend the beautiful work of ecological philosopher Henryk Skolimowski (1993) to further explore these concepts.

Here are a couple of little tangents that prove very interesting in terms of spiritual beliefs. The first story involves potatoes. The potato used to be considered evil because it was not mentioned in the Bible. The potato originated from South America and was known at least 8000 years ago. It was brought to Europe by Spanish conquistadors who found it growing high in the Andes mountains. The Europeans had a great fear of the potato because of its evil connotations. Interestingly, the church removed this worry by imposing a tithe which permitted parishioners to use the potato after they had made a payment to the church. The potato has carried many of these connotations with it over the centuries and still has a certain bad and unfair negative nutritional reputation, with many claiming "too high a level of carbohydrates," *etc*. This reputation, which is even clung to by some dietitians and nutritional advisors, can be traced to the old negative religious views about the potato. In reality, the potato consists of 80% water with the remaining 20% being packed with vitamins B1 and C, useful amounts of minerals, carbohydrates as well as proteins – I believe second only to soybean (National Museum of Science and Technology, Government of Canada, 1991).

Likewise, cats were considered evil. They were thought to be an animal manifestation of the devil, so were slaughtered by the hundreds of thousands. The result was a population explosion of rats and their inhabitant fleas, carrying the Black Plague. "When those fleas infested homes throughout Europe, much of the European population died a slow, grisly death. Feline retribution perhaps?" (Kilcommons & Wilson, 1995, p. 45).

People with strong and stable spiritual beliefs are not threatened by new ideas. Their own spiritual base is strong enough to withstand critique and exploration. Those who are rigid in their beliefs are insecure and have not integrated their belief system into their life, heart and soul.

A CAUTION – MODERN TRENDS: SOME CONCERNS

Much of what I am dealing with here in relation to an holistic approach to healing is simultaneously arising time and again in both modern mental health professional literature and "new age" thought. On one hand, it is good that we are expanding our concepts in the healing professions. But I do have serious concerns about certain aspects of the "new age" movement. One concern is that many people are being drawn into some very serious processes with no meaningful depth. They are touching deep issues in a superficial manner. It is vital to ground oneself scientifically. Many "new agers" are referred to by some grounded professionals as "white lighters" because all they seem to think is needed to fix the world is surround everything in a vision of white light. I sometimes refer to this superficial approach to healing as the "butterfly syndrome" in reference to those who flit from seminar to seminar, method to method, trying out everything in sight but never settling anywhere.

> An emphasis on spirituality at the expense of wisdom and knowledge was a root cause of the Dark Ages.... Schools were closed, books and libraries were burned, the quest for empirical knowledge was condemned as devilish (Walker, 1989, p. 4).

I believe there is some cause for serious concern about how the direction of certain present spiritual beliefs lead us away from centuries of scientific knowledge. Walker (1989) notes some modern trends of a new barbarism that should cause at least a moderate apprehension. These trends include the spread of illiteracy, religious fanaticism, indifference to proven facts, and irrational beliefs. I would add to this list a lack of consumer protection, with charlatans preying on the gullible and vulnerable.

1) *The Spread of Illiteracy.* Unfortunately, worldwide, illiteracy is on the increase.

2) *Religious Fanaticism*. Also on the increase worldwide. *Exodus* 20:13 says "Thou shalt not kill." Yet, even in our own North American countries certain anti-abortion crusaders in their own brand of fanaticism have taken justice and the law of God into their own hands and have killed doctors with alleged abortion practices.

3) *Indifference to Proven Facts/Irrational Beliefs*. An example of a valuable tool or method taken to ludicrous extremes is the use of stones and crystals in new age healing work. Many "New Age" practitioners have adopted the ludicrous belief that this or that stone cures this or that physical illness. This is beyond silly. It is downright dangerous. Stones do not cure illnesses. A stone or crystal may be extremely valuable in the therapeutic process, but only in the sense that it may be symbolic of the healing journey in general or it may be a focal point for a storytelling exercise of a tool to meditate on. Therein lies their value.

There is a great deal of disciplined study required of a healer, whether one is a medical doctor or a herbalist. Much of the training is tedious and mundane. A scientific study and approach to healing demands such discipline. Yes, learn to center and to heal. Examine, explore and critique modern views of people like Larry Dossey. Begin to understand the power of prayer, the power of the spiritual. But never lose sight of all that we have learned through painstaking efforts and research to date.

> Nature is a great teacher, but she instructs only those who come to her with honest humility, ready to labour at assimilating earlier lessons. Knowledge of nature does not come to the mentally lazy, who prefer subjective imagination to disciplined study (Walker, 1989, p. 9).

Each day I like to sit and spend time with minerals of the Earth. They have great sensual characteristics. Each one feels and looks different. The fact that I am aware that the beauty and healing qualities in them is metaphoric, not literal, does not take away from their value. They are symbolic of the sacred. There is nothing more reflective of the symmetric, rhythmic and cyclical nature of life than an optical mineralogical view of a mineral. There is a truly a "magical" subtlety to the healing powers of stones, but it does not lie in the direct methods that "new agers" believe.

> Probably there is a healing force within the human spirit, but we don't yet know how to tap it deliberately, without delusion. Study of this subject is a challenge for the future. Meanwhile, let us not confuse this force – whatever it is – with external objects. It does

> not dwell in external objects. It is part of the self. Popularized crystal lore too often converts spiritual needs into tools of exploitation, rather than developing the impulse toward enlightenment (Walker, 1989, p. 65).

A useful technique designed by Viki Takacs, both an IBECPT and CACPT Certified Child Psychotherapist and Play Therapist, indicates how nature and stones can be used within a therapeutic process. It is called *Talking with Rocks* and is found in *Chapter 11, Nature... Working with the Earth: Plants/ Rocks/Animals in the Healing Process.*

Another excellent source for the use of stones is Barbara Walker's *The Book Of Sacred Stones*. She does not take "new age" crystal mysticism seriously. In fact, the book serves to thoroughly debunk the ridiculous myths coming out about the "healing powers of stones." Walker recognizes stones solely for what they are—wonderful and natural creations, nothing more and nothing less.

Despite the wonders of geological knowledge, the discoveries of optical mineralogy and general mineralogy, crystal mystics make bizarre literal claims concerning the use of stones and crystals in healing. I believe that there is great room for the use of crystals in the healing process, but as metaphoric tools for meditation and storytelling, not for antibiotic or cancer curing properties of their own.

> Crystal mysticism can be a valid and rewarding study, potentially rich in appreciation of our Mother Earth; but not as it is being disseminated at present. The current level of crystal mystics' comprehension of their subject signifies a deplorably lazy attitude toward learning. Ignorance may feel comfortable, but in the long run it hurts. Much knowledge has been gained about minerals and crystals in the last two centuries or so. This knowledge should not be ignored or falsified. We can hardly expect to understand our Mother Earth by rejecting what has been discovered about her so far (Walker, 1989, p. 4).

4) *A Lack of Consumer Protection*. Another concern about the "new age" movement is a lack of consumer protection and the high number of gurus and self-proclaimed "experts" in the field. There are those

who take a couple of workshops, read some books and then set themselves up in practise as "experts," "healers," whatever, in some specialty. I realize that this concern should by no means be limited to the "new age" field. It is also an issue in certain areas of mental health, especially sexual abuse and the phenomena of dissociative identity disorder (formerly identified as multiple personality disorder). There are a number of practitioners ("psychotherapists"—a totally meaningless term in regard to the consumer of services as there are no restrictions on who can call themselves a psychotherapist) who have little or no legitimate professional training in the area in which they "specialize" but take workshops in the field, do some reading and then set up shop as experts.

With regard to physical issues, when there are such concerns, I strongly advocate that mental health practitioners always request a medical opinion of a person's condition. Emotional metaphoric healing should be an adjunct to medical treatment, not a replacement. An unqualified practitioner could be the cause of a patient neglecting a serious disease in an early recognizable stage and only reporting for professional diagnosis and treatment when past the point of no return. There is also a tendency in many new agers to see every disorder of the universe, physical, emotional, spiritual—as being an indication of some kind of personal imbalance that individuals are responsible for themselves. With that kind of attitude, the polio vaccine would never have been developed. Cures for many diseases would still be unknown. Antibiotics would never have been developed.

> Bacteria, viruses, environmental toxins, parasites, genetic defects, the inevitable deteriorations of old age, and similar disease producers are not, however, widely recognized in the [new age] mystics' world. The general theory is that all illness is caused by wrong acts and attitudes, anxieties, fears, and unresolved conflicts. Physical "imbalance and disharmony" result from conflict between the personality and the soul; but by understanding this, we are told, we may cure our own diseases. Such may well be the case with emotional illnesses, but most physical illnesses are not to be so simplistically dealt with (Walker, 1989, p. 57).

Given such seemingly clear criticisms regarding "new age" methods, I must also note that I have learned methods of using stones in my own healing processes. I learned much from my grandmother and my Irish Celtic past where stones were used as healing focal points. They serve as meditative devices in the healing process. The stones do not do the healing. They simply serve as devices to focus on while doing the energy/emotional healing. Do they work in and of themselves? Would the healing be just as effective without their presence? Honestly, who knows? There is some recent pioneering scientific work in the area of stones and crystals which leads me to believe that they may be effective in a very subtle manner for reasons we do not yet understand. There is especially fascinating material coming out on the fields of chemistry and archaeology in the areas of electron spin resonance and energy anomaly research (Robins, 1988).

Despite my criticism of "new age" issues, we should also be careful about what we discard or scoff at simply because we do not presently have concrete data to prove effectiveness. If we were to do this we would have to abandon most psychotherapeutic methods, for there is little proof of the effectiveness of any of our modern psychotherapy treatment techniques.

SELF CARE FOR THE HEALER

HEALING OURSELVES IS A VITAL PART OF OUR PROCESS WITH OTHERS!!!!

I have been asked the following kinds of questions time and again in lectures I give:

> "How do you give your mind a rest and keep the problems of your clients from intruding into your life outside the work setting, especially at night?"
>
> "Could you talk some about care for the therapist? Do you have any techniques that help you leave the children and their family problems when you go home?"

I have tried to think of some polite way of phrasing it but my daughter, Erin, says what I am trying to say is "Get a Life." I had hoped to be able to say it a little more politely, but have yet to find any phrase that describes it as clearly as that one.

Therapists need work boundaries. They need to set limits on

the amount of time they put into their clinical work, the amount of work they do, the number of clients seen. Don't become obsessed. We all need vacations, physical activity of some kind and a full and rewarding life outside the workplace.

If each of us in the role of healer does not take care of ourselves, we will not be of any use to those we hope to serve. I have seen many very good healers burn out because of a lack of their own self-care. Their rational for entering the downward spiral is truly noble and honourable, yet without taking a step back and looking at themselves and gaining perspective, they enter a self-imposed trap from which it is increasingly difficult to escape.

How this usually comes about is in the form of an initial "crisis." I will use arbitrary numbers here for the purpose of illustration. A therapist may regularly see ten people a week in the therapy process. Then, one week 5 people are in crisis and "need" an appointment. However, the healer never returns to his or her own original baseline of service. It's now a year later and fifteen appointments a week has become the norm. But now there are more crises. So one week the therapist sees twenty people. Three months later it's twenty-five, plus two community board meetings over four nights a month, the monthly agency board meeting, reports on twenty five clients, the grant proposal, the accreditation report, the extra half day on weekends for those three families who just can't come any other time, the therapist has a partner and two kids of their own, one of whom is having nightmares and doesn't want to go to school (maybe by this point they just want to stay home and have some real time with mommy or daddy)...and the spiral is complete. Now the therapist starts to resent Mondays, a lack of energy Monday mornings and a resentment of the director or the job...and next it's a resentment of clients and their "resistance"...and so on....

Self care and the ability to both know one's limits and be able to say "no" are vital for an effective healer.

I maintain that anyone involved in a healing profession needs a bare minimum of four weeks vacation a year, though six would be preferable. I say this in training programs sometimes and hear gasps as if this is asking the impossible. I think this is because we have a sociopolitical arrangement where many agency executives and managers push staff to the limit and beyond to try to get every possible morsel of therapy energy out of them. It is the wise therapist who gets out of this environment as soon as possible. Agencies need to function as healing spaces and offer a supportive environment for their staff. Training, staff development, in-service education, consultation and supervision need to be built in, during regular work time, to the ongoing agency process.

Footnotes

[1] Some aspects of the natural world can, at times, seem supernatural. One of Carl Jung's (along with Nobel prize winning physicist Wolfgang Pauli) great contributions to modern thought was the concept of synchronicity. He defined it as an "acausal connecting principle." I maintain that this is one of the more important concepts in the healing arts and sciences. Within synchronicity lies such depth. The fact that synchronistic events even occur points to the existence of worlds/times of which we have only fantasized. An example of a very clear and concrete synchronistic event would be a situation where a person goes to bed, dreams that a loved one who lives thousands of miles away has had a heart attack and awakens in the morning to discover that the loved one has, in fact, had a heart attack. A less concrete example of a synchronistic event would be a situation where a clock stops at the exact time of someone's death. Or, to use the previous example of the loved one, a synchronistic occurrence would be that the power fails as soon as the phone is hung up with bad news. There was certainly no cause and effect there, but it is like a parallel world has been tapped. There is an "otherworld," one which only some have glimpsed. Synchronicity is not supernatural. It simply lies beyond our present wisdom to understand it.

[2] I am quite aware that the very word "magic" seems to scare some people who feel that it has negative and sinister connotations. My first thought is a professional perspective and is concern that such people who fear the word "magic" would be working with children and the poor children who have to see such non-playful therapists. My second thought is that such people must

lead very boring lives. Imagine never being able to have fun going to *DisneyWorld* because it features *The Magic Kingdom*. I guess these same people must be the ones who consider *Barney* to be evil since magic and magic wands are used on the *Barney* show. I think such attitudes result in a bizarre hunt for sexual images and words in the dust of Disney's *The Lion King*. These are people with too much time on their hands, too few brain cells in their heads, and too little meaning in their lives.

In a similar situation, a colleague/friend, Bridget Revell, and I were presenting a training program in St. Louis, Missouri under the auspices of an organization called Mandala Therapeutic Services. The program was called *Play Therapy and Child Abuse*. One of the participants approached us during a break to tell us how much she was enjoying the program. She also noted that she had been forced to pay her registration fees on her own since her employer would not approve funding for her because a cheque had to be made out to Mandala Therapeutic Services, the sponsor, and the word mandala had "new age" overtones and was, therefore, unChristian. This was a frightening misuse of power by her employer based solely on his religious beliefs. As mentioned previously in this text, the word *mandala* comes from sanskrit and means circle. I found it absolutely disgusting and degrading for this poor woman to be at the mercy of her power hungry director who was imposing his values onto a clinician's right to receive training.

This is not in any way meant to negate the effects of abuse on a person who is abused in situations where someone pretends to be invoking magical elements and so on. However, this does not mean the concept of magic is bad. People warp many wonderful ideas and processes in their abuse of others. For example, the fact that many people have been sexually abused by their ministers does not mean that their particular religions are bad because of this. Similarly, we should not condemn the concept of magic simply because of how some "wackos" may have related to and used the concept.

[3] Some descriptive terms may be slightly confusing for readers from different areas of the world. Typically, the inhabitants of a region who have been present for the longest period of time are referred to as aboriginal. In North America there are two descriptive terms for such people. In the United States, aboriginal people are referred to as Native Americans. I have two problems with such a phrase. First, anyone born in the country is a native of the country. To call them otherwise would seem to make them second-class citizens. Second, it is never clear if the term Native American refers to inhabitants of Canada or not. Being Canadian born and living in Canada, I am never sure if the term American in actual use refers to North America or to the United States of America. In Canada, aboriginal people are known as First Nations people since they have been present as a nation long before anyone else arrived. In my discussions here, I will be referring to both First Nations people and Native Americans interchangeably to refer to the aboriginal population of North America.

CHAPTER 5

Symbolism and Metaphor in Play: The Child's Inner World

SYMBOLS
METAPHORS
FANTASY

SYMBOLS

In discussing symbols it is important at the outset to have an understanding of what exactly is meant by the term. A symbol is some conceptual form that has a greater depth than its obvious outward meaning. A symbol is more than just a sign leading directly to some specific thought or action. Signs are clear and direct. For example, I am a pilot and fly a great deal. In landing I am given instructions by the control tower directing me to a specific runway. If I am told I am cleared to land on 01 I know that I will be viewing the numbers 01 as I land on the runway. Once on the ground, I may see a number of indicators with numbers, arrows, directions, colours. These are all signs with one direct message leading me to specific thoughts and procedures. They are important concrete messages. Another example is the stop sign at the corner of many streets. It, too, has a clear and direct meaning.

On the other hand, a symbol has a depth far beyond its

external form. An image of a lamb may take me deeply into the unconscious. The crocus and other spring flowers may be a simple indication that spring is on its way. However, they can potentially also lead to a great symbolic significance. They may take someone to an internal psychological processing of death, rebirth, redemption. A truly powerful symbol is unlimited in its depth. It leads to many thought paths.

In some training programs I have run with Bridget Revell we show several slides with different images on them. We ask participants to focus on the image and we give specific directions on what kind of concept to associate with the image. For example: we show a skyscraper and ask them to think of a person; a box...a message; an ambiguously coloured wine glass...a colour; a rose...an animal; a hook on a door...an emotion; a lamb...an experience; a teddy bear...a setting or place.

Although we are limiting the kinds of potential thought processes, there is still a wide variety of individual responses. If we had gone in with a checklist, we would have told the audience about our own symbolic meanings to each of these items and learned nothing of theirs. The above images lead to so many symbolic explorations. For example, I have heard a variety of meanings ascribed to the skyscraper. Some people think of someone rigid who they don't particularly like and we hear them say "Oh gawd, that's my rigid supervisor." Others see power and endurance and might say "That's superman." Yet others see an omnipotence and strength and say "To me that is God. Always there, always strong, always my link to heaven." You see how easy it would be to miss the meaning behind any particular individual if we were to go in with a prefabricated idea on the meaning of symbols.

I do not believe in providing you with a cutesy "dictionary" of symbols. There are too many such "dictionaries" out there where the meaning of a number of symbols is given. Such an approach is treading on extremely dangerous clinical territory entering the realm of science fiction.[1] It sets us up to take power away from those we are supposed to be helping. We imply that we know more than they do about themselves and their own inner world. This applies to all types of creative therapies. We cannot assume that a symbol takes on a limited meaning for all people and that we know the personal meaning of the symbol for someone other than ourselves.

Thus, in this text, you are not being given a reference listing or checklist as to what the meanings of different symbols, drawings or toys are. Therapy is not about checklists. I do not think that we can pretend to have this knowledge. This has been, historically, one of the major downfalls of the mental health field and one of the reasons we are too often less than credible. We read too much of our own stuff into what we see. We are always looking to define and encapsulate in far too simplified terms. Our knowledge base is still very limited and regularly borders on science fiction[1] rather than hard scientific fact. I cringe when I hear some court proceedings where a so-called expert is diagnosing based on his or her own narrow interpretations of a child's play, art or dreams. All too often there is, in fact, excellent diagnostic material present, but it is diagnostic of the therapist, not the child.

We must tread very carefully in order not to find ourselves interpreting the inner world of another person based on our own preconceived set of symbols. There is an extreme danger of misunderstanding and misdiagnosing. In training residents and interns, I have often given them art, play situations, dreams and other creative scenarios to explore. Invariably there have been numerous diagnoses and big word jargon thrown around to impress. Always, there is a great deal of silence and hopefully humility in the room when they learn that their great clinical extrapolations and fantastic diagnoses have been based on the work of normal, healthy, well-functioning children, or, even better, my own drawings or scenes in a sandbox.

In searching for the meaning in a child's (or adult's) inner world, it is safe to assume nothing. We must enter that person's world with a very open mind. Rather than assuming a preconceived set of symbols based on your own inner world or based on some ridiculous checklist,[2] you may find that if you enter with an open mind you discover many different meanings to symbols for many different children and different cultures. One of the finest examples of this is the snake. The serpent, a symbol of the Celtic healer, of wisdom and of rebirth (it sheds its skin and is born anew) is similar to the Celtic knot which represents the spiralling toccata of infinite knowledge and the total relationship of every atom, quark and molecule in the universe. Irish crosses, so to speak, were alive with twining serpents (Bonwick, 1986). As Condren notes:

> The image of the Serpent, because of its association with life, rejuvenation, fertility, and regeneration, was a symbol of immortality...creation and wisdom (1989, p. 8).

This serpent symbolism is important in our work with children. I have met many therapists who assume that any child who draws a snake has been sexually abused (thanks again to the intensely destructive Freudian influence on the field of mental health). Such interpretation is first, ridiculous, and worse, racist. It does not account for the impact of culture. We know that the

> Greeks had it [the serpent] as a symbol of Apollo, Minerva, and Juno. The Ophites, of early Christendom, saw in it a symbol of Christ, or the mundane soul (Bonwick, 1986, p. 179).

In Egypt, it has been both an evil spirit as well as a positive symbol of new birth and rebirth. Cultures of Assyria, India, China, Aztec, many First Nations (Native North American), Scandinavia and numerous others hold the serpent with distinction and great respect. Many cultures, professions and national symbols include the snake, dragon or other serpent form. One prime example is the universal symbol of the medical profession, the physician's caduceus. This symbol of the healer, intertwined snakes on a staff, has been found in many cultures including Mesopotamia, Greece, India, Aztec and North American Indians (Walker, 1988, p. 85). So does this mean that if a child draws a picture of a snake we should assume it represents the healer, or wisdom? Of course not. We should explore the snake symbol exactly like any other symbol and find out what it means to the child.

As another example, I have seen wolves represent aggression and terror to a child. I have also seen them represent nurturing and family life. Had I gone in with a list of "what wolves mean" I would have missed the whole process involved with the individual. Checklists are for insecure therapists who lack knowledge and skills in the deep healing process and who, in fact, may be frightened by the depth, intensity and passion of the healing process and therefore they rely on checklists to deal with the unknown. Try to avoid both such checklists and therapists. They are not healers.

A useful method in finding the meaning behind individual

symbols is the rather obvious method of asking people what the drawing or toy means to them...are they like that in any way...do they ever feel like that...what does the person in the drawing need...do they ever need that...always bring it back to the individuals' own lives and experiences.

To discover what the inner process that is underlying a symbol for any individual, I would "play" at exploring the symbol as follows:

> In this scenario, the child has had a dream the night before. In the dream there was a wolf that scared the child. Rather than make any assumptions about what a wolf means in a dream or what the child may be feeling in order to have the symbol of a wolf arise, I would simply play an exploring game with the child (I would also recommend this same method with adults).
>
> Therapist: Johnny, let's pretend that I come from another planet and I've never seen a wolf before. How would you describe a wolf to me?
>
> Johnny: Well, a wolf is an animal.
>
> Therapist: Johnny, on my planet we don't have any animals. What's an animal?
>
> Johnny: It's, ahh, it's like this thing that lives in nature.
>
> Therapist: Guess what? Where I come from we don't even know what nature is. How would you describe nature to me?

It doesn't usually take more than two or three of these "bluffing" kinds of questions until you come to some meaningful process or issue. In the example there are a couple of paths which might emerge. I will give you an example that may be predictable. Then I will tell you the actual words from the little boy.

> Johnny: Nature is, well, it's scary. It gets dark at night and there's no one there to help. You're lost out in the forest....

Obviously, there is an issue of fear or maybe even being overwhelmed in such a description. What Johnny really did say was:

> Johnny: Nature is, well, remember how I talked with you about going for picnics with mummy and daddy before they got killed in the car accident. Well we used to go out to the park every weekend and have a picnic out in nature. That doesn't happen any more.

For Johnny, there are unresolved issues of loss and grief. Much mourning remains to be done. But where's the wolf? Truly, who cares? The actual symbol is irrelevant. What is important is what emerges from that symbol for the individual. If I'd gone in with some preconceived notion that whenever a child has a dream with a wolf in it he or she is feeling...nurtured, overwhelmed, angry, hurt, or whatever, I may have missed what was actually happening for the individual with whom I am working in the here and now. That is why I always recommend assuming nothing with regard to symbols; always explore the symbol for its meaning instead of telling someone what that symbol means. This also holds true for choices of colours. I do not assume that any given colour means any general feeling. I have witnessed so many variations that long ago I realized that any kind of generalization is very dangerous.

I would like to point out a dissenting opinion from mine on this issue of interpretation of symbolic meaning. I particularly admire Byron Norton, and his opinion on this issue differs drastically from my own. We both agree that there is meaning to symbols, but Byron's view suggests that we can easily determine, as outsiders, just what the meaning is behind the symbolic representation. An upcoming text by him will expand on this and explore the issue.

Such varying opinions are the main reason that I suggest that anyone interested in therapy with children and play therapy attend as many training programs as possible in order to hear a number of views. As I so often state, there is no one correct approach. Explore many approaches to determine what is right for you as a professional. I strongly suggest your guideline in decision making be empirical research to support your intuitive sense.

METAPHORS

Like symbols, metaphors have a greater meaning than their outward image. *Webster's Dictionary* defines a metaphor as "a figure of speech in which a word or phrase literally denoting one kind of object or idea used in place of another to suggest a likeness or analogy between them." The word metaphor comes from a Greek word meaning to transfer, implying that when we use a metaphor we are transferring meaning.

I think the understanding of metaphor can be really mystified by and in the mental health field to the point where the process of its use seems like some complex and earth shattering experience. A metaphor is simply a symbolic phrase or story, an anecdote which is meant to convey more than its direct and obvious meaning. The metaphor contains alternate storylines which take the beholder deeper than the story itself.

Metaphors can be very useful in the teaching and learning process as well as in the healing process. They aid everyday communication. The following are examples of some common metaphors.

A mother may be trying to convey to her family physician how sick her child is and how high the child's fever is. The mother expresses: "Doctor, my daughter Katie is so sick. She's burning up." Obviously, the child is not literally on fire, but this phrase, this metaphor, gives a clear image to the receiver of the information that this child has a high fever. The image is clear without the use of numbers.

Susan may have had a hectic and busy day and felt like whatever she did, it didn't get the job done. Chaos was the order of the day. When she arrives home, she says to her partner: "The whole day I felt like I was running around like a chicken with its head cut off." This is another very clear metaphor to describe the experience of the day. The image negates the need for a lot of description. Images remove the need for a reliance on words.

One final example: Billy is visiting Auntie Jill. He is outside playing, but steps on a thistle and runs into the house crying. Jill is later describing the sight to Billy's mum and says "Billy took off like a bat out of hell."

These are each examples of metaphoric communication. They

are not necessarily therapeutic in any way, but they are great aids in communication.

A metaphor tells the child with whom you are working that you do understand what it's like to be in his or her position. It says, "Hey, I understand. And, guess what, you're not alone in that feeling." There is an increasing amount of research that points to the fact that

> the right hemisphere [of the brain] is activated in processing metaphorical types of communication. Since the right hemisphere is also more involved than the left in mediating emotional and imagistic processes, it is believed likely that psychosomatic symptoms are processed by predominantly right-brain functions. In other words, the right brain may be the "home" of both metaphoric language and psychosomatic symptomatology (Mills & Crowley, 1986, p. 17).

Cowan notes that

> mythopoetic language, specifically metaphor, has the ability to heal mental and emotional pain because the metaphor mediates the contradictions of life, thus providing a solution that appeals to our deepest hope that it is possible to transcend the human condition (Cowan, 1993, p. 97).

Mills & Crowley (1986) describe some interesting research (Rogers, TenHouten, Kaplan & Gardner, 1977) involving the study of language. The Hopi and English languages were compared in terms of hemispheric activity of the brain. A story was translated into both the Hopi and English languages and was told to bilingual Hopi elementary school children. EEG measurements were recorded. The results indicated that higher right-brain activity was involved in processing the story in Hopi than in its English version. The Hopi language is a much more contextual and involves greater metaphoric usage in communication.

FANTASY

Fantasy is a vital aspect of a human's life. It is one of the abilities which seems to separate us from much of the animal kingdom.[3] Through fantasy, children learn to test out the world of day to day life. There have been some rather negative views of fantasy in both the fields of mental health and education. Rather than viewing fantasy as a positive normal expression and part of a healthy life, Freud saw fantasy as a mechanism to compensate for some earlier harm, wrong or pathology. Even worse, Maria Montessori, who has had a profound influence on the field of education, considered fantasy to be "a somewhat unfortunate pathological tendency of early childhood that encourages defects of character" (Mills & Crowley, 1986, p. 38). This is hardly the kind of attitude that results in a positive influence on education. Montessori only provided opportunities for structured play that would promote certain intellectual and cognitive skills,

> considering there to be no value in imaginative play.... The rigid structures built in by Montessori did not allow for [spontaneity and individuality] (Meighan, 1994, p. 317).

Little wonder that the early childhood education approach of many Montessori schools seems rather rigid and overly structured, with no room for the imaginative aspects of a child's life that are so vital to emotional well-being and psychological growth.

Fortunately, in more recent times fantasy has received its due positive regard. Certainly, very few still maintain the absurd and negative views of Freud or Montessori. Thanks to extensive research in developmental psychology we now know and understand that children need to enjoy, squirm around in, and passionately embrace the world of fantasy, not follow some rigid, predetermined method of learning devoid of playful fantasy, spontaneity, passion, and life.

The Fantasy of Fairies

Fairytales and fantasy allow us to end the realm of the "otherworld," the land of fairies. This is the world between the worlds —the world between day-to-day reality and fantasy. Fairytales and fantasy can promote psychological growth through metaphoric processes involved in healing and recovery. In the fairy tale there is a happy ending. I have heard fairy tales receive outright condemnation. Some professionals and teachers argue that fairytales are bad because they give the child an unreal picture of the world. I would argue that fairytales are not dealing with reality. They are dealing with fantasy and the world of the unconscious mind. The happy ending of the fairy tale gives a child an image of positive possibilities. The fairytale encourages hope. Difficulties can be overcome. Evil can be defeated. After a period of challenges and difficulties, good effort is rewarded. Loneliness, rejections, and devastation can all be overcome. It is bizarre that anyone in the human services fields would consider these kind of messages to be negative. These are all positive messages that every child needs. By giving children a new picture of the world through fairytales, we can help them develop a positive outlook.

Fantasy and fairytales can be nothing more than stories for children, or they can serve purposes of psychological healing, growth and joy. To be emotionally useful, a certain sense of "distance" from the story is required. This can be accomplished by simply using words like "once upon a time" or "a long time ago, in a land far away." With those words you remove a sense of direct confrontation with the child. You begin working parallel to his or her world. The child is able to watch what is going on rather than feeling directly in the spotlight. The focus is removed from personal issues and worries.

Other aspects necessary for psychologically productive fantasy include a temporary sense of danger, a period of desolation followed by eventual growth and recovery, and, finally, consolation and success—a rebirth through the happy ending. These factors in children's fantasy stories and fairytales allow a sense of hope to be experienced. What is happening in the fantasy story appeals to the internal emotional processes of the child.

Although I think that the most powerful stories and fairytales come through their own telling or reading, I would not rule out the advantages of some movies. For example, the movie *Never Ending Story*[4] fulfils all of the requirements for a psychologically positive fairy tale. In this movie, there is a young boy, Bastian, whose mother has died. His father doesn't understand the boy's grief and the child becomes enthraled and entwined with a story he is reading. The story in the movie begins with "It was midnight in the howling forest." Thus, a sense of otherworld fantasy, one of the main requirements for a psychologically beneficial fairy tale, is immediately created.

In the movie, a land called Phantasia is in danger of complete destruction. The wise one of the land is a little girl, known as The Childlike Empress, and she is deathly ill. Her illness began at the same time as the destruction of the land. No one knows for sure what is happening, only that something called the Nothing is causing the destruction. The Childlike Empress calls for a little boy named Atreyu to help save the land. Along the way of trying to save the land from the Nothing, Atreyu has to deal with a number of personal battles (such as his own fear and self-doubt), as well as external battles with strange beings. He must go on a great quest. Atreyu is told it will be a very dangerous journey and certain conditions are placed on his quest: he must go alone and he must leave all weapons behind. Along the way, he has the assistance of certain natural creatures. Success in his journey comes through getting in touch with nature and these creatures, as well as realizing his own personal worth.

Finally, in a battle with an evil animal called a Gmork, which has been chasing him, Atreyu feels like he has failed. Most of the land is destroyed. Immediately prior to the battle, the Gmork reveals the basis of the problem: "Phantasia has no boundaries. It is the world of human fantasy. It is dying because people begin to lose hopes and forget dreams. The Nothing is the emptiness that is left. It is like despair destroying the world. People who have no hopes are easy to control." This is so like the modern struggles of the world. A battle occurs and there is great destruction. The Gmork is destroyed, but all that remains of the land is a grain of sand. Atreyu then reports back to The Childlike Empress. The movie ends with words of wisdom from the little girl. Her young face graces the screen as she speaks words of deep awareness to the despondent Atreyu: "In the beginning it is always dark." There is such wisdom in her words, hope in her face, and encouragement in her voice.

We should aim to incorporate such hope to all of our fantasy stories for children. It is quite clear the

> fairy tales assure the child that every evil phantom has its opposite which is more powerful in doing good than the evil figure is in doing evil, something the child may not be able to imagine all on his own when overcome by what, at the moment, seem to him the overwhelming difficulties of his life. It is the subtle balance between good and bad powers that is finally tipped in favour of the victory of virtue which gives the child the hope that in real life, his misfortunes will not only be limited in time, but will completely

> disappear, to be replaced by his elevation to a higher plane of existence where he will be secure for the rest of his life. While in reality there is not always a happy ending to our travails, it is the hope that there might be which sustains us, while without it we may fall into despair (Ehrlich, 1985, p. xi).

Surely, hope is one of the greatest gifts we can give to a child. Perhaps this is why Lewis Carroll referred to the fairy tale as a "love gift" to a child and C.S. Lewis felt that they were spiritual explorations, life felt, or divined from the inside (Bettleheim,[5] 1977).

Footnotes

[1] I am a very big fan of science fiction. Let's not confuse it with fact.

[2] I am not referring here to legitimate psychometric tools. My criticism is not aimed against such well researched tools as the Achenbach Child Behaviour Checklist, the Conners Rating Scales, and other similar tools.

[3] This is a disputable statement on more than one level and is certainly not the last word on the subject. I have tried to temper the statement by saying "*seems* to separate us from *much* of the animal kingdom." I believe that some animals do, in fact, actively fantasize. But since we do not, at present, have some common language, we do not know this. I can only say "I think" about this.

[4] Based on the book of the same name by Michael Ende. The book and movies are considerably different. There is only one book. There are two movies, *Never Ending Story* and *Never Ending Story Part Two*. I have not seen the Part Two version, but kids I know who saw it were fairly consistent in their disappointment. On the other hand, I was personally very impressed with the first movie and I have only heard rave positive reviews from both children and adults who saw it.

[5] I realize that all may not be well in the Bettleheim camp. Szasz (1994) relates that "After Bettleheim committed suicide in a nursing home in the spring of 1990, survivors of his (mis)treatment came forward to set the record straight.... Bettleheim lied and abused children: [quoting Pekow] *While publicly condemning violence, [he] physically abused children.... Bettleheim called us crippled in the mind.... [He] used all-school assemblies to tear people down*" (p. 85). Given this new information I find it unfortunate to be quoting Bettleheim. However, his theory on the benefits of fairytales is quite valid, despite other problems with his approach and in his life.

CHAPTER **6**

Developmental, Cultural and Political Considerations

DEVELOPMENTAL ISSUES

In our contact and work with children it is important to take their developmental level into consideration. This may sound like stating the obvious, but, time and again, I have seen parents, teachers and therapists with good intentions demonstrate very unrealistic expectations of children in their care. As Greg Lubimiv notes:

> Understanding the nature and processes of normal child development is essential to working with children and families.... By understanding what is normal behaviour, affect and thinking of children, you will better be able to understand and deal with what is considered abnormal or problematic behaviour. As well, you will be able to keep problems in perspective for yourself, the parent(s) and other concerned adults. There is a balancing act for all of us to accomplish in working with children and families. How do we keep from making a mountain out of a mole hill—while ensuring we don't make mole hills out of mountains? Having a strong background in child development will not guarantee this will never happen—but you will certainly be better prepared (1994, pp. 17-19).

From a holistic perspective, we cannot separate biological influences from environmental ones. It is foolish to try.[1] All children have certain biologically controlled potential, but without proper environmental stimulation, they may be deprived of reaching their own potential. Biology and environment are intertwined in any individual's development.

> The competences that are dependent upon growth of the nervous system can be affected, often seriously, if animals or children are deprived of stimulation or an opportunity to act (Kagan, 1984, p. 5).

I think there is a trend in the modern world to promote premature physical and intellectual growth. The child's physical and cognitive growth, especially in the Western world, is promoted at the expense of social, psychological and creative development. Children are provided with an endless stream of physical aids, upright bouncing devices, and so on that promote an upright approach to the world, potentially undermining the important crawling and rolling stage of development. Children are encouraged, pushed even, to walk, to learn to read, write, spell, identify words, and be mini-intellects at the expense of an imaginative approach to the world where fantasy, fairies, magic gardens and daily life coincide.

In making decisions about the kind of play interventions to make with children, keep in mind that treatment needs to be geared toward the level of the child's emotional and cognitive functioning, not chronological age. In this way, you do not put the child in a position of feeling like a failure.

BELIEFS ABOUT CHILD DEVELOPMENT

Until the 1600s, there was not much interest in how or why children develop as they do. The general view of the time was that

> children were miniature adults, with small-scale adult traits, virtues, and vices. They were cared for until about the age of six, when they could care for themselves. Thereafter, they were dressed like adults, put to work alongside them, punished like them for wrong deeds or disobedience to authority, and even hanged for thievery (Hunt, 1993, p. 352).

This all changed in the 1600s with Locke's view that the child is actually born as a blank slate. This gave us the notion that the environment may play a role in the outcome of an individual's life. Slowly the field of child psychology would develop from this base. The first known documentation of longitudinal development in children was published in 1787 by Dietrich Tiedeman. The study, entitled *Observations on the Development on Mental Capabilities in Children*, "can be viewed as the back bone and initiator of empirical research in this field" (Yavari, 1995, p. 2).

One of the most significant contributions in developmental psychology came at the turn of the 20th century from Stanley Hall who "steered what was then known as *the child study movement* toward experimentation and data gathering" (Hunt, 1993, p. 353). Through this "child study movement" came a blossoming of the scientific approach to the understanding of children.

The Western psychoanalytically influenced psychotherapeutic model places intense importance on the early development of a child. We must keep in mind the key sources of such beliefs: S. Freud and

Jung, neither of whom had any direct experience with children. Freud was responsible for his psychosexual theory of child development, despite not working with children. This oft-quoted, unscientific theory, based on Freud's philosophy rather than empirical evidence, will not be outlined here. As noted by Szasz, Freud was "a domineering founder of a religion (or cult), rather than a dispassionate scientist or compassionate therapist" (1988, p. 155). Eysenck takes it even further and details the damage done by Freud's approach. He notes that Freud, by refusing to follow scientific empirical standards, set the science of psychology back at least 50 years and that we

> will have to abandon the pseudo-science of psychoanalysis [which] will remain forever one of the saddest and strangest of all landmarks in the history of twentieth-century thought.... [Freud's] place is not, as he claimed, with Copernicus and Darwin, but with Hans Christian Anderson and the Brothers Grimm, tellers of fairy tales (Eysenck, 1984, pp. 207-208).

I believe the same can be said for Jung.[3] In 1954, Jung published *The Development of the Personality.* This was a philosophical exploration and a strange "contribution" to the field, given that Jung did not work with children. Although given immense credit by religious followers, I do not believe either of these influential thinkers of the twentieth century offered any great contribution to the field of child psychology.

It is well past the time to turn away from the psychoanalytic theories of childhood and turn our efforts to true scientific research. Unfortunately, it is next to impossible to find a play therapy text which does not make reference to Freud's theory in a manner implying some legitimacy to—even reverence for—as in any cult or religion—his thinking.

A truly great pioneer in the field of child development, who actually worked with children, was Jean Piaget. He, like Freud and Jung, has had a strong influence on our modern views of children.

> While Piaget was not psychoanalytically oriented, he agreed that infants and very young children are totally "egocentric," explaining the world in terms of their needs and its reaction to them, and he believed that child development involves an increasing understanding that the world functions according to logic and laws

> that exist independent of the self. The acme of human development—which occurs through a process of assimilation, incorporating what is "out there" as part of the self, and accommodation, changing the self to be compatible with the world out there—is to appreciate objective reality by thinking like a scientist.... Subsequent research has demonstrated that this progression is far from orderly and that Piaget may have confused an appreciation of the world as it is with an ability to verbalize that appreciation. Very young children who are not supposed to understand the permanence of objects, for example, find magic tricks based on defying this permanence surprising and amusing (or distressing).... Nevertheless, both the psychoanalytic and the Piagetian beliefs in the importance of childhood-to-adulthood movement from primitive egoism to reality testing had a profound impact on professional psychology, reinforcing the belief in the overriding importance of childhood experience and the view of adult psychopathology as resulting from an inability to grow up, a view that is consistent with paternalism. Childhood became not just an experience, but a tyranny with the result that not only clients but everyone is considered fragile—what Paul Meehl (1973, pp. 252-255) has termed the "spun glass model" of the human adult (Dawes, 1994, pp. 265-266).

From the above, one can see that many of the early mental health field's beliefs relating to child development may need refinement or even a complete revision. This is not meant in any way to discredit the painstaking efforts of Piaget. He was a pioneer and we must take the beginnings that pioneers offer us and develop from there. This is what is occurring in child psychology today. We are finding ourselves outgrowing our "founders." Nor is this, in any way, meant to compare Piaget and Freud; Piaget was a scientist, Freud was not. Piaget's work was a catalyst for the field of child psychology. Freud's work was a hindrance. Piaget's great contribution to developmental psychology was his conception that intelligence is "a form of biological adaptation of the individual to the environment" (Sattler, 1992, p. 53).

Since the 1940s, developmental psychologists have made great gains in understanding the development of children. Given the rapid growth of this field, it is vital that our knowledge base be as up-to-date as possible. To still be referring to the work of Piaget, a great pioneer, as fully descriptive of our present knowledge base is foolish; to refer to the work of Freud is inexcusable.

PLAY AND DEVELOPMENT

Play and fantasy are crucial for all humans as well as many other species.

> Animal play clearly serves several purposes: learning of social rules in a nonserious atmosphere where mistakes are tolerated, mock hunting if the animal is a predator, mock evasion if he is a prey animal, mock combat if combat is part of his species-society means for establishing hierarchies, mock mating or preliminary sexual play before full sexuality emerges. All these are necessary to the animals survival learning (Pearce, 1977, p. 142).

Play serves many important functions in the development of a child. Being able to play allows a child to participate in what I would all "social theatre." Children can try out different roles. They may play and act at being a mummy or daddy, a pilot, a letter carrier, a doctor, a gardener. Each time they try out a new role, children are training in social skills and vocational skills, getting a feel for what it would be like to be in the position they are playing.

Play promotes a social competence and a "readiness to engage with peers, ability to sustain give-and-take with them, and popularity with or acceptance by them" (Hunt, 1993, p. 375). Earliest involvement in social play activities necessitates the learning to "take turns."

There is more to all of this than simply social issues. Play has a deep biological function that, I believe, is either ignored or completely misunderstood by the mental health professions. In both animals and humans,

> play offers a way by which the young can learn the social rules and adapt to them with minimum risks. In both, play offers a chance for the child to learn to use tools without economic pressures. Vigotsky gets close to the matter in his observation of play as a "pivot between the real and the imaginary." But he misses the point by not understanding the difference between the world and reality. Almost unanimously, psychologists fall into the error of

> considering the child's play to be wish fulfilment at a fantasy level.... Beneath all the studies and comments about animal and child play runs a central, if unrecognized, thread: Play serves survival. But our notions of survival are so grim, so opposite to play. The very word conjures up pictures of a gray, marginal existence, hanging to life by a thread, down to the last tissue or tank of gas. Instead, consider survival to be the victory of life over death, a cause for celebration. This victory is what constitutes most animal play (Pearce, 1977, p. 141).

Young healthy animals of all species play with a reckless abandon, frenzied in their passionate play activities. This is not wish fulfilment, it is the ecstasy of experiencing life to its fullest, living absolutely in the moment. Play is not, as many think it is, a denial, an avoidance or escape from reality.

> Nothing of the sort is involved. The biological plan is vastly more intelligent and skilful and the purposes of play and imitation are light-years beyond these paltry, facile, impotent, and deadly unimaginative academic notions (Pearce, 1977, p. 145).

Play IS a testing of reality in the service of full participation in life. Through their play activities, humans and other animals have an opportunity to experience many situations without actually involving the risks that the literal or symbolic "life or death" situation would entail.

IMPORTANT ASPECTS OF CHILD DEVELOPMENT

Having a good grasp on child development helps us understand our own children and maintain realistic expectations for them as parents, and in our professional work to: conduct accurate assessments; plan appropriate interventions; evaluate the child's progress and effectiveness of interventions; make predictions about future development. The following are important aspects of child development that caregivers and play therapists need to understand to fulfil their roles properly.

Bronfenbrenner's thesis (1979) maintains that

> a critical factor in a child's development is the active involvement of at least one adult who is simply crazy about the child. I am raising this issue of someone being totally in love with the child here because of its importance for children of all ages. Clearly, a grandparent can be that person, and facilitating such grandparent-grandchild relationships may be an important preventive measure in fostering children's mental health.... The available research is consistent with the view that grandparents are an extremely valuable resource in promoting infant mental health (Cited in Crockenberg, Lyons-Ruth & Dickstein, 1993, pp. 47, 49).

I think that grandparents are a badly neglected lot. Their positive value in a child's life cannot even begin to be measured.

> Evidence that grandparents serve as backup socialization agents and contribute in significant ways to the development and mental health of their grandchildren comes from several sources (Crockenberg, Lyons-Ruth, & Dickstein, 1993, p. 47).

I am using grandparents as an example here, but it need not necessarily be a grandparent. Many other significant people in the child's life can foster their social and emotional growth and adjustment by being "crazy" about them. Maybe their aunt, uncle, minister, or grade one teacher sees something very special about this child and is just "crazy" about them.

The Kauai Longitudinal Study (Werner & Smith, 1992 cited in Mrazek, 1993) has been described as one of the most comprehensive prospective studies of risk and resiliency. This particular study followed hundreds of individuals from birth to adulthood and monitored a number of significant biological and psychosocial risk factors, stressful life events and protective factors in individual's lives. One of the most notable findings was that

> the support of alternate caregivers, such as grandparents or siblings, was a protective factor that gained importance as the children got older (Mrazek, 1993, p. 164).

Mrazek (1993) points out that protective factors can exist within the individual, family, or community. If they are missing from one domain, it is more critical that they occur amply in another.

That grade one teacher who thought the world of little Suzie and gave great emotional strength to her may never know the results of her attention to Suzie. Yet, that teacher may be the one who allows Suzie to see herself as a worthwhile, even an amazing, person. Without ever knowing the result of his or her positive approach to little Suzie fifteen years previous when she was in grade one, that teacher may have saved this child's life. Despite tragedies or even abuse in her life, setbacks and difficult times, Suzie may have learned early through the caring efforts of just one individual that she was a worthwhile person. Instead of another name at the morgue following a suicide when she was eighteen years old, Suzie is a physician at the local hospital or the chief supervisor at a well-known engineering firm.

No one should ever underestimate his or her influence on the life of a child or fellow human being. People who care about others and give to others and who love children have serious, positive long term effects on the lives of those children.

EARLY BONDING

Since the 1940s and 1950s there has been an intense interest in the earliest years of human development. The most popular topic to emerge from this era would appear to have been mother-child attachment. Fathers, grandparents and other potential caregivers have largely been ignored by the early research, and even most modern research. Fortunately, babies don't care about research and have just kept right on forming bonds and attachments with all kinds of significant people in their lives.

There have been positive and negative consequences from the work of attachment theorists (Bowlby, 1969, 1980; Ainsworth, Blehar, Watters & Wall, 1978; Stern, 1985). On the one hand, these theorists have contributed a great deal to our understanding of early child development and the consequences of trauma at different stages of development. Unfortunately, some of these theorists have attempted to lock us into a view that the first 3 years, or one year, or 3 days or 3 minutes, predetermine the remainder of our lives (Chess, 1978,

1979; Chess & Thomas, 1982; Chess, Thomas & Birch, 1959)—a silly assumption at best.

> We know a great deal about the importance of a positive parent-child relationship. We know a great deal about many of the specific factors that promote or deter such a relationship, and how these factors in the child and in the parent interact in a mutually influential developmental sequence. But just as the child's nutritional requirements can be met successfully with a wide range of individual variation, so can his psychological requirements.... As we grow from childhood to maturity, all of us have to shed many childhood illusions. As the field of developmental studies has matured, we now have to give up the illusion that once we know the young child's psychological history, subsequent personality and functioning is ipso facto predictable. On the other hand, we now have a much more optimistic vision of human development. The emotionally traumatized child is not doomed, the parents' early mistakes are not irrevocable, and our preventive and therapeutic intervention can make a difference at all age-periods (Chess & Thomas, 1982, p. 221).

Whatever biological influences and maturational effects exist in a child's world,

> environmental conditions play a crucial role in fostering enthusiasm for learning and providing the child with an opportunity to develop fully. A supportive and stimulating family environment is needed if each child is to realize his or her maximum potential (Sattler, 1992, p. 62).

Early Bonding and Substitute Care

Research into attachment issues should raise a certain amount of concern about abdicating caregiving responsibilities to others, including day-care settings. Dual working parents'[4]

> diminished contact with their infants may deprive them of opportunities to fine-tune their relationship, potentially contributing to less comfortable and possibly less secure parent-infant relationships (Sroufe, 1988 cited in Barton & Williams, 1993, p. 447).

As a result of rapid changes in our culture in terms of child care arrangements, it is yet possible to determine the long term societal effects of such changes. We know that in the United States

> in 1972, 24% of mothers of infants under the age of 1 year were employed; by 1987 that figure had risen to 51%, and the increase is expected to continue (Barton & Williams, 1993, p. 445).

The unfortunate aspect of such research is that it relates to working mothers rather than working caregivers.

We have all heard the propaganda about how good day-care can be for children. Studies have been cited that "prove" this. However, there are certain flaws in the arguments. First, the studies which have shown that children appear to benefit from *high-quality* (and high quality is a key) day-care have been done with children from economically impoverished homes. It is a major error to generalize such studies. The second major flaw in the thinking about "benefits" from day-care is that almost all studies have been focused on cognitive development. Well, of course, if you take a child from a non-stimulating and impoverished environment and provide intellectual stimulation, nutrition, and positive social contacts, you are going to see an improvement in cognitive development. It shouldn't take a rocket scientist or millions of dollars of taxpayers' money to figure that one out. Again, the very research typifies our focus on intellectuality rather than the world of emotions, personality and spirituality.

When it comes to emotional development, early studies which studied attachment and showed positive effects from extra-familial child care were flawed and have been strongly criticized on both philosophical and methodological grounds. Samples used were small, only high quality daycare settings were studied, and the ratings of attachment-related behaviours and similar issues were very narrow.

Over the past several years, there have been great improvements in research endeavours. As a result, the findings that have emerged are much more accurate, reliable, and frightening. The findings of these studies have not been hitting the headlines, nor have politically correct (but factually wrong) social workers, other mental health professionals or child-care workers been quick to quote from these more up-to-date and more accurate studies.

> Clearly, there is an impressive and increasingly incontrovertible body of data suggesting that nonmaternal care in the first year of life is associated with infants' classification as insecurely attached, and perhaps specifically with the insecure/avoidant classification (Barton & Williams, 1993, p. 448).

Most studies have looked at lengthy periods (more than 20 hours per week) of time spent in outside "care" settings. However, it has been found that as little as 5 hours per week of substitute care can result in insecure attachment. Interestingly, there does not appear to be any consistent increase in insecurity as the amount of substitute care increases. Fortunately, in modern years, some "brilliant" person realized that children also have fathers in their lives so studies are starting to emerge on infant-father attachments. These studies are coming up with findings similar to the infant-mother studies. Children in substitute care arrangements have also been found to have insecure attachments with their fathers.

Since the 1960s, there has been a positive philosophy and attitude among professionals toward substitute care settings. As discussed, some of their arguments about the benefits have focused on cognitive skills of children in such settings. Another argument has focused on the positive social benefits for children enroled in day care. The variables to which they glowingly refer have included things like increased frequency of social interactions (again, did we really need to waste any time and finances on studies that concluded that children in large groups of other children are going to have more social interactions than children raised at home—well, duh), increased confidence, more advanced play, more positive affect exchanges between day care children and adults, and advanced language development for children in day care settings. As noted previously, the studies have largely involved high quality day care settings and children from impoverished environments. Unfortunately, we now have a culture which has erroneously generalized these findings to all day-cares and all children. However, an equal number of studies, which champions of day-care choose to ignore, have revealed

> an association between early day care experience and negative social-emotional development, particularly increased aggressive or noncompliant behavior (Barton & Williams, 1993, p. 454).

Such aggression and noncompliance have been found in both verbal and behavioral areas. Studies have found day care children to be rated more aggressive and more socially isolated by their peers. Interestingly, and perhaps indicative of a lack of awareness or sensitivity, such children were not rated differently on either dimension by their teachers (Barton & Schwartz, 1981). Also of interest are modern studies which find that youngsters attending cognitive oriented programs[5] have more elevated levels of aggression than those attending non-cognitively oriented programs.

> The ratings of aggression for these children were greater on every variable than for children enroled in day care for longer periods of time (Haskin, 1985 cited in Barton & Williams, 454).

Particularly frightening from a societal perspective are findings such as those from Belsky which note that

> non-maternal care in the first year of life is related to subsequent social maladjustment, and particularly to an increased incidence of aggression and noncompliant behavior (1988 cited in Barton & Williams, 1993, p. 453).

On the other side of the coin from all of these arguments, though, are children who do have early insecure infant-mother relationships. High-quality substitute care settings may actually help ameliorate the long-term consequences of such insecurity. Most psychoanalysts and many early attachment theorists have attempted to give the impression that insecure attachment in the first year of life automatically means insurmountable negative consequences. Such a belief is far from true. As Kagan (1984) notes:

> I am not suggesting that it is irrelevant how adults care for infants. It does matter! But an insecure attachment during the first year need not always lead to adult pathology, and a secure attachment is no guarantee of future invulnerability to distress (p. 254).

Given that so very many children are now placed in substitute care arrangements on a regular basis and the fact that we now fairly conclusively know that children from high-quality substitute care arrangements do much better than children from low-quality care arrangements, at the societal level and academic level it is imperative that we begin to optimize substitute child care arrangements and settings. Now that we know what makes a good substitute care arrangement, we need to determine the best possible methods for training those involved in substitute care and the best kind of atmosphere within which to provide such care.

I cannot emphasize strongly enough that if you can't afford for one parent or consistent family member (do not ignore the importance and potential of a positive grandparent, aunt, uncle) to stay home with your child, don't have children. I am told that I am far too often an idealist. So, to take reality into account, if you already have children and are looking for daycare arrangements for your child, there are certain things to look for. First, since regulated settings provide a higher quality of care than unregulated settings (Fosberg *et al.*, 1980, cited in Barton & Williams, 1993, p. 459), you should be looking for a regulated setting. Important aspects of a substitute care arrangement include things like small size, well-trained staff, low child-to-staff ratios, and as little structure as possible, but as much as necessary. The environment should be very clean, have lots of well cared for creative supplies, and have time devoted to children rather than routine. Openness is crucial. You should be able to drop in at any time for any reason and be a totally welcome guest/observer of the setting. Thus, an ideal setting would include caregivers as part-time volunteers in the daily routine as well as parental involvement at the decision making level.

> Parents should be told that the decision to use substitute care represents the formation of a partnership for parenting, not an abdication of parenting (Barton & Williams, 1993, p. 459).

The importance of quality child care cannot be overemphasized. Ellen Galinsky, Co-President of the Families & Work Institute, comments that

> "you either pay now or pay later, that what we're beginning to learn about brain development, what we're beginning to learn about the impact of bad quality child care on children will show that there will be a cost to us later." Unfortunately, a lack of available quality care combined with parents' vested interests in finding a place to keep their child, make parents poor judges of

> level of quality in daycares. Further, Galinsky notes that "parents can be very satisfied with child care that observers rate as not being good for kids learning, not even being safe" (Galinsky on *CBS*, February 21, 1996).

As well, "a study of US day-care centres released last year found that only one centre in seven provides high-quality care; 70 percent provide mediocre care, which may hurt a child's ability to learn; 40 percent of centres that care for infants were judged unsafe" (*CBS*, February 21, 1996). This latter 40 percent was not just an inadequate or low quality rating, it was a rating of downright unsafe. This means that millions of North American children are spending the bulk of their childhood waking hours in unsafe care environments. Surely, we can find the funds to improve this situation. Here is another way to use wasted mental health money. Transfer it to child care settings.

INFANT PLAY: SENSORIMOTOR DEVELOPMENT (BIRTH TO 2 YEARS)

A child's early play is motivated by the senses and movement. First, everything is simply experienced by the senses. Soon, with the development of early physical skills, body movement comes into play: The child reaches for a toy, mouths it, looks at it. To try to experience the world solely from a sensorimotor perspective, hold and touch, look at, smell, taste, intuitively sense, and listen to a herb (try lavender and spearmint, they each speak very clearly). Now describe it to a partner using your eyes only. Now, use only sounds (no words) from your mouth to describe it. Next, simply hold your hands up to your partner's hands (do not actually touch), only come close enough to feel the warmth of energy from the other's hands—one partner's hands on top, the other on the bottom allows a greater distance than hands outstretched facing each other—using this energy only, try to describe to your partner what the herb is like. Now use your hands and arms to describe it. Now use your whole body to describe the herb. Now, whoever is the partner, sense a different herb, describe it in a similar manner as above. This is the realm of the sensorimotor.

The primary mode of play over the first 18 to 24 months of life is sensorimotor (Piaget, 1962). Early orientations are all sensory oriented. Jernberg (1983) defines sensory-motor play as

> the play of the concrete, self-centred, predominantly biological infant. Sensory-motor play permeates both the baby's own movements through space and his or her handling of objects in the outside world. Both large- and small-muscle movements over this first period of life progress from crude and undifferentiated to directed and refined.

In the second half of the first year the infant has begun to attempt to control the surrounding world. Attention and focus is increasingly oriented to exploring and influencing. This new process is referred to as *mastery motivation*. "Mastery is considered to be intrinsically motivated and self-reinforcing" (Lyons-Ruth & Zeanah, 1993, p.26). Mastery refers to a child's present attempts to master the world around him or her. Also toward the end of the first year of life, early forms of pretend play briefly emerge. However, the child is still sensorimotor oriented.

This sensorimotor stage *sets a path* for future development. However, unlike early psychoanalytic, attachment and some developmental theorists, I do not believe that it predetermines or even determines the path of future development. This is a very important philosophical point. Psychoanalysts, attachment theorists and some developmentalists have placed such an emphasis on this early development that it is seen as determining all that unfolds afterwards. This has never been shown to be true. We do know that delinquents can choose to stop stealing cars, a person who abuses a child can choose to nurture instead of abuse that child, and that human beings can make minor and major changes at any point of their choosing in life. Yet, the Western world view prefers a focus on stability after initial development. This applies to many areas, not just child development. It differs considerably from many Oriental views.

> Classic Chinese premises form a compelling contrast to those of the West, for an emphasis on change, rather than on permanence, has dominated philosophical writings during most of Chinese history. An important third century essay – the "Chuang-tzu Commentary" – captures this theme: "Of the forces which are imperceptible forces, none is greater than that of change.... All things are ever in a state of change...therefore the I of the past is no longer the I of today" (Fung 1973, cited in Kagan, 1984, p. 12).

I think the view that considers the perpetual potential for change is the optimistic view that educators and mental health professionals need to take. Otherwise, if all is predetermined by the past, there truly is no possibility for change, why bother to educate or to conduct therapy?[6] The absurd contradiction of doing therapy despite a predetermined outcome never seems to be addressed by analysts and "destiny" attachment theorists.

As noted, this sensorimotor stage does have significant *implications* for future development. Attachment, bonding and trust all have their beginnings during this stage. However, if there are disturbances during these first couple of years of life, it in no way means that an individual can never attach, bond or learn to trust. It does mean that an individual may need to work on these issues later in life than a person who had an ideal childhood. In studies looking at different cultures and different species we find that humans, regardless of their culture, are cognitively the most highly evolved life form on the planet. As such, we have greater adaptability and greater ability to repair old personality wounds. Whereas a member of another species who suffers early maternal deprivation may not have the ability to make up for this early metaphoric "wound," humans do seem to have a capacity to heal from even some of the most severe traumas. We must be very careful in some of our cross species comparisons. A *Nova* documentary (*WGBH*, December 9, 1980) reviewed a number of experiments involving other species, especially primates, and showed that primates separated from their mothers suffered actual brain damage (for those completely deprived of touch) or physiological damage in the form of immune system suppression (for those temporarily separated). What we don't yet know from these studies is: 1) if such early infantile needs are met later in life, does this repair the physical damage? For example, if these primates were given extra doses of touch later in life, would their immune systems return to normal, and 2) do these studies really describe the human condition? I believe (but do not yet know this) that we humans can make up for early lacks, even deprivation and abuse, later, by returning and meeting the early needs in appropriate ways.

The work of Gina O'Connell-Higgins focuses in this direction. Her work on resiliency (1995) clearly indicates that

> those of you who touch the life of a child constructively, even briefly, should *never* underestimate your possible corrective impact on that child. The more resilient the child, the more mileage he or she will gain from your help.... Furthermore, never forget the immense contrast between simple, *sustained* kindness and horrendous abuse.... Enormous reparative potential resides in the bread-and-butter basics of caring about the young and listening closely to their lives. You can do this in *any* capacity: babysitter, teacher, therapist, neighbour, relative, clergy, coach, butcher, baker, or candlestick maker.... Remember, too, that surrogates of the resilient were generally available for only small amounts of clock time, and some faded after a limited developmental exposure. Yet their positive impact persisted for life. Just as abuse poisons by small acts in brief moments, so can we sow antidotal seeds through our gestures of caring concern (O'Connell-Higgins, 1995, pp. 324-325).

I think the work of O'Connell-Higgins emphasizes what I am saying here about reparative work being done at any point in a human's life. We truly can make up for past neglect, old wounds and trauma of the past.

One of the most important principles from *Developmental Play Therapy* (Brody, 1993) states that "A child feels seen first through touch." To be touched, along with feeding and breathing, is one of the earliest needs in a human's life. After our life sustaining biological needs of food and shelter are met, the next most important need is touch. A trauma early in life may involve negative perceptions of touch.

> Attachment- and trauma-related problems often involve past negative experiences with touching, and children who have these problems must learn through experiencing it that intimate touching can be a safe and pleasurable means of communication as well as intrinsically rewarding (James, 1994, p. 76).

Psychological work with children who were emotionally wounded at an early age will likely need to involve some reparative component relating to touch. Caregivers may need to be encouraged to positively touch their children. Teaching the caregiver some practical aspects of infant massage or shiatsu (Japanese pressure point massage) may be quite beneficial. Perhaps simple tasks such as rubbing baby lotion or hand cream on the child's hands or arms can be built into ongoing therapeutic work.[7]

The primary work with children actually in the sensorimotor stage must be with the caregivers of such children. Appropriate therapeutic interventions for children with issues arising from problems during this stage are those designed to take developmental considerations into account. The use of touch such as through massage, nurturing holding and cuddling, the use of the other senses and motor activities: all these give children new opportunities to make up for what lack may have existed in their lives. I would especially recommend storytelling for this age group as well. This may seem odd since the wee ones will have no idea of what is being said. However,

> storytelling, more than a transmission of characters, plots, and themes, is a unique form of communion between two people. What is valuable in the early years of storytelling is for the child to become accustomed to an adult's voice, especially a parent's voice, and to associate it with a peaceful time of day (Maguire, 1985, p. 80).

A further benefit is that story time often involves cuddling and other physical closeness. Alternately, if facing the child, there can be soothing, playful and joyous eye contact as well as body movement with gestures to accompany the stories.

If your work involves children under the age of one and a half or two, you need a great deal of sensory oriented toys—things that can be felt, squeezed, pushed, tugged at, stroked, mouthed. Many different textures are recommended—soft, rough, smooth, silky, hard, squishy. Toys that make sounds are useful with this age—rattles, boxes, things to put inside one another, toys that squeak or make other sounds when squeezed, touched or pulled.

IMAGINATIVE PLAY (2 TO 7 YEARS)

After the second year, the child is no longer so sensorimotor focused or motivated. The imagination has started to develop. During the imaginative stage of development, the child "engages in role play and weaves a magic web of fantasy around everything in his orbit" (Masheder, 1994, p. 129). In the second year, especially toward the end of this year and into their third year, children increasingly participate in pretend activities. By two and a half and three, children have become fully involved in pretend play, cooking, serving, pretending to drink from a makebelieve cup. The land of makebelieve is a very real place for the three year old. Children pretend to cook with utensils and pots and pans, they pretend to talk on a telephone. By three and a half the child is fully able to use one object to represent another in many play situations. In this early stage of pretend or symbolic play, you should have fairly realistic toys available for children: domestic type toys that are quite literally representative. These may include things like dolls, mini appliances, table and chairs, telephone, kitchen and bedroom toys, and a doctor's kit. At every stage of development it is wise to have creative arts and crafts supplies available. This should include things like crayons, construction paper, non-toxic glue, safety scissors, egg cartons, pipe cleaners, odds and ends and scraps of material and paper.

All higher animal species play in order to learn and to gain mastery. The symbolic play of human children is fairly unique. The child is actually able to symbolize, something largely absent from the abilities of most animals. In other words, the child can play assuming

> an "as if" stance, using one thing to "stand for" or represent (symbolize) another, to which it may be vaguely, accidentally, perhaps unconsciously, related (Irwin, 1983, p. 151).

The pretend play stage of development is based on a child's development of symbolic play and is the "primary type of play behavior observed in children between the ages of two and six years" (Shaefer & O'Connor, 1983, p. 93). Time after time you will hear the five year old say things like "let's say this is the zoo" while pointing at the living room. "I'll be the tiger, You be the lion." The child is his or her own director of this play, the producer of the story, the director of the action as well as an actor in the story. Children, in participating in this kind of play, imitate others (many animals do this). In addition, they "put real and imagined experiences together in new combinations" (Irwin, 1983, p. 151) (which most animals do not). The child imitates and pretends. This play is not goal directed. It is spontaneous and self-gratifying. It is fun for the child. This is truly the land of make-believe.

The play of this period occurs after a certain developmental process involving both cognitive growth and environmental stimulation. There are many children who simply do not know how to play. Unfortunately, there are also many adults in the same position. One reason for such an inability to play can be difficulties experienced by the child during the ages of two to six. Another reason may be developmental delays due to cognitive impairment, or from a lack of stimulation or opportunity to be involved in pretend play.

For children with impairment in the area of pretend play, toys like the sandbox and puppets offer great opportunities. The use of a sandbox allows for stories to unfold using a three dimensional format. Words are not required to tell the story. The use of the sandbox offers an added feature: the sand is very tactile and can also assist a child who suffered harm or deprivation during the sensorimotor stage of development. Puppets offer "symbolic, nonverbal, and interactional data" (Irwin, 1983, p. 159). Please refer to *Chapter 7, Puppets* in this text for ideas on methods for working with puppets.

Choices

A note of interest regarding this age range concerns the issue of tantrums. These are so common in this age range in our culture that they have come to be considered a normal part of child development. I am not convinced that this is the case. There have even been suggestions by a number of authors that such temper tantrums are really the result of premature or sudden weaning.[8] Whatever their origin, they are definitely a sign of intensity. I think that part of their function may be to display an attempt to gain or regain power in the world. I do not believe children want to misbehave or tantrum. Children—more specifically, secure and attached children—want nothing more than to please their caregivers. "Toddlers, in Kagan's view, once aware that standards (qualities of goodness or badness) exist, are intrinsically motivated to meet them" (Lyons-Ruth & Zeanah, 1993, p. 27). A method that can be quite helpful for children who apparently are "out of control" (I do not really believe a tantrum is a sign of being "out of control") would involve the empowerment of giving them choices. As children enter the age of about two, they may become "difficult" to deal with at times. They may not seem to know what they want and any suggestions are met with a resounding and often quite loud "NO!" Any attempts at communicating seem futile. The following is an example of this kind of scenario:

Parent: Johnny, it's time for supper.

Johnny: No, I don wawn supper.

Parent: Come have your supper.

Johnny: No.

Parent: Johnny, now you listen to me, you have to eat....

Not only does the conflict escalate, but such battles often involve meals, methods of clothing oneself, and bedtime routines. So, not only are you establishing major conflict times, you could also be laying the basic groundwork for lifelong eating problems, sleep disorders and bizarre fashion statements during adolescence.

Rather than little Johnny being given no choice and a supreme battle emerging as a result, I think at this very early age, you can begin to teach the child decision making skills. Instead of being stuck with a "terrible two," you are presented with another golden opportunity to help the "terrific two" grow and develop. This is not to say that the average two year old does not become obstinate. They do. However, it is just a phase, and if the caregiver wisely teaches skills of empowerment it need not lead to total frustration for all parties involved. So how to deal with this? First, don't wean early or abruptly. There is nothing wrong with a child continuing to nurse well past the age of 12 months or even 24 months.... Next, when the child starts to appear as if he or she is entering the "no" phase, teach "yes" as well. Two year olds are very fragile and vulnerable creatures. They are at the mercy of the decisions of others and yet they are becoming individuals of their own, though individuals with no power. They need their caregivers, yet are maturing and developing as individuals. They are beginning to feel themselves as separate from their caregivers and this is very threatening. The added anxiety of the separation process can promote wild tantrums for the child who is also feeling powerless. To get through this phase, my strongest recommendation is to offer the child choices, and live with the choices you offered. When "no" seems to predominate, make sure you also teach the child the word "yes." For example:

> Parent: Johnny, it is time for supper. We'd really like to see you. Would you like to join us, yes or no?
>
> Johnny: No.

That should be the end of the discussion. He doesn't eat, he gets hungry and eats later. So what? Healthy children will not starve themselves to death. It is indicative of the emotional state of the family if Johnny would rather eat alone later than with the family at the dinner table. It is definitely a sign of trouble. Make some changes. Making Johnny come to the dinner table will not change anything. Being a pleasant family that is fun to be around and who love and respect children will attract Johnny to the dinner table.

Suppose Johnny does come to the dinner table. In serving, Johnny should be respected and his choices should be respected. "You eat your potatoes right now young man or...bleah bleah bleah" is not a respectful statement. Again, physically and emotionally healthy children will not starve themselves. They need to be allowed choices. They need the right to say "no" and go at their own pace in these matters. There are enough areas where they don't have choices, and should not have choices, at that age. Don't make dinner time a disaster due to power conflicts. Handle meal time like this:

> Parent: (passing the carrots) Johnny, Dad made some real yummy carrots today. I bet even the bunnies are trying to sneak in the house to have some with us, would you like to try some, yes or no?
>
> Johnny: Yes.

Honestly, with this approach, Johnny is much more likely to say yes and eat them than if you try and force them on him. Your relationship will be that much better and Johnny will begin to learn to make decisions.

Let's use another example of bedtime. You may take my rationale to the extreme and think you should let the child decide when to go to bed. I do NOT advise this. Caregivers set the crucial limits and the time for bed should be one of them. A tired child is more miserable than a briefly hungry child. So it's bedtime. You can still give the child choices in certain areas:

Parent: Johnny, it's bedtime, would you like some stories tonight, yes or no?

If Johnny does want a story, let him pick his choice of story(ies). Bedtime needs to involve more than just a quick story, getting tucked in, a peck on the cheek and light out. Bedtime should be a time of cuddling, closeness, chats, and storytelling. I can't see a soothing bedtime taking less than half an hour. Make sure that time is available for your children. This may well be the prime quality time in the day that children get. Don't steal this time from them by trying to make it brief because you haven't yet been able to read today's paper. Many children act up at bedtime because they realize on some level that the only way they are going to get any more attention today is by being naughty. If they are not naughty, they are ignored and abandoned. This desire for attention will be most noticeable when the child enters the "twos." It will become particularly intense if you also have another child enter the family scene at this time.

The storytelling of four year olds often causes concern for caregivers, raising fears that the child has been abused or somehow traumatized in the past. There are even ridiculous checklists out there that tell you that if your child tells certain kinds of stories, then he or she has definitely been abused in the day care setting. The people who create these absurd glossaries should quietly be put out of their misery. They have done much harm and no good in their quest for quick answers and solutions to the problem of child abuse. The idea that everything a child says is true (in terms of literally everything said being absolutely a literal or symbolic reflection of reality) has only become popular among child abuse pop experts over the last decade or two. This is a belief that is not based on reality, nor is it supported by empirical evidence. It is a very dangerous political view to think that everything children say is true and factual.

We know that children often have trouble separating fantasy

from reality. Normal, healthy, well-developing children often tell stories filled with cannibalism, mutilation, dismemberment, murder and other horrendous things. Children seem to find these kinds of stories and fairytales gratifying because they on some level represent the child's own fears of being overwhelmed, abandoned or devastated. These stories serve the function of bolstering children's egos by reassuring them that the threat can be overcome.

Children around the ages of three to five are particularly fascinated by some of these gruesome tales because this is a time in their lives when they are haunted by fears and anxieties of being alone, separate from their caregivers. A great deal of four year olds' storytelling may be rather unpleasant. They can be creatures of considerable unconscious violence. Their stories should not be taken literally, nor should they be taken to represent abuse. However, things like "abuse checklists" that identify items like unusual storytelling as indicative of abuse try to simplify very complex issues and, in doing so, do a great disservice. The result can be that when a child shows up who has actually been cruelly abused, she or he is not taken seriously because a number of "wackos" and self-proclaimed experts have discredited the field. Such self-proclaimed experts and authorities are usually severely lacking in training in normal child and sexual development.

THE PLAY OF LOGIC AND ABSTRACTIONS (FROM 6 YEARS)

During this phase of development, children come to find joy in structure. Games that can be played with others—games like "hide and seek" and "Pooh sticks"—come to be enjoyed within the structure they provide. Children in this phase are excited by playing within a scheme of pre-ordained guidelines. However, at this stage, it is still the fun of playing for the sake of the process involved alone, rather than for any outcome-oriented reason, that provides fun for children. This does not mean that fantasy disappears. During this stage, fantasy play becomes more internalized.

Due to the fun of play,

> it is self-motivating. the very essence of play is not taking it "for real" (*i.e.*, too seriously). And so, though play is part of the serious business of childhood by which a child learns to handle the environment, it need not be taken excessively seriously by the

> child. In playing games, children can feel relatively spontaneous and free to be themselves, to have fun "trying things out". Usually we do not have to work at getting a child to play. Play and games are, hence, an educational and therapeutic medium which is naturally attractive and important in the overall development of children (Nickerson & O'Laughlin, 1983, p. 175).

The use of games with children can open many doors for dealing with emotions. Obviously the game must fit the child and the situation you are attempting to work on. For example, if a child needs very infantile sensory stimulation, games which promote such stimulation would be advisable. If a child has trouble with make-believe, games involving role plays would be appropriate. The average child begins this stage of development after the age of six. This does not in any way mean that you do not use methods suitable for the sensorimotor child or symbolic play with children over six. The child over six who is in treatment likely needs to return to an earlier stage of development before progressing. Even the adult may well play (and need to play) in the sandbox or with puppets.

EMOTIONAL DEVELOPMENT (The bulk of the following material is based on B. Revell, in M. Barnes & B. Revell, 1994 – Revell's background material derived from S. Harter, 1980, 1982, 1983; R. Selman, 1980)

Simultaneous Feelings

Children's understanding of multiple/simultaneous emotions goes through three distinct phases. Initially, a child has no concept that two emotions can co-exist. In the second phase, children come to understand that two feelings can exist sequentially. Finally, children reach an awareness that they can simultaneously experience two feelings at the same time. In their developing understanding of emotions, children's understanding depends on both the mood of the emotion and the object of the emotion.

The easiest thing to understand and the earliest awareness to develop is that one can have two different feelings of the same mood toward the same recipient. For example, love and happiness are both experienced in relation to the mother.

Next would come an understanding that one could experience both love toward mother and happiness about having a picnic. Here we see different emotions of the same mood but different objects receiving the feelings.

Finally, and most difficult to understand, would be two emotions of differing mood directed at the same object. For example, feeling love for mother and being angry at her at the same time.

To help children begin to understand things like different mood feelings, it can be helpful to use two dolls back to back to express the different feelings. A feelings pie may also be useful. In the feelings pie, children show on a pie chart the different feelings they are experiencing. They indicate the greatest feeling experienced with the largest slice of pie. This can help them understand different emotions within the same person.

Inner Feelings vs. Expressed Feelings

Prior to about the age of 5, children perceive their emotions as being obvious to the outside world. Asking 3 or 4 year olds why they did something is a developmentally ridiculous question. At that age they assume they did it because they did it. "Why did you hit Billy?" is most likely to receive the response "Because I hit him." Children do not recognize inner feelings. This does not mean that they should get away with hitting or any other negative activity. But you are wasting your time in any discussion on inner motivation with young children. Instead of asking "why" they did it, it would be effective and more appropriate to ask what the results of what they did were (for example: Johnny cried; I got in trouble; I wasn't allowed to go outside to play that evening; and so on). In that way children can begin to learn consequences without needing the cognitive skill necessary to understand their motivations.

Beginning around the age of 5 and continuing until somewhere between the ages of 7 and 9, children come to believe that inner feelings are the same ones that are expressed outside. What is expressed is what is felt. This is why it is difficult to get 6 year old Billy to act positively toward Auntie Susan who always pinches Billy's cheek (and he hates this) when she arrives for her visits. Average 6 year olds do not realize that they can hide their inner feelings. This ability begins to develop around the age of 7, but may not be fully developed until the age of 10. Like the 4 year old who hit someone should learn not to hit, the 6 year old can and should be taught that rudeness will have serious negative consequences. Children may not understand that they can hide their feelings but they can learn that being polite has rewards and being rude results in punishment. This should not mitigate the fact that someone should speak with Aunt Susan and let her know that what *she* is doing is not welcomed by Billy.

Between the ages of 10 to 12, children begin to recognize that they can put their feelings aside and express something other than what they are feeling. Finally, in the early to mid teen years the child comes to realize that some feelings can be hidden even from oneself. To try and work on unconscious motivation with a preadolescent is developmentally inappropriate.

> For many clinicians, an important therapeutic task is to aid the child in understanding the motivations underlying his or her behavior. Selman's formulation implies that it is not until...somewhere between the ages of 10 and 13 that the child has the cognitive capacity to engage in the type of self-awareness typically associated with insight therapy (Harter, 1983, p. 108).

CHILD SEXUAL DEVELOPMENT

An understanding of this aspect of development is crucial in assessments involving the child who is considered to have been sexually abused. In our work with children it is important to respond as therapeutically as possible. We need to be aware of our own attitudes and what we are comfortable with. When I talk about normal sexual development, I am referring to the context of a broad cultural scene and the kinds of development and behaviours that can be expected in "normal" children, *i.e.*, age appropriate development in children who have not been overly negatively stressed or traumatized. Within such a framework and perspective, we must remember to allow considerable flexibility in our interpretations of what we are seeing. Within any broad territorial "culture" (*e.g.* Canada, America), there will always be a wonderful mosaic of subcultures. The overall context of any broad culture strongly influences any given individual's development (sexual, social, etc.) within his or her respective culture and subculture.

History of Values Regarding Sexuality

It is important to understand the history and development of certain values which you may see in your office or classroom on a daily basis in terms of a child's sexual development. It is not uncommon in Western cultures to hold a view that sex is bad or dirty. This belief can be traced back many centuries to the writings of St. Augustine (353 - 430 C.E.), who significantly influenced Western beliefs and Christian doctrine on sexuality. Augustine went so far as to argue that women do not have souls (Cabot & Cowan, 1989, p. 59). His battles with sexual desires were described in his text entitled *Confessions*. It was Augustine who associated guilt, rather than pleasure, with sex. Following his conversion, Augustine became a leading proponent of the anti-marriage/anti-sex movement. He equated sex with sin. Since in Augustine's mind, intercourse was an act of sin by its very nature, any child conceived was sinful and baptism was, therefore, needed to wash away the sin of sexuality, the "original sin." Since the time of Augustine, lust has been declared to be the original sin of Adam and Eve. This idea of sex as sinful persists even today, toward the end of the twentieth century.

Another highly influential writer on human sexuality was St. Thomas Aquinas (1225 - 1274 C.E.) who, in *Summa Theologica*, a massive work of several volumes, outlined the Church's position on sexual and moral issues in minute and extensive detail. Aquinas was highly influenced by "natural law," believing that God created the rules of nature and, therefore, if something occurs in nature it must be good. Aquinas did not have much of an awareness of ethology and the principles of animal behaviour, or "natural law" would not have formed the basis for his views of morality. For example, since a number of species eat their own young, this is hardly a basis for establishing rules of human behaviour. Aquinas, like many other early theological writers, believed that women were inferior and weak and wrote that

> Woman is in subjection because of the laws of nature, but a slave only by circumstance.... Woman is subject to man because of the weakness of her mind as well as her body (Cabot & Cowan, 1989, p. 59).

Gratian, a Church Canon working with Aquinas, wrote that:

> Man, but not woman, is made in the image of God. It is plain from this that women should be subject to their husbands, and should be as slaves (Cabot & Cowan, 1989, p. 59).

During the Renaissance, which began in Italy in the fourteenth century and spread throughout Europe, continuing into the seventeenth century, a contradictory process developed. On the one hand, we had a blossoming and full expression of love, sex and humanness. At the same time, we had the ugly holocaust of the Inquisition under way. For an understanding of the Inquisition, the reader is referred to a stunning documentary produced by the Government of Canada's National Film Board, *The Burning Times*. The "Burning Times" refers to the execution of an estimated 9 million people, predominantly women, as witches. The political situation behind this indescribable horror is ugly but fascinating, and a reflection of the misogyny which has existed in the Western world for centuries. There were both political and economical influences underlying the development of the Inquisition. As Christianity spread, indigenous people who did not convert were accused of devil worship.

In addition, there were conflicts between traditional healers and the medical profession, a male profession. Women were the primary healers of the rural folk society. Anyone who practised medicine without a degree was considered guilty of witchcraft. Yet, women, who were the main healers of the time, were not allowed into medical school. Many women were arrested for practising medicine without a license and, despite many medical talents and skills, were declared guilty of witchcraft and burned alive (or hanged, or crushed to death with stones). It was stated that "If a woman dare to cure without having studied [in university], she is a Witch and must die" (Cabot & Cowan, 1989, p. 70).

In 1484 Pope Innocent VIII declared witchcraft heresy and instructed two Dominican monks, Kraemer and Sprenger, to publish a manual for witch hunts. The published manual would become the *Malleus Malleficarum*. The writers of the *Malleus* believed that the end of the world as we know it was approaching and would involve a desperate battle between Satan and the followers of Christ. This same viewpoint still fuels the fires of televangelists on modern television. The writings in the *Malleus* told of how female independence is evil: "When a woman thinks alone, she is evil." The same description used for witches had been previously used for Jews and Christians by previous persecutors in earlier times—the possession of horn, tail and claws, the stealing of babies for worship ceremonies, and so on (Cabot, 1989, pp. 62-63). Now these descriptions were used for women.

The witch hunts were really about sex roles, greed and power, not spirituality. Economic issues were intensely involved as a prime motivator. When someone was accused of being a witch, her property was confiscated (regardless of an eventual outcome of innocence) in order to pay for the trial, jail keeping and so on.

King James fancied himself an expert on witchcraft and the Bible was retranslated to suit and please King James. One major change was implemented to facilitate the witch hunts. *Exodus* 22:18 had previously read "Suffer not a poisoner to live" but was retranslated for King James to read "Suffer not a witch to live,"[9] thereby contributing to an estimated loss of 9 million lives. It wasn't hard to prove that a person, especially a woman, was a witch. With regard to women, all that had to be proved was that she was capable of healing. Cabot and Cowan (1989) review a 1322 trial of a woman accused of witchcraft. She was tried by the medical faculty of the University of Paris. She was found guilty because she was "wiser in the art of surgery and medicine than the greatest doctor in Paris."

During this time, no one could question authority. The teachings of the Bible were deliberately kept hidden from the masses. The Church forbade research and reading of the Bible by lay persons. The possession of the Bible written in the vernacular of the people was a crime punishable by burning at the stake. With knowledge hidden, it is much easier for authority to be absolute and to fully fit the needs of greedy oppressors (like King James).

In more modern times, Sigmund Freud held a rather dogmatic and misogynist view which has insidiously poisoned the mental health field. When his own daughter, Anna Freud, the future child analyst and ego psychology theorist, was born, Sigmund Freud sent out letters of announcement and noted that he would like to have sent a telegram had it been a boy, "but it was a girl." Need more be said about his views on women, and female children?

Values

The previous discussion may seem only vaguely related to children and work you may do with them, but that is an illusion. Such values and ideas mentioned concerning sexuality and men and women have highly influenced today's sexual attitudes. All of these views and influences still creep into the lives of many children that we see in our therapy offices, classes, sports teams, clubs and so on. Such views have deeply influenced perceptions of child sexual development and our expectations of how children should behave.

To explore some of the influences on your own sexual development, sexual attitudes and beliefs, Bridget Revell recommends the use of a drawing she calls a *Sexual Influences Pie* (unpublished exercise, 1991). This involves making a circular diagram and then drawing lines within the pie to break it into pieces. For the influence you feel had the greatest impact, use the biggest slice of pie. You can use this to visually describe and understand the many different influences that have existed on your own sexuality and sexual development. Bridget and I have used this exercise in training programs with professional therapists and have consistently found people amazed by how much they learn about themselves when they visually describe their own historical influences through this simple drawing. We have also seen a great deal of impact that first "loves," boyfriends and girlfriends have had on the developing sexuality of many individuals. This is also a very useful method with someone who may have been sexually abused in the past. The drawing helps give some perspective. Instead of viewing oneself as solely a "sexual abuse survivor," this drawing can help capture a greater fullness.

Sexual Development

With regard to the earliest development in life, we still know very little about life in the womb. Although not in abundance, there are certain good works studying life before birth, for example, *The Secret Life of the Unborn Child* (Verny, 1981). We do know that the unborn child is influenced by the outside world. I will primarily deal here with life after birth. The main thing to note is that attitudes are influenced by those closest to us and begin to develop very early, probably prior to birth, or even conception.

Very early in their development, babies learn the names of eyes, nose, mouth, fingers, toes and many other parts of the body as parents tell them these names. Children's concepts of themselves develop as they learn about their own physical selves. In a happy, loving, nurturing and affectionate setting, children will feel good about themselves and their bodies.

Despite learning the real names of many body parts, when it comes to sexuality, children tend to be given "cutesy" names rather than correct names. A nose is a nose, not a "snuffer," a "sniffer," an "air grabber" and so on. However, when is comes to penis or vulva, children get a myriad of cute names and often are not told the actual name for this part of their little bodies. This creates an unnecessarily mysterious aspect to sexuality very early in life for children. It seems that there is an assumption that "if we don't name it, they won't notice it." Some children I have worked with actually have referred to their genitals as their "mussentouch." I kid you not, I thought they were referring to some new Muppet character the first time I heard this.

It is a wise parent who gives children the names of all of their body parts and who permits babies to explore their own bodies. Such an approach promotes an increased knowledge of the world, a clear body image, a positive self concept and future positive adult sexual adjustment.

There is something unique about a child's sexual development compared to all other areas of child development. In general, as children develop, they reach new levels and complete new tasks. For example, developing children move from mother's breast to mushy foods that are fed to them, to beginning to eat with their hands and fingers, to using utensils, to eating more solid food and, finally, mastering adult techniques of dining using knife and fork, spoon and even different utensils that look similar (some of us have never reached the epitome of development—give me more than one fork or spoon and I just reach for the one that's closest, start from the outside...or was it inside...all too confusing for some of us adults!). On the other hand, with regard to sexual development, a child is simply supposed to "stop" or "give it up." They are often not presented with more mature forms of behaviour—for example, touching yourself is something that should be done in private, not in front of other people.

Genital awareness can be very confusing for young children. They have become aware of sensations that make them feel pleasure, yet adults seem to think that these penis or vulva things are not very important—"they never talk about them, don't even give them a real name, and sometimes I even get scolded for paying any kind of attention to them." This is all very confusing for young children of limited cognitive skills.

An area of great concern for many parents is children fondling their own genitals. The fact is that all young children, including infants, do a certain amount of handling or rubbing of their genitals. Caregivers, teachers, and professionals need not worry about casual, infrequent masturbation. I would only be concerned if this were practised with frequency, and to the exclusion of play with peers. Then we may be dealing with a troubled child. My concern would be if a child is using the pleasure of masturbation to ward off deep seated anxiety. However, my concern would not be with the issue of masturbation but with the underlying anxiety. Normal, non-anxious kids may masturbate because they are bored, or unhappy, or just because it feels good. In public this can be embarrassing. It is the parents' responsibility to divert their four year old before it becomes a habit.

Contrary to some popular notions, children exploring their own bodies, including genitals is not, per se, a sign of any problem. It is interesting to note that genital play will result when there has been optimal parent-infant encounters and bonding in the first year of life. Such children naturally explore themselves. Part of their explorations includes genital play. If early bonding and relationships were problematic, early genital play is much rarer and other activities tend to replace it. If infant-caregiver interaction was very poor or absent, early genital play will be completely missing. It will arise later and have more of an obsessive quality to it. So early (infant and toddler) self sexual exploration is obviously not a bad sign at all.

Another area of concern for many caregivers occurs when they see their young children using some inanimate object in what appears to be sexual activity. For example, toddlers may rub their favourite "blankeys" against their genitals when going to sleep at nap time. Again, this is not a cause for concern. This object, sometimes referred to by certain theorists as the "transitional object," seems to be used to blur a distance from the caregiver. Between about 18 and

36 months, the wee one's ego is developing. The child is becoming an individual, separate from the caregiver. The awareness of this separateness causes a certain anxiety. A sense of being alone can be terrifying to a vulnerable little child. This object may be a representative reminder of the person to whom he or she is close. Now this kind of theoretical thinking arises from theorists in a culture where children are largely deprived of early tactile and closeness needs. It would be interesting to compare the need and/or use of a transitional object from an anthropological perspective and look at cultures where there is a great deal of physical closeness with children, where they are carried everywhere by their caregivers, sleep with their caregivers and have a large amount of early physical closeness compared to cultures where children are placed in cribs, playpens, nurseries and generally deprived of a large amount of touch. We do not yet have this information.

Toilet training can cause great anxiety for many parents. The fact is that the less parental anxiety there is around toilet training and the later it is begun, the less time it takes for the child to master this skill. Children will be ready for toilet training only when they are physiologically able to control themselves. You can start whenever you bloody well please. They won't be trained until they are physically ready, no matter what you do. By the age of about two, children can begin to perceive signals of elimination, they can hang on long enough to get to the toilet, and can learn to release their sphincter muscles at will. This does not mean that toilet training should automatically be started at the age of two. Some kids learn at two, some at three. It should not be left much later, or you are probably going to have a child where nothing is ever expected of him or her. In a desire not to push children, they may be left too much on their own.

Toilet training should be started by about the age of three. Then, with relaxed guidance, children can take pride in their new accomplishment. When parents are comfortable and relaxed, body image and self-esteem can be positively influenced. This is a very big accomplishment for the child. It is not that the toilet training, in and of itself, is the biggest issue for the child. However, this is one of the earliest major developmental accomplishments and how caregivers handle this learning seems to reflect their general future approach to child rearing—relaxed, supportive and playful, or anxious, threatening and worrisome.

By the age of four, children's sense of self has expanded and they have images of their own homes and personal territories. By this age, when in groups there will tend to be a boy/girl division in teams and roles. When anxious or socially stressed, four years olds may grasp their genitals and feel the need to urinate. At this age, you may expect to hear a great deal of verbal play about elimination and hear name calling like: "you old poopoo," "you shit," or "you fart face." It's not exactly pleasant, but neither is it abnormal in any way. It's just four year old stuff. The four year old may also take an interest in other people's bathrooms and bathroom activities. Games of "show me" and other sex play between children is not uncommon for the four year old.

By about the ages of five to seven, children start to want direct and brief answers to their questions about sex. I must emphasize the words direct and brief here. They don't want to spend hours on the issue, or even minutes. They just want some of their confusion cleared up.

Their interests in sex differences may show up in the form of sex play, including the handling of each other's genitals and hospital play (in which rectal temperatures may be taken). It takes no great interpretation to realize that children who have had their temperatures taken by insertion of a thermometer up their rectum may repeat this behaviour in their own play. It certainly is not an indicator that there has been abuse. I have heard many professionals state that this is so. All I could assume from their statements was either they had no training in child development, or, perhaps, they themselves had abused children in this way so that's how they came to believe this was indicative of abuse. It is also wrong to assume that this sex play is in any way erotic. It may only be serving an educational purpose as children learn about each other's bodies. This is one reason that children may perceive adults as overreacting to this type of play. It was not serving the function or purpose that the adult beholder had assumed.

By the age of seven or eight, children become ashamed of their fears and mistakes. They become self-conscious about their own bodies and are quite sensitive about being seen in the buff. They have usually become quite modest in both their personal hygiene, dressing and toileting habits. This is a good sign of developing personal boundaries. In contradiction, at this age, during unsupervised play, the cuddling, fondling and handling of genitals of others is not uncommon.

Healthy sex education should be carried out in the home rather than in the school, playground or washroom. Children need to learn from their parents about the functioning of their bodies. They also need to learn about self respect and respect for others in their home situation. It is a sign of dismal child rearing failure in our culture when the only education of this nature children get is at school.

THE SIGNIFICANCE OF EXTREME STRESS AND TRAUMA IN DEVELOPMENT

I will not deal with prenatal influences here. Excellent material is available elsewhere on this issue (Pearce, 1977; Verny, 1981). Contrary to early psychoanalytic beliefs, the birth experience itself is a natural, not traumatic, event. Anything which disrupts the natural process may be stressful or traumatic. For example, studies show that the lack of stimulation during caesarian section births results in babies that require an increased amount of "regular concentrated periods of hugging, rocking, and stroking after birth, perhaps to replace what they missed in prebirth *hugs*" (Davis, 1991, p. 30). Please keep in mind as you read this material that there are many things that can stress a child. There are many sources of trauma. The child may have been in a car accident at the age of 6 months or 3 years. The family home may have burned down when he was two months old. A five year old may see her beloved dog run over by a car. These are all stressful, potentially traumatizing events. Unfortunately, many now deem these insignificant. We seem to have globally come to the conclusion that only the child who has been abused in some way is stressed and traumatized.

When there is extreme stress or trauma in a child's past,

> myriad small acts of protection and kindness are needed to erode a child's negative stereotype of adult caregiving from previous traumatic experiences (James, 1994, p. 73).

Regardless of the age at which the traumatic event occurred, a rebuilding of a secure world will be important. Nurturing, consistency and constancy lead to the experience of a predictable and safe environment. Early severe stress or trauma occurring in the life of a child under the age of 2 will mean that early needs will need to be met or re-met. Loving touch, holding, and positive physical contact will be important at some point of involvement with the child. It is crucial for the very young traumatized child that a stable, nurturing and protective environment be available as soon as possible after the trauma. We also know that, whatever the age at which the stress occurred, the child may appear to remain a child for considerably longer than expected. He or she may still be playing fantasy games and be involved in pretend play well into teen years. You may also find that individual or overall developmental level regresses following severe stress or trauma. For example, a six year old who was beginning to be able to draw people with round circles for bodies with armlike protruderances, but, after severe stress, goes back to drawing stick figures typical of a much earlier age.

I have been particularly fascinated by a set of drawings by a young child. He was drawing a picture of himself before and after the abuse he had suffered. In a stunning example of regression, his picture from before the abuse reflected his present art skills. However, his picture of "after the abuse" revealed severely regressed skills. The picture was entirely comprised of stick figure representations of people. So, he did not just regress following the abuse. He also regressed when dealing with the abuse in his mind. This was one of the clearest examples of trauma implicated regression I have seen in my career.

You may be working with an adolescent who was physically abused as an infant. At some point in the treatment process with this young person, he or she will need to experience positive touch. Your work may involve helping the present caregiver positively nurture this young person as if he or she was an infant. For example, perhaps at some point every day, plan for this child to have 15 minutes of completely unconditional nurturing time together with the caregiver (Theraplay activities would work well here) rubbing baby powder or baby lotion on the hands or feet of this child. The child may well benefit from many periods of cuddling on the caregivers lap.

If you know that the stress occurred between the ages of 2 and 7, you can model nurturing for the child through scenes of kindness, gentleness and nurturing play with dolls and stuffed toys, in the sandbox and in storytelling. You are using the "as if" stand-ins appropriate to the developmental level.

Children over the age of 6 and under 12 who have been severely stressed or traumatized may be more amenable to playing it out and acting it out. Nevertheless, remember to make sure resolution is built in, or you run the risk of promoting post-traumatic re-enactment.

We also know that one method that can help make up for early unmet needs is through nurturing others and acts of generosity and kindness to others. By giving, one sees that there is goodness in life. This is an excellent way for adolescents to meet old needs in a constructive manner, by giving to others: participation in peer counselling; volunteer work with animals, the elderly, the hospitalized. A great deal of healing occurs through giving rather than taking.

There is a dangerous myth that a child who has been emotionally wounded only needs love in order to recover.

> They also need limits, guidance, courage, time to heal and to accept the realities of their experience, and an enormous amount of parental patience (James, 1994, p. 199).

Ignoring or hiding from a painful past will not make it go away. It will more likely just make it harder to deal with later. This is why it is so important to help children come to terms with painful events by talking openly about them and allowing a full expression of feelings. There is another all-too-common myth that

> children's early abuse histories will fade in memory if they are allowed to forget them. Children don't just forget pain and terror. They may hide from their memories, but their behavior is often directed by unexpressed feelings. Ignoring what is known to be true about the child can lead the child to believe that her past is shameful or too overwhelming for even the adults to mention (James, 1994, p. 199).

One of the most helpful and hopeful pieces of advice for both caregivers and professionals who are working with emotionally wounded children comes from Beverly James:

Messages Children Need To Hear

You are likable.
You cannot overwhelm me.
Others have been there too.
There's hope.
You have choices.
You are needed.
You make a difference.
This is a safe place.
It's not your fault.
You are not a bad person (James, 1994, p. 200).

These messages are important to keep in mind in working with the child of severe pain and stress, trauma, and abuse. These messages are just as important in working with all children.

CULTURAL CONSIDERATIONS

In working with children, an awareness of their cultural background is crucial for a better understanding and fuller view of the child. We have to account for the effects of culture and race, racism, language, parenting patterns, socioeconomic status, sex role expectations, cultural rules, extended family and kinship bonds. The religious beliefs and even methods of entertainment—for example, musical indoctrination to a lifestyle typical of a culture—can have significant impact on the behaviour of both an individual child and his or her caregivers (Sattler, 1992). Failure to take cultural contexts into account can result in an ineffective therapeutic process.

> Studies with African-Americans (and more recently with Hispanics and Native Americans) have found cultural mistrust to explain high dropout rates from counselling with white clinicians, lower expectations for the counselling process, and lower performance on intelligence tests (Terrell & Terrell, 1981, cited in Garcia Coll & Meyer, 1993, p. 65).

All comments I am making here in this section on cultural considerations must be taken as very cautious generalizations, and we need to remain alert to the fact that there is considerable variation within any given culture. An excellent assessment tool for exploring and helping to understand the issues from the family's perspective, regardless of culture, is to ask the family the following kinds of questions:

1. What do you think has caused your child's problem?
2. Why do you think it started when it did?
3. What do you think the problem does to your child? How does it work?
4. How severe is your child's problem? Do you expect that it will have a short- or long-term course?
5. What kind of treatment do you think your child should receive?
6. What are the most important results that you hope to have your child receive from intervention?
7. What are the main things that the problem has caused for you and your child?
8. What do you fear most about your child's problem? (Kleinman, Eisenberg, & Good, 1978, cited in Garcia Coll & Meyer, 1993, p. 63).

This kind of questioning allows the family perspective to emerge and be shared. It also gives a great deal of information on family expectations about the healing process and outcome.

It is generally accepted by play therapists that play therapy can have benefits for most children. Despite this professional belief, cultural issues may override this consideration.

> Recommendations for play therapy, or for working with parents to facilitate parent-infant play interactions, may be...regarded as inappropriate by some cultural groups...because these are roles relegated traditionally to siblings, other children, and occasionally grandparents (Rogoff, 1990, cited in Garcia Coll & Meyer, 1993, p. 64).

I think it needs to be acknowledged that it is a possibility that play therapy is not for all children. It is definitely not appropriate to impose the values of the play therapy field on those who do not wish to share such values.

If play therapy is culturally appropriate, it may be necessary to adapt methods in order to take culture into account. For example, in traditional Hispanic-American culture, it is preferred to solve emotional conflicts within a family context. As well, the pride of the family may make it difficult to engage the family in any kind of mental health service (Sattler, 1992, p. 584). In such situations, it might be wise to make use of *cuento therapy* which

> incorporates the traditional Puerto Rican medium of telling folk tales that serves to transmit cultural values, to foster pride in Puerto Rican heritage, and to reinforce adaptive behavior. These folk tales have been adapted to convey the knowledge, values, and skills useful in coping with the demands of being raised in inner-city neighbourhoods. The medium of telling folk tales to address problems of childhood may represent a more culturally familiar and acceptable treatment approach for serving Puerto Rican children and their families (Garcia Coll & Meyer, 1993, p. 64).

Considering the importance of storytelling in many cultures, this may be a useful approach that can be used in more situations than just those therapeutic encounters involving Puerto Rican children and families. I can see an adaptation of this approach being invaluable with: Irish Celtic culture where the role of the storyteller is revered; Black culture where verbal abilities are highly prized, and; Native culture. There is an interesting adaptation of this within a Native community in southern Ontario in Canada. Ganohkwa Sra[10] has published books by Sandra Montour that are designed to help children understand the dynamics of sexual abuse from a traditional Native perspective. *Eagle Child* illustrates how two Native children come to their own understanding of sexual abuse under the guidance of their wise and loving grandmother (Montour, 1992, p. 3).

Regardless of culture, there are some similarities in child development. In all cultures, the child rearing trends within the culture are thought to be for the benefit of children. Children in all cultures show consistent tendencies in certain areas of development, for example, the development of communication skills, cognitive, intellectual and social skills. Furthermore, all children form primary attachments, although the expression of affection as well as how much separation or closeness is valued may differ between cultures (Sattler, 1993). Finally, "gender differences seem to be universal. Boys and girls tend to be treated, responded to, and socialized differently" (Garcia Coll & Meyer, 1993, p. 59).

I will now focus on three specific cultures: Celtic, Native American and Black American. I believe that each of these is seriously misunderstood by many medical and mental health professionals. Each is remarkably similar in beliefs and in healing traditions and practices. Due to living it and being most familiar with it, my examination of Celtic Culture will be most detailed.

IRISH CULTURE/CELTIC HEALING

In most articles or texts on culture, ethnicity and therapy, there is a complete absence of any reference whatsoever to Celtic culture and influences. For some reason, this culture is completely ignored.[11] This is particularly peculiar given the significant impact of the Irish Celtic culture on Western contemporary habits and beliefs (O'Driscoll, 1981). In Canada, in some parts of the province of Newfoundland or the area of Cape Breton, there are residents whose first language or only language is Gaelic. Millions of the inhabitants of North America have an Irish (or Scot or Welsh) Celtic heritage. During the famine known as The Great Hunger in the late 1840s, while an estimated two and a half million people died, another two million emigrated from Ireland to North America in a four year period alone. Throughout my travels, in most cities I visit, I find a fairly large Celtic population, Celtic specialty shops, festivals, architecture and music clubs. From Orlando to Boston, St. Louis to New York, and Kentucky to California there are Celtic influences.

In training programs around North America, I have occasionally presented a workshop on *Holistic Healing from a Celtic Perspective* as part of an International Child Therapy Seminar Series presented by the Canadian Play Therapy Institute. Although a number of the exercises I present in this workshop are quite adaptable to our work with children, the presentation is not specifically geared toward child therapy. At the beginning of this workshop I always try to be very clear about this and ask participants what brought them to the program. Most are exploring their own Irish, Scottish or Welsh cultural heritage or, if not, they are interested in Celtic beliefs. Many are on their own spiritual quest. It is a wonderful discovery to find how many people are looking to this path as a route for themselves. I will present here an overview of Celtic beliefs as they impact on healing processes. As there are a number of texts covering Celtic history itself (Bonwick, 1986 [originally published 1894]; Sharkey, 1979; O'Driscoll, 1981; Condren, 1989; Matthews, 1991; O hOgain, 1991), it will not be discussed here.

What I say about Irish culture fits many Earth oriented cultures, especially those where both water and agriculture play an important role in the economy. As well, there are striking parallels between the patterns of Celtic tribal life and healing methods and those of Native Americans (Cowan, 1993) and Black Americans. Following the workshop that I present on Celtic healing, I am often approached by Native healers who tell me that the healing processes of our respective cultures are almost identical. The endurance and wandering spirit of the Celts is another aspect of the culture that resembles certain Native cultures, such as the Hopi. Similarly, after a training program on play therapy (in which I made reference to traditional Celtic healing) in Lexington, Kentucky, I was approached by a psychologist[12] who shared with me her sense of how both modern as well as traditional ancient African practices and an Afrocentric world view correspond closely to the Celtic view. Two dear friends, David Shah from India and Soraya Yavari from Sweden but of Persian descent, each tell me our world views and the healing processes and rituals of each of our cultures overlap far more than they differ. I think what we are discovering, as various Earth and nature oriented cultures and aboriginal peoples of their respective lands come together, is that we all walk on the same path.

Celtic culture considers spirituality, nature and healing to be inseparable.[13] The use of plants, stones and herbs are an essential part of Celtic healing. Celtic healers, mystics, bards, Druids and priestesses, poets, and artists are all connected by

> solid spiritual values that have remained constant over the centuries. That rich strain of mysticism, which the Romans labelled superstition, was in fact the backbone of Celtic spirituality. It is also the philosophical basis for shamanism, a feature that makes the Celt, ancient or modern, a prime candidate for shamanic experiences.... There was probably never a time, nor will there ever be, when the true Celt does not believe in the unseen Otherworld and the possibility of journeying there to discover the mysteries of the divine universe (Cowan, 1993, p. 7).

There are similarities between Celtic beliefs and certain Eastern views concerning the transmigration of souls. The soul is considered to be imperishable and undergoes transmigration – passing from one being to another upon death (or passing into certain animal guides during shamanic states). Celestial beings aid us in development. "Ultimately all will be happy and evil finally extinguished" (Bonwick, 1986, p. 63). In fact, the belief in transmigration is so much a part of Ireland that it "has led some to assert their conviction that Buddhist missionaries conveyed it" (Bonwick, 1986, p. 67).

Nature and all of her reflections are considered sacred to the Celt. This does not mean that nature is directly worshipped. It is believed that there is one Divine Spirit. There are five sacred elements – Earth, Air, Fire, Water, and the Heavens (Bonwick, 1986, p. 63) – Air provides an entry point to the land of the spiritual. Fog and mist open the door to the Otherworld. Water, and wells that tap this element are essential. The sea gives the Celt food. Rivers bring food and water and are reference points for travel.

> Rivers were a crucial source of life throughout the Celtic world.... Sacred temples were often situated near these sources of life, and this was certainly the case with Brugh na Boinne, the present day Newgrange, in the Boyne Valley (Condren, 1989, p. 26)

A central feature of many holy sites was the never ending fire. For example, a

> central feature of the monastery of Kildare [Brigit was historically associated with the foundation of a convent of nuns in Kildare] was the preservation of the sacred fire (Condren, 1989, p. 66).

This site of Kildare was an ancient sacred Druid fire location prior to becoming a convent. Bonwick (1986) notes that the ancient lighting of fires was attended with solemn ceremonies and how these are similar in other cultures, particularly Native American and Persian. It is also believed that the Divine can be found and related to in trees, forests, bushes. To spend time with the Divine Creator was as simple a task as going into the forest. Even in our modern age, trees are revered by the Celt. A 1995 recording by the Celtic musician Enya is entitled *In Memory of Trees*.

To the Irish, and to Celts from many other nations,

> this world and the world we go to after death are not far apart.... Indeed there are times when the worlds are so near together that it seems as if our earthly chattels were no more than the shadows of things beyond. A lady I knew once saw a village child running about with a long trailing petticoat upon her, asked the creature why she did not have it cut short. 'It was my grandmother's,' said the child; 'would you have her going about yonder with her petticoat up to her knees, and she dead but four days?' (Yeats, 1893, p. 86)

It may be that, in spite of our modern interest in a holistic focus and our rediscovered understanding of the importance of bodymind connections and even the beginnings of a spiritual emphasis, we are still children of our modern age of rationalism, and

> feel more comfortable 'explaining' [spiritual phenomena] in psychological terms (archetypes, collective unconscious, the active imagination) rather than in the older framework of spirits and spirit world. But in so doing we are underestimating [the experience and ourselves] (Cowan, 1993, p. 27).

To the Irish Celt, the Divine is omnipresent and we are all intimately connected with the Divine. All is one. This is evident in much Irish poetry such as Amergin's[14] incantation:

> I am a wind on the sea,
> I am a wave of the ocean,
> I am the roar of the sea,
> I am a powerful ox,
> I am a hawk on the cliff,
> I am a dewdrop in the sunshine,
> I am a boar for valour,
> I am a salmon in the pools,
> I am a lake in a plain,
> I am the strength of art
>
> (cited in O'Driscoll, 1981, p. 207).

The Celtic knot is very descriptive of the culture. In the knot's intertwining spirals, all is connected with no apparent beginning or end—a perpetual continuity and a connectedness. This describes the "web of life" concept that is so important in Celtic healing processes. Through a full and dedicated participation in nature's flow of life, we heal. When we become a part of the forest, a piece of the Earth, a drop of water, and we give ourselves up to the Divine omnipresence, we tap the wisdom of the forces of healing and magic.[15] The knot, the spirals, and the intertwined snake all typify the cycle of life of the Celt. Belief in the permanence of life have been evident in Celtic culture as far back as it has been studied. The

> most outstanding stone temples in Malta and at Newgrange in Ireland, with their giant spiral capstones and corbelled stone roofing, were built over five thousand years ago.... However, their symbols are unmistakable. The curving loops of the great spiral show the journey of the soul moving through death to find rest and rebirth (Sharkey, 1979, p. 78)

For those with a Celtic heritage, the Otherworld, the world of spirit and Divine presence, is always close to ordinary consciousness and could appear at any time—while walking the dog, lighting a candle, planting a garden. This nonordinary reality, in Celtic terms, is often represented as a fire in the head. This fire is a "source of enlightenment, illuminating visions of other realities. The shamanic journey begins and ends in the mind" (Cowan, 1993, p. 8). A belief in fairies, the "little people" and spiritual guests is not an indication of mental illness but an indication of a deeply spiritual culture.

> To the Celtic peoples, magic was as common as breathing. It was not something set aside for special occasions anymore than was their beautiful twisting artwork. Like their intricate designs that decorated even ordinary utensils, magic was a part of everyday life (Conway, 1990, p. 5).

Life at the Edge: Betwixt and Between

To the Celt, places of change or transition hold an enchanting and mystical appeal. It is felt that at such places exists wisdom. Such a place might be a sea shore, the edge of a lake, a riverbank, where plains turn to mountains, a full moon, the new moon, a solstice, an equinox, dawn, twilight, a bridge, the entrance to a church, the entrance to anything, doorways between rooms, windows.

> The area where different worlds meet, such as the act of dying, the mist between sea and air...the shore at the river-ford, was of special significance for the Celts (Sharkey, 1979, p. 20).

Any such situation where differences or opposites meet holds magic in the Celtic imagination, and

> the Celts had no difficulty reconciling materialism and spiritual insight because they clearly understood that each is present in the other, that matter is only solidified spirit (Conway, 1990, p. 5).

Even modern physicists seem to be arriving at the same conclusion.

The Web of Life

It is a Celtic belief that the human soul, the human being, the potato, the tree in the forest, the water in the ocean, the dew on the grass, the bee in the hive, the bat in the darkness, the faeries in the world between the worlds, the pebbles on the beach, the air we breath, the fire in the fireplace which warms us and the cotton in the shirt that I wear are derived from the same source, Divine energy. Nature, the soul, human beings, the spirit are all one. Even in modern times

> the Web of Life has been preserved. If both God and the human soul are to be found in the ocean, a lake, a flame, a spark of light, the Celtic mind [is] still viewing creation from a shamanic perspective (Cowan, 1993, p. 45).

The Creator and the creation are one. Thus, all life is sacred. The entire universe is filled with life, the Divine is accessible to each of us and we are each responsible for the well-being of the natural world around us.

> W.B. Yeats maintained that this single energy, and the great memory of nature herself, could be evoked by symbols. The

> greatest symbols of the ancient sacred tradition of magic and religion in western Europe are the mysterious megalithic monuments (Sharkey, 1979, p. 24).

Over a number of centuries, with the advancement of so-called civilization, the beauty and wonders of nature came to be considered dirty, evil, something which must be conquered, even destroyed. The magic has slowly been abandoned from our lives, the passion displaced. Now, many exist as if they are separate from nature. Yet there is always a yearning; the desire for a hamster, a canary, a cat or dog, a few plants in the house, maybe a fireplace. The yearning tugs at us. It pulls us back. We can never completely separate from nature. Cowan (1993) says that the world was disenchanted over the centuries. But it can never become completely distant from us. Nature leaves us with nagging doubts, the desire for an enigmatic "more" when we are too far from our source, from the Creator.

> We seem to have lost the ability to even imagine a culture that lives by the belief that human consciousness can participate in the natural world and that the natural world responds to the will of human consciousness.... Celtic belief nurtures an intensely magical, mystical life with nature, grounding their work in the community (Cowan, 1993, pp. 118-119).

Celtic Culture and Healing

There is a time and a sacred place for healing. It may be a concrete reality, such as a clearing in the forest, or it may simply be a creation in one's mind. Each time I, as a healer, cross over into the healing place I sense (imagine, if you will) that I am entering sacred space. This may be with a young child entering an office, or it may be with a loved one entering a healing place in the forest. In either situation a sense of the sacred is projected from the mind onto the environment and the mind and nature become entwined, like a medical doctor's healing symbol of the entwined snakes.

In the Celtic worldview humans have an intimate relationship with nature and all its unseen forces. There are many of a Celtic background who believe in fairies, but it is unlikely many, or any, of them will be admitting this in a clinician's office. "Many people still have the fairy-faith but do not wish to invite ridicule by talking about it" (Leslie Shepard, in the *Foreword* to Evans-Wentz, 1966, p. xiii). For example, it is believed that at the Celtic new year—a time betwixt and between two years—the entrance to the fairy world "would open for a time and it would be possible to walk again with the loved ones and, in some cases, lead them to safety" (Condren, 1989, p. 52). It is believed in Celtic culture that as long as one is in balance with nature, if we are in "harmony with this unseen fairy-world in the background of nature, all [will be] well" (Evans-Wentz, 1996, p. 278).

In Celtic healing, nature and natural cycles are of the utmost importance. Sacred are the trees and forests, wells, rivers and water in all its forms, stones, and fire. These are all considered to be potential sources of deep healing. Animals may act as spirit guides. The healing process involves being in tune with nature and the earth, with the rhythms of life and the natural world. It also involves being in touch with the Otherworld, and the world between the worlds.

> Perhaps more than any other people, the Celts have always cherished the country of their true home – the Otherworld [which] in Celtic myth is an inscape of or overlap upon the land. It has its special gateways or crossing-places but it is not conceived of a being "up or out there." Rather it is contiguous with every part of life (Matthews, 1989, pp. 63, 8).

In terms of active healing processes, the daily and monthly cycles would be more important than the seasonal cycles, which were largely oriented to the world of work, not healing. The healer is not one who uses words (like the modern therapist). The respected healer is one who is in tune with nature, nature's gifts and cycles, and who is in touch with the spiritual. To be a Celtic healer means to be able to live between the worlds. To be effective in a healing process with a person of Celtic heritage means to get out of the head and into the heart and soul. It means entering and connecting the realms of earth and angels.

FIRST NATIONS/NATIVE CULTURE

It is necessary to keep in mind in working with any First Nations child that each subculture's primary identification and influence is with and from its particular group. The many different tribes/groups are not homogenous and should not be treated as such.

> You must learn about the history and traditions of the particular [North] American Indian community that you are serving if you are to achieve success" (Sattler, 1993, p. 587).

Despite the idiosyncratic history and traditions of individual groups, there are some common values to consider in clinical work with members of the different First Nations communities.

Across different Native American groups, whether it be Navajo, Hopi, Iroquois or Cree, there is a general desire to live as part of a natural flow in harmony with the natural world. Controlling nature is an absurd concept in First Nations' thinking. One lives with power by working with nature, not by trying to have power over nature.

There is a fairly consistent desire to follow in "the old ways," respecting the wisdom of the elders and honouring ancestors who have gone before. This value of the importance of the family as noted in the respecting of the "old ones" is also reflected in the high value given to the extended family. The extended family, childhood and old age are given great importance. In many training programs I have been involved in with First Nations healers, I have been touched by the closeness of the extended family unit. In some exercises we look at where one goes to heal, where one goes to feel nurtured, how one has fun. So many times the healing journey of First Nations healers involves connecting with "my grandmother," "my mother," "my uncle," "my father," "my great grandmother," "my brother." The wisdom of relating to the family as a healing process in and of itself cannot be overemphasized.

The concept of time is oriented in the present. The future is not of great concern in the here and now. This is related to the existence of a nonlinear time sense.

> Like others living in close harmony with nature, the Native person has an intuitive, personal and flexible concept of time.... The Native people developed the concept of "doing things when the time is right"—that is, when the whole array of environmental factors converge to ensure success. The concept remains in play today [but now] seems less a principle for living with nature and

> more of a manifestation of the need for harmonious interpersonal relationships.... Given the universality of the concept of time in Native society, Native people never seem to be inconvenienced or annoyed if social functions and other meetings start hours after the scheduled time" (Brant, 1990, p. 536).

An important factor in Native lifestyle is the principle and practice of non-interference. This principle

> promotes positive interpersonal relations by discouraging coercion of any kind, be it physical, verbal, or psychological.... A high degree of respect for every human being's independence leads the Native to view instructing, coercing or attempting to persuade another person as undesirable behaviour (Brant, 1990, p. 535).

This can cause considerable conflict and confusion in intercultural relations with the wider Western society. An example involves school attendance. I was consulting with a school board where there was a great deal of absenteeism by Native children. Teachers, school social workers and other personnel were gritting their teeth in frustration about this situation. There was obviously also a clear resentment toward the children's parents. I heard comments from staff like: "The parents are no help, they're just as bad as the kids," and "What's the use, the parents aren't going to make them come to school no matter what we do. They can't be relied on for support." There is great disrespect in these statements. What has happened here is that the principle of non-interference is at play.

> It is one of the most widely accepted principles of behaviour among Native people. It even extends to adult relationships with children and manifests itself as permissiveness. A Native child may be allowed at the age of six, for example, to make the decision on whether or not he goes to school even though he is required to do so by law.... Native parents will be reluctant to force the child into doing anything he does not choose to do (Brant, 1990, p. 535).

I tried to phrase my response to the school board staff in a way that was respectful, but what was really needed was to make school attractive and interesting enough to make the child want to attend. If the child feels respected, the educational material is interesting and fun to learn, and the child sees benefits from attending, then you will not have absenteeism. In working with any culture it is essential to build on the culture's traditions. For example, something that has been used with great success is to incorporate classes in the Native language, classes on history of the Native culture, and activities that draw from the culture's beliefs, traditions and celebrations. With this approach, you will have low absenteeism. I suspect that a great many more Natives know who Stan Jonathan[16] or Ted Nolan[17] are than who the fourth prime minister of Canada or 7th president of the United States was.

In working with a Native child, there are two other factors that can cause misunderstandings with the dominant White culture. These both involve the Native approach to showing approval and methods of teaching. If one is expecting a parade of thanks for one's work with a Native child, you are in the wrong field. Approval is not likely to be given. Gratitude is not seen as important. It is assumed that "the intrinsic reward of doing the deed itself is considered sufficient" (Brant, 1990, p. 537). I know of many non-Natives who have gone in to work with Native children or in a Native community and constantly sensed that they had a thankless job and felt ignored, unnecessary, and rejected because no one ever thanked them for the work they did. The message they inferred may not in any way have been the one the community was feeling.

Two issues that may arise from this lack of showing approval may be the Native child's difficulty in accepting any praise, and a reluctance to try anything new.

> Native people have a great deal of difficulty accepting praise, reward and reinforcement. Native children who are praised by their teachers will often deliberately do something to reverse the teacher's opinion the next day (Brant, 1990, p. 537).

This even applies where the praise was quite warranted. Children do not want to stand out from their peers nor "embarrass their peers who have not done as well" (Brant, 1990, p. 537). Excellence is expected at all times. Because of this they "generally are reluctant to try new things [and they] experience a great deal of performance anxiety about making mistakes" (Brant, 1990, p. 537).

A last comment on a unique feature of Native culture involves methods of teaching. The dominant learning models of the world today are based on lectures, the passing on of knowledge, and, basically, telling someone how to do things the right way and rewarding them for doing it the right way. This does not fit many traditional and earth oriented cultures. It is definitely out of place in working with Native children. In Native culture

> one is shown how rather than told how.... The teacher does not purport to know more than his student, but through his actions conveys useful and practical information which the student then has a choice of adopting or rejecting. The student is never placed on the spot and required to perform before he has been adequately trained. This reduces his performance anxiety and increases his loyalty to his teachers, who usually are parents and older members of his extended family. Modelling seems to increase attachment to the older members of the group, promoting group cohesiveness and continuity (Brant, 1990, p. 537).

In other words, what you want the child to know and learn, you must show. This obviously will necessitate an extremely high level of integrity and patience on the part of teachers. This method of teaching applies to a Native child in school and to a Native adult learning any kind of skill. Extended lectures only show disrespect. What you wish to convey must be shown, lived. A Native therapist's best learning will occur through watching another therapist, by role playing and by experiential *exploration*, not from listening to the "Psychology 101" professor talk *about* the way to do things. A Native child will learn by seeing and feeling. For example, classes on self esteem and self respect will be in vain if the teacher "teaching" about these issues does not express esteem and respect for the culture with which he or she is working. This respect demands an understanding of the dynamics of the culture.

Native Culture and Healing

The process of all healing in Native Cultures, whether it is physical, emotional or spiritual healing, involves a return to balance — with Nature, with spiritual forces with the most important factor

> in Medicine [being] the importance of balancing the human being as he should be governed by the laws of nature...in order to keep

> peace of mind, one must keep balance with nature. The minute we become out of balance with nature, we are in trouble! Even if you live in a large city, you can still keep somewhat in balance with nature. You can know what foods are best for you. You can know how much sleep you need, and how you can best adjust to your individual cycles... (Steiger, 1975, p. 197).

Clinical approaches will have to be adapted in working with this culture. It may be considered quite rude, or even incompetent, to be asked direct questions by a clinician. Self-disclosure by the clinician or other interviewer will model that it is acceptable and even desirable to share aspects of oneself.

In clinical work with Native children or families, there are important cultural considerations. Communication styles are significantly different from the predominant culture. Things like eye contact, a firm handshake, and direct questioning may be a sign of sincerity to the clinician unaccustomed to First Nations culture. Unfortunately, these very behaviours may be perceived as very rude, or even incompetent, by the First Nations culture with which you are working (Sattler, 1992). Everett, Proctor & Cartmell (1983) note that Native American children may approach non-Native clinicians with apprehension. They are likely to be more sensitive to a clinician's non-verbal behaviour than the average child in the general culture. It is recommended that sincerity and patience will be of the utmost importance in working with First Nations children.

Silence, something that can drive many clinicians nuts, may be a place of solace for the Native child. Intuition and spirituality are highly valued in Native culture and both may be completely misunderstood or, worse, discounted by many clinicians.

> Both play therapy and parent counselling tend to stress linear logic in organizing and discussing behavior and interactions. Some other cultures, such as those of American Indians, value intuitive and holistic approaches, often placing much more emphasis on the spiritual components of human existence. The play therapist may become frustrated with the caretakers' and child's apparent inability to focus on the particulars of an event, while the caretakers and child are confused by the therapist's seemingly endless preoccupation with insignificant details (O'Connor, 1991, p. 53).

I would argue that far too many therapists really **are** preoccupied with insignificant details and have no conception of magic, intuition, spirituality, or the holistic. I think it is also a sad comment on the field of play therapy when those in the field do not see a need, or even the potential, for it to operate within a holistic model that can have an emphasis on spirituality.

The spirituality evident in Native healing processes includes:

> The vision quest and the emphasis on spiritual discipline through a minimalist approach to the self. Through the vision quest come the wisdom of body and soul.
>
> A belief in the essence of the Divine presence in everything. This results in a deep reverence and a passion for the Earth Mother. Each living thing is considered to be a part of the web of life and humans have a responsibility toward all plant and animal life.
>
> A total commitment to one's beliefs that pervades every aspect of one's life and enables one truly to walk in balance (Steiger, 1975, p. 13).

When our activities help the Native child focus on a return to balance, then we are in the healing realm with them. All children need our respect and understanding of their uniqueness. The Native child is no different from any other child in this respect. Once we are able to comprehend the unique features of the culture, then we can truly *be* with the child.

BLACK CULTURE

There may be significant cultural differences between Black culture in the United States, Black culture in Canada, and elsewhere in the world. The historical roots of each culture differ drastically. Many people of Black heritage entered Canada through different regions of Ontario and points further east as part of the "underground railroad." Canada was the door to freedom from slavery. Thus, a different Black subculture originally developed than in the United States where the dominant culture remained the oppressor rather than the liberator, or at least an illusion of a liberator. Today, on a larger scale, there is so much geographic movement that this historical influence has decreased considerably. Worldwide, Black culture has less opportunity than White culture. Black culture in North America has had to be very adaptive to survive (Sattler, 1992). The culture has endured generations of slavery, then oppression and humiliation.

Many Black Americans have cultural traditions that are founded upon and reflect or are influenced by those found in traditional African societies. The core of ancient African and the Afrocentric world view include: spirituality, harmony, balance, interconnectedness, authenticity, and cultural awareness (Phillips, 1990, p. 56).

Spirituality in Black culture implies a Divine influence in life's issues. It means that there is a belief that appeals to the Divine will be heard. It is considered proper and noble to govern oneself with the knowledge that a power transcending the human exerts power and influence in our everyday lives. Something, some greater power, is always at play in our lives and it is wise to always maintain a relationship with this Divine essence.

Harmony implies a certain oblivion, a blending. An individual does not stand out from the environmental background. Rather, it is seen as important to blend in with the whole. Linked to all his or her surroundings, an individual gains a sense of safety and belonging. The aspect of harmony involves a spiritual connection.

> The overriding focus of life and, indeed the goal of the mentally healthy person, is to be in harmony with the forces of life.... When we are harmonious, we are "at peace" (Phillips, 1990, p. 57).

A further reflection of this view relates to the concept of balance. Life is perceived, much like the oriental view, as a "dynamic process of energy fields and forces" (Philips, 1990, p. 57). An important process in one's life is the balancing of these forces, with the end result being wholeness. This whole concept of balance also ties in with Black community values as healthy Black behaviour is seen as

> being in harmony with the authentic needs and social priorities of the African community, i.e., towards it affirmation, enhancement, survival, positive development, and fulfilment of its potential as a community (Philips, 1990, p. 57).

An example of culturally appropriate healing can be seen in NTU psychotherapy. NTU (a Bantu concept referring to a Divine-like unifying force of existence) focuses on spirituality, with the therapy process being viewed as both spiritual and sacred. The task of therapy is twofold. The therapist must have integrity and live within the principles professed. The therapist works with the client to allow natural healing forces to emerge. In other words, the therapist acts as a catalyst.

Life being a dynamic interweaving process, movement, rhythm, and the cycles of life are vital. Respect for this view is seen in the high value placed on music and movement. Both are forms of a

> rhythmic orientation toward life.... Music and dancing are ways of engaging life itself that are life-sustaining media, vital to one's psychological health (Boykin, 1983 cited in Sattler, 1992, p. 581).

Also indicative of a high respect for nature and natural rhythms of life is the value placed on orality by Black culture. Like the Native American and the Celt, Black African culture had an oral approach to both history and traditions. The elders responsible for maintaining this knowledge were revered members of the society.

> The value of orality is maintained in Black American culture today. Being able to rap, sound, or run it down is a prized oral skill. This holds not just for the street culture, but for every level of Black culture (Sattler, 1992, p. 582).

This is seen throughout Black culture in verbal routines, song, preaching, ritual insults, jokes, and storytelling.

Given the status given to orality, there is an important educational and clinical issue which arises. Many children from an African influenced culture speak a dialect of English best described as Black English. Such a dialect has its own set of highly developed rules and usages. In a classroom, therapy, or testing situation, children who speak Black English may have come to feel that they are

> inadequate and inferior to other children who speak standard English.... You should recognize that those children who can speak both Black English and standard English have a highly developed bilingual skill (Sattler, 1992, p. 582).

Professionals who work with West Indian families would be wise to develop their chatting skills. It is quite polite and expected to engage in social chatter prior to getting down to the business at hand. Children of West Indian families, especially those newly arrived to North America, are expected to have a deep respect for both neighbours and authority figures. Part of this respect means avoidance of direct eye contact. This can be misperceived by the dominant culture, one which highly values direct eye contact, as indicative of evasiveness, fearfulness, or guilt.

> Children who have recently arrived from the West Indies, acting out of customary good manners, may not speak up in class discussions or in conversations with professionals. Unless children are asked direct questions, and shown, through kind attention, that it is permissable to speak, they may remain silent (Glasgow & Adaskin, 1990, p. 226),

and this may be misinterpreted as ignorance, lack of intelligence or passivity. A professional working with such a child may develop a completely erroneous picture of the child simply due to a lack of understanding of the culture's values.

Black Culture and Healing

Healing in Black culture involves being in tune with the flow of life on earth and in heaven. A friend, Rose, from the Caribbean Islands, spoke with me at length about the healing practices from within her culture. Like other cultures that honour nature and natural cycles, Afro influenced cultures have healing methods that depend on a positive relationship with the earth.

> When we would play as children and someone didn't feel well, we caught a flu or cold and were all stuffed up, there was no running off to the doctor. My mum took good care of us. Sure, if the regular stuff wasn't working, then she would make sure we saw a doctor, but I can hardly remember a time when that was necessary. The first thing mum would do was pick some leaves. Picking some leaves was most important. She'd grind them up and give us some liquid to make us better. Now I remember it didn't all taste that good. But it did always seem to make us better pretty quick.

Obviously, herbal preparations came first. Rose describes it as more than just the plants at work: "It's not just the plants. The timing is so important. It's important to do things to respect nature, to keep in tune with natural cycles." She described how the planting and harvesting of substances used in healing were done at prescribed times according to different natural cycles.

There is also a time for cleansing, purifying—physically, spiritually. At the end of each season and beginning of another, a person would be cleansed, ready for the next cycle in the natural flow of the year. If one is not in touch with the natural flow, healing of any sort, be it physical or emotional, will be hampered.

Without an awareness of the spiritual nature of life, there is no healing. The traditional healing practices include an awareness, respect and acknowledgement of the role of the Divine in all healing. Physical, emotional, and spiritual healing are not separate. They are reflections of different sides of the same process.

> Religion has always been central to West Indians [and most people of Afro heritage]. In the difficult times of slavery, and even now, religion has provided an avenue for optimism, hope for the future, and a means of social control to protect the society (Glasgow & Adaskin, 1990, p. 216).

Many professionals of Afro heritage in the healing professions are very aware of the need for balance and being in tune with nature and of acknowledging the role of the Divine in everyday life. Like the person from a Celtic background, many have learned to keep certain ideas quiet, private from the scornful eyes of the rational world. But the healing works more quickly if we are not fighting against our own natural tendencies. The healer in Black Culture is intensely aware of this.

POLITICAL CONSIDERATIONS

On the political front, there is much to be done with regard to the well-being of children. For example, we can push for stringent and enforced handgun safety.[18] It seems clear that if every handgun in every community was properly locked and stored, and handled safely when not stored, there would be few, if any, suicides,[19] murders, or accidents involving handguns. The same applies to proper handling of rifles and shotguns. Taking the issue further, maybe we should give up destructive sports. Is it really that important for our culture to ensure that members of our society have the right to kill other species for sport (please be clear that this is a comment on killing for "fun"—killing simply for the sake of killing. It is not a comment on respectful hunting for food, clothing, and so on)? The films *Planet of the Apes* and *Beneath the Planet of the Apes* (and some of the sequels), although at times silly, were very relevant and meaningful social commentaries in the 1970s and have just as valid a point going into the turn of the century as they did in their own era.

We can help provide our children with a better world by recycling all we can; by walking or biking instead of driving; by walking up stairs instead of taking an elevator. Each of these acts is a political statement that has impact on our environment. In our own immediate environment we can make a difference. I know that The Canadian Play Therapy Institute, on more than one occasion, has been encouraged to change its advertising methods and go to glossy paper or heavier grade paper for its professional brochures and advertising flyers in order to have stronger commercial impact and first impression impact on potential consumers of their services. However, this would mean the Institute would be using a product that is less easily recycled and recyclable. Thus, this approach has been rejected. Perhaps there is some cost to the organization, maybe even a great cost. However, in the long run, there would be a far greater negative environmental impact if they changed their advertising and went with the "glossy" approach.

You can work to make your own home and office recycle in the optimum range. Anyone with a house and yard who is not fully recycling kitchen and garden waste is essentially raping the Earth. They are making the political statement that the environment doesn't count.

There are reprehensible and horrible national and international situations such as the nation of France conducting nuclear testing in the Pacific. This was a profane act against all nature. Likewise, China's weapons testing off the coast of Taiwan or U.S. missile testing over Canada are powerful metaphoric rapes.

Vote with your feet and wallet. Make political statements through consumer preferences. As a way of protesting the nuclear testing by France, I refused to buy any product made in France. It was important to make sure letters went to the French government and the makers of products. This adds considerable impact to the behavioral statement being made in avoiding such products. Two million people making such statements could seriously and positively alter the future for our children in terms of the environment in which they will be living.

Working in a garden and planting a potato plant or a tree outdoors has an impact on the lives of children. First, it gets you working outdoors with your child. Second, instead of sitting indoors using up electric energy by having the television or audio system on, you are providing cleaner air outdoors by planting a tree or plant, each of which serve to filter pollutants from the environment. When you spend time with a child in nature, it models a belief that nature is important.

> The conventional belief that "man" is separate from nature – that we were created to be masters, not caretakers, of the earth and are therefore given license to do as we please with what the father-god has given us, has left us with a legacy of acid rain, dwindling groundwater, and the extinction of species every day. Honoring the earth is not simply a romantic thing to do – it is our children's survival (Carson, 1989, p. 173).

In Ontario, Canada, as in many other areas of the world, there are considerable government funding cutbacks going on as we approach the end of the century. I am yet to be convinced that this is a bad thing. There is far too much government involvement in our lives and far too much individual dependence on government. This is especially true in Canada, where through about five decades of more and more socialist style governments, the population has been increasingly spoon fed. Now, recently, in some of the economically richer provinces such as Alberta and Ontario, there has been an awakening to the fact that there is not an endless pit of money going around to dish out left, right, and centre. Many programs are being eliminated. Some of these are valuable programs. My concern about a lot of the criticism about cutbacks is that people forget how much individuals have to give. Do we always have to rely on "government?" In reality, the so-called public service is a terribly wasteful enterprise that is serviced by the public pocket.

I was speaking with some people recently and they were

ranting and raving about government cutbacks and doing the "ain't it awful?" routine. I asked them what they were personally doing to make the world a better place. First, they didn't even know what I was talking about, but when I expanded on my question and stated that perhaps we can't rely on some ambiguous big-brother government to do all the care-giving and caretaking in society and perhaps, if every individual who proposed to care socially about the world around them personally expended a significant amount of effort in volunteer work and charitable giving, we wouldn't need any government support.

Probably needless to say, these individuals were not participating in any community volunteer work, they were not tithing any of their own income (10% given to worthy causes is not an unreasonable expectation of a socially responsible individual), they were not committed to any child caring of their own and really had no excuse for their complaining when not actively participating at a personal level. If you care about your world, stop whining about government, and contribute a significant portion of your own energy to some volunteer endeavour. There are certainly enough worthy causes—positive religious organizations, wildlife organizations, humane societies, Meals On Wheels, hospitals, Big Brothers/Big Sisters, War Amps, nursing homes. Skip a movie or a sports event and give the money to a worthwhile cause. Go out and give.

Footnotes

[1] I am not critiquing legitimate research that examines biological influences and environmental influences. We need this information. The foolishness to which I am referring is in the day to day misapplication of this kind of information.

[2] The word treatment arises from the medical model of therapy and I simply cannot accept it. It implies an illness, a pathology. Its use grew directly from a Freudian psychoanalytic approach. Such an approach belongs in the historical curiosity pile.

[3] To his credit, Jung largely accepted that psychotherapy was "merely a new name for the cure of souls" (Szasz, 1988, p. 172). This

critique of Jung is not meant to take away from some important philosophical contributions of Jung's pioneering efforts in the mental health field. However, we must keep in mind that philosophical contributions are not identical to scientific or clinical contributions. Two important philosophical contributions of Jung were his emphasis on the importance of spirituality in the life of humans and his understanding of "the metaphorical nature of mental illnesses and mental treatments" (Szasz, 1988, p. 171).

4 I use the phrase "dual working parents" here. However, the research overwhelmingly relates to "working mothers." I take great exception to the lack of consideration for the importance of fathers and other extended family members.

5 I have previously noted the negative Montessori view toward the inner world and fantasy life of a child. Such a cognitive approach can certainly be critiqued based on this research as well. Clearly the research indicates that a cognitive approach to child care and education is predictive of an elevated level of aggression.

6 Along these same lines, I do not think that "insanity," an "abusive past," and so on should ever be an excuse for present behaviour. This belief needs to be applied in courtrooms throughout the world. "Sorry you had a bad past, bud, but it's not an excuse for hurting someone else in the present. Welcome to prison/the electric chair. End of discussion." I heard a funny, and very astute, monologue by a stand-up comedian that went, "some of these idiots want to use insanity as an excuse for hurting children, raping, and so on. It wasn't their fault, they didn't know what they were doing. Well, tell them the electric chair is just a ride, strap them in and pull the switch. If they don't know what's happening, they won't know it's not really a ride" (apologies, comic's name unknown).

7 An all-important consideration here is that you must determine, before recommending any touching activities, that the

caregiver is not potentially someone about whom you need to be concerned with regard to personal boundary issues and sexual abuse of the child. You do not want to be encouraging a potentially exploitive touch relationship with the child.

[8] In a tantrum the child is raging at the world. It is a reflection that things are not flowing well. There is a battle going on. This may sound like just another bizarre psychoanalytic concept, but the suggestions have not come from the psychoanalytic field. They have arisen from the field of anthropology.

[9] In some translations it reads "Suffer not a sorceress to live." In an interesting patriarchal twist, men were considered to be sorcerers who performed sorcery. Women were sorceresses or witches who practised magic, and magic was considered evil. What was the difference between magic and sorcery?—only the sex of the practitioner. It was an attempt to eliminate women healers.

[10] Ganohkwa Sra is taken from the Cayuga language and means "love among us." It is the name for the family violence program in the Ohsweken community because "it is a goal we seek for all families, and it is through love among us that we, as a community, can put an end to family violence" (from a statement provided by Ganohkwa Sra).

[11] Perhaps we are still suffering the remnants of the penal laws of England which attempted (literally) to create a situation where the Irish did not exist. The penal laws stated: "Only Irish Catholics are subject to these laws.... Education of Irish children is forbidden by law.... Use of the Irish language is forbidden.... None are qualified to own or lease land.... All are excluded from official stations, without exception..." (O'Toole, 1990, p. 8). The penal laws of England as applied to the Irish go on and on, but the previous should give some clear idea of the intense oppression of a culture. Further, during the Great Famine of 1845-1849, Sir Charles Edward Trevalyan, who despised Ireland and the Irish, was placed in complete charge of the Irish relief fund. The result was "the appalling fact that

during the four years of the Great Hunger, 25 million pounds sterling worth of wheat and beef were **exported from Ireland to England**.... In Ireland today there is a saying, *If Trevelyan is in Heaven it is an infallible proof of the infinite mercy of God*" (O'Toole, 1990, p. 8). It is time to start paying due respect to some of the greatest healers, philosophers, writers and artists the modern world has known. In this section on cultural considerations I mention the Celts out of respect and honour to my own heritage and out of respect to those so terribly wronged not so long ago. The world is largely unaware of this holocaust, as the Irish Celt is a survivor of incredible endurance who simply gets on with bringing joy and laughter to the world and living a life of passionate involvement with the world around him or her.

[12] My thanks to Dr. Betty Smith Brown, the psychologist who approached me, for her kind consideration in making available to me the article *NTU Psychotherapy: An Afrocentric Approach* by Dr. Frederick Phillips.

[13] Many authors and patriarchal historians consider the Celtic races to have been very war-like. However, it has been noted that "by the time Celtic societies are recorded in history, hostile patriarchal states had arisen around them, the most powerful being the Roman Empire. Like earlier Goddess peoples, the Celts were pressured into adopting organized warfare, proving the old adage that if you have to fight a bear, you will grow claws" (Cabot & Cowan, 1989, p. 41).

[14] Amergin was the chief bard of the Milesians, who, legend tells, invaded Ireland and, according to the *Book of Invasions*, battled the Tuatha De Danann. Milesian beliefs continue "to haunt the Celtic imagination" (Cowan, 1993, p. 28) in a positive way, I must add.

[15] Keep in mind I do not place any "occult" or esoteric overtones on the word magic. There is nothing "supernatural" in magic. Magic implies being in touch with nature and being able to alter consciousness and life processes by understanding natural processes.

[16] Stan Jonathan was a Native hockey player on the Boston Bruins in the 1960s. He was noted for his small size and big spirit and heart.

[17] Ted Nolan is the coach of the Buffalo Sabres NHL hockey team. He is a Native Indian from Northern Ontario.

[18] I do not support highly restrictive legislation. This is a political hot potato. It is questionable whether restrictive control does anything to prevent violence in society. What is needed is early intervention and prevention in the lives of children. In the long term, we need to work towards the creation a society that abhors violence rather than one, like the present, that worships it. In our present milieu, what is needed is careful handling of guns. We need mandatory safety courses for anyone wishing the privilege of purchasing or owning a firearm. On the other hand, restrictive registration is a frightening political tool. A prime manipulation of a fascist police state is gun "control." One political leader was quite aware of that: "This year will go down in history, for the first time, a civilized nation has full gun registration! Our streets will be safer, our police more efficient, and the world will follow our lead into the future!" (Adolph Hitler, 1935). Today, many political leaders who want to score points in the public eye start whining about gun control. They need to stop the rhetoric about gun control and start putting funding into social and educational early intervention programs.

[19] Contrary to a public opinion, most firearms deaths are not murders, they are suicides. In fact, 80% or more of firearms deaths are suicides (Minister of Justice and Attorney General of Canada, 1994, p. 2-1).

CHAPTER 7

Puppets

Puppets are wonderful and natural tools to use in working with children. In fact, they are one of the most useful tools in playful therapy or just simple playful contact with children, adolescents, adults, and families. Puppets can be found to be an extremely effective method for getting at material deep in the psyche. In their day to day use, they serve many different functions: regression; projection; modelling boundaries, and; an intermediate step toward increased verbal communication.

REGRESSION

Puppets have quite an ability to take us back to an earlier developmental stage. There were some very interesting first hand situations demonstrating this in my own home recently. In the training programs that the Canadian Play Therapy Institute holds throughout

North America, they have a display involving large numbers of hand puppets and full body puppets. One summer's day, a large shipment of these "creatures" had arrived in my own home. The result was a living room full of cuddly, soft, fluffy "beings" sitting around. Late in the afternoon, my teenage son, Rory, arrived home with his friend Andy. I was in the den at the far end of the house. I heard them carrying on and, basically, they were pretending to hold up the house in a robbery. Andy's voice deepened as he loudly said, "alright, everybody down on the floor, this is a stickup. Nobody move, this is a stickup. Give us your money. Nobody move." At that point, they walked into the living room and the faked deep voices suddenly took on a high pitch and, instant regression, "oooooo, look at the bunny wabbiiiits!" Now we would really be making social progress if full body puppets could be used in preventing real robberies.

Interestingly, not half an hour later, my older teenage daughter, Erin, and three friends arrived home. The two young men and two young women entered the house being very "cool" and "like, that new CD by Nirvana is like, really like, truly digital, and like it is so like rad" and so on...until they hit the living room and it was an exact repeat of the previous scenario. Down went the male voices as they saw the puppets first – "oooooo, bunnies, cool!!!" – and suddenly I had a house full of 6 year olds instead of teenagers.

Now, I must be honest about the final outcome of all of this. Within half an hour they were still playing with the bunnies, but the voices were again deeper and the bunnies were flailing their heads up and down singing "We're Nirvana, we're Nirvana" (for those of you not familiar with the context here, Nirvana is the grunge band from Seattle. Kurt Colbain, their lead singer, was the "superstar" who committed suicide in 1994. The band is noted for passion and intensity, to put it mildly).

PROJECTION

It can be difficult and feel treacherously vulnerable for young children to express their feelings directly to an adult authority figure. Far less threatening is the expression of issues through use of a puppet. I might ask a child how he or she is feeling and not get any real response. Maybe the child is shy or maybe it is just too scary to say "I'm really scared. Mummy and Daddy have been fighting a lot lately and making lots of noise at night yelling at each other."

On the other hand, asking the child how "bunny" feels today, may indirectly and safely lead to the real issues weighing on a child's heart. Perhaps I hear that bunny is scared at home because his mummy and daddy fight a lot. Although it is not safe to assume literal interpretation of what the puppet says or direct representation of the child's life, it should cause you to reflect on the relationship, literal or symbolic, between the puppet's expression and the child's life.

If the child expressed that bunny is scared because his mummy and daddy have been fighting, rather than directly say to the child: "That sounds an awful lot like what's been going on at your house." I would rather explore the issue in more depth indirectly. I want to know what "bunny" needs when he feels scared. Who can help when bunny feels scared? What other things make "bunny" feel scared? The way a session might be processed follows:

Therapist (holding a puppet): Holly, have you ever met my friend?

Holly: (whispers) No.

Therapist (Facing Holly): Well Holly, this is Jerome, my bunny friend.

Therapist (Turning and facing the puppet): Jerome, this is Holly. She comes to visit me every week. When she was real little, the judge at court decided that Holly needed a really good home where she would be safe all the time. So she went to live in a new home. She still lives there with her new mummy and daddy. Sometimes, she needs someone to play with and talk with about things that are bugging her and giving her very strong feelings. You will probably see her coming into the play room every week.

Therapist (Again facing Holly): Holly, what do you think Jerome is feeling today?

Holly: He's feeling scared.

Therapist: I wonder what's making him feel scared.

Holly: His mummy and daddy fight at night.

At this point you may be tempted to say something like: "Has that happened to you lately?" However, I think it is too soon and defeats the use of the puppet. Keep exploring the issue through the puppet, rather than bringing it back to the child too soon:

Therapist: What does Jerome do when mummy and daddy fight?

Holly: Sometimes he cries. (This statement is followed by a long silence as the therapist says nothing but just sits with Holly.) Sometimes he hides under his covers in bed.

Therapist: What might help Jerome when he feels that way?

Holly: I don't know, maybe he could sleep over at a friend's house.

Therapist: What do you think Jerome needs when he feels scared?

Holly: He needs somebody to talk to.

A little further into the conversation, it may be appropriate to bring the issue directly to Holly.

Therapist: Holly, can you think of a time when you ever felt scared?

I think that taking the conversation directly to the issue of Holly's home on the previous night is too much of an intrusion and too directive. For example, I would never say to the child: "Were your own mummy and daddy fighting last night?" Better to always go safely around the issue, circling it, until the child is able to handle the strong feelings that are entwined with the issue. If Holly next said, "Yeah, last night when my own mummy and daddy were fighting," then you are given that material by the child and it would be very appropriate to deal with it.

Note that in the above example the therapist is talking to Holly about how the puppet, Jerome, is feeling. It is assumed that Holly is simply projecting her issues onto Jerome. An alternate way of doing this that is even less direct would be to ask Holly to talk for Jerome and to hold Jerome. Then the therapist is talking to the puppet. There is no eye contact between the therapist and Holly. The therapist speaks to and looks directly at Jerome. By using the puppet, some space and distance are built in for the child. This serves as a safety valve and prevents you from forcing things directly onto the child which he or she may not be able to handle at the moment.

A clear example of the process of projection came while listening to a colleague, Cindy Taylor, several years ago. It was in the middle of a Canadian winter and Cindy had just returned to work after a relaxing southern vacation in the warmth and sun. The first appointment she had upon her return was with a seven year old girl, Mandy. Cindy looked quite relaxed and refreshed following her vacation. I heard the two of them chatting as they walked up the stairs near my office. Despite how relaxed Cindy looked, I heard the little girl:

Mandy: Do you ever look tired.

Therapist: Why might I be tired?

Mandy: You might have been up all night.

Therapist: Why might I have been up all night?

Mandy: Your mummy and daddy might have been fighting.

Therapist: Has that happened to you lately?

Mandy: (begins to lightly sob) Last night.

That was the last thing I heard before Cindy's office door closed, but it certainly proved to highlight the issue of projection. Cindy could have ended the meaningful conversation very quickly had she initially said, in response to the comment of looking tired: “No, I've just returned from vacation and I'm feeling great.” Stop, end of conversation, no doors opened. Handling it as she did took her into the realm of the child's world. The therapist could also intervene immediately (and too quickly) by saying: “No, I'm not tired. But I am wondering if you are tired.” To this, Mandy is just as likely to have said “No.” Time to explore must be built into such processing. Therapy should not be rushed or treated like a head-on collision.

This discussion on the process of projection should in no way be used to imply support for “projective techniques” as described in the section entitled "Major Flaws in Our Present Work" in *Chapter 3*. In this present discussion I am referring to a process where we follow children's play to get at their issues. This differs radically from taking children's play and interpreting it, analyzing it, and dissecting it while assuming we can discover hidden issues based on our interpretations.

MODELLING

Puppets can be used to model behaviours and boundaries. You may be holding a big cuddly full body puppet while sitting with a child. The child is likely going to take an interest in the puppet. You could say to the child: “Would you like to hold the puppet?” Before the child can reach out, you could next say: “Just a sec, let's ask bunny if it's okay if you touch him.” You can then turn to the puppet on your hand and say: “Bunny, is it okay if Suzie holds you?” Now, you as the therapist may know exactly what bunny is going to do, but that is irrelevant here. The point is to acknowledge the right to personal space. So, the bunny nods yes. The child can then hold or touch the bunny. An interesting twist here: the child is now holding the puppet while you, the therapist, are asking questions. You are in an ideal position to explore the child's inner world. It is often possible for a child to speak while using a puppet when he or she is otherwise finding the expression of something too difficult.

In using puppets, it is important to consider the developmental stage of the child. For example, with preschoolers, puppets are best used as a general aid to communication. I have heard some people who think that this is the best age with which to use puppets therapeutically, but that is not the case at all. In fact, their main use with the preschooler is as an aid to facilitate communication. To try and develop intricate stories or puppet tales with the young child is a misunderstanding of child development. The preschooler is too easily threatened by anxiety and doesn't have the same kind of ego defenses and psychological protection that an older child or adult would. When an issue is tapped which provokes any kind of anxiety in younger children, they are likely to resort to silliness or a distracting and increased motor activity level. This does not mean that we should not be using puppets with the preschooler. This is a population where puppets may be the only way to get beyond resistance. Simply be aware that we should not expect more than is realistic given the developmental stage of the child.

On the other hand, older school aged children have more resources and an ability to tolerate both ambiguity and anxiety provoking situations. Their use of puppets is more complex and more revealing of their own inner psychological processes. Storytelling with puppets is ideal with this age group.

APPROACHES TO THE USE OF PUPPETS

In working with children through puppets I suggest you not distance yourself from the process. There are a number of different approaches to puppetry with the older child:

Adult/Therapist Holds the Puppet. In this method, the therapist talks to the child indirectly via the puppet, which the therapist holds. Make sure that the puppet is not dangling off to the side while you look the child in the eyes and talk. It is supposed to be the puppet talking here, not direct communication from the therapist. If you aren't going to use the puppet, don't bother putting it on your hand. This is one of the areas where people beginning to work with puppets have trouble. They put the puppet on and then act as if it isn't there. Let it become real. If you have trouble not being the one to look at the child, hold the puppet in front of your face as you talk with the child so the child can't even see you. They only see the puppet. This is a good way of getting over the tendency to want to maintain eye contact.

Child Uses Puppet. The child holds the puppet and the therapist is talking directly to the puppet. Again, like when the adult or therapist uses the puppet, a problem with this method is that I have seen many situations where the therapist is actually looking at the child or looking into the eyes of the child rather than at the puppet. The puppet is just kind of there with no apparent purpose. In this case, why bother using the puppet? Make sure if the child is using the puppet that you look at the puppet, not at the child.

Both Child and Therapist Use Puppets to Communicate. Here, the real fun (and hard work) begins. In this arrangement you give the child real safety. Not only is the child not confronted directly, but there is no direct interaction between anyone but two puppets. This puts the child in a very safe position. He or she is likely to feel far less vulnerable than when forced to directly address personal problems. The puppets hold the conversations and deal with issues. There are many different kinds of conversations and questions which can be developed using the puppets.

Puppet as the Participant. Children who are reluctant to do some exercise or who seems particularly anxious may be able to use the puppet for an exercise. For example, rather than drawing a picture of how they feel, they can have a puppet on their hand and the puppet can hold the crayon and do the drawing exercise. The puppet can answer questions about feelings and issues.

Puppet Shows. In puppet shows the child gets to create as much as possible—the stage, the background scenery, the characters of the puppets. I have seen many very well equipped settings that I could only long for. On the other hand, such settings with wonderful wooden puppet stages, curtains on the stage, elaborate puppets and so on, take away from the child's ability to become part of the creation. I believe it is more in the child's interest to do as much of the creation as possible. To boost self esteem, children should be encouraged to accomplish as much as possible with regard to their own creations. Help them by providing cardboard boxes, fabric, paints, crayons, glue and other creative arts supplies. Work with them to help create the stage, the scenery and so on. The older the child, the less you should be helping. In designing and performing puppet shows, you allow children to be artistically creative, as well as giving them a forum for dealing with their own internal conflicts and issues.

YOUR PUPPET COLLECTION

There are many views on the kinds and numbers of puppets you "need" in order to be doing puppetry with children. I try and remain flexible with regard to such details. I have worked in a situation where I forgot to have my puppets with me on a certain day, so I used a marker and painted a face between my thumb and fingers and used my hand as the puppet. That is probably a rather minimalist approach. I have also used a legal sized business envelope as a puppet when no puppets appeared to be available. Simply put your thumb inside one end of the envelope and your fingers at the other end. Fold the envelope in half, and now you have a puppet with a very large mouth. You can colour in the mouth, nose, eyes, and children can really make this a part of themselves, as it is completely their own creation. Another way of creating puppets with minimal supplies is to use old socks as the puppet. You can sew or glue on the eyes, ears, mouth, hair, nose and other special features. The truth is that you don't need a huge budget in order to be doing puppetry with those with whom you work. I realize manufacturers and distributors may not want you to believe that, but they are not necessarily working in your clients' best interests.

If you are determined to have a large collection of puppets I would recommend certain types to include in your collection:

Full Body Puppets. There are, at times, concerns about the message children get when they are given the visual image of an adult's hand up the rear end of a puppet. In general, I am not too concerned about this, as I tend to use many hand puppets. If I know the child has been abused I am likely to be careful and will probably want to give safe and clear images. I would like either use a hand puppet where the child clearly sees my hand and the giraffe's head is simply the puppet on my hand, or use a full body puppet where my hand goes in the back of the puppet or in its head. The puppet then sits on my other arm. I would probably not be using a puppet where my hand appears to be going up the "rear end" of the puppet when I know the child has been sexually abused.

Cuddlies. Always, some soft and cuddly, fluffy looking bears and cute animals can create a soothing image in your office. I have a couple of big fluffy full body bunny and teddy bear puppets. I also have a little cute teddy bear in red overalls.

Sillies. Try and have some goofy or silly looking hand puppets. I have a giraffe, a crocodile, a wolf and horse hand puppets. I also have two bizarre and completely off-the-wall looking creatures. They can say all kinds of goofy things at times.

Magic. A wizard, a witch, a dragon, unicorn and other symbols of magic from the fantasy world.

Popular Trends. I usually have a few that younger children will find familiar and these seem to depend on commercial marketing of the day. The ones I use are not nasty or macho in any way. Things like Beethoven (the dog), Barney (the dinosaur), maybe Bert and Ernie or Kermit, Winnie the Pooh, and other non-aggressive popular characters.

Protective Shells. I always include things that have shells to hide in my collection. The interesting thing about things that have shells to hide in is that they often go really slow, too. I'm thinking of turtles and snails specifically. These can be very representative of the healing process in general. When the stresses are too great, one can withdraw for a while and one certainly never moves along too quickly.

A WORD OF CAUTION

Never have the puppet make teasing or degrading comments or comments you would not want to make directly to the child. Many adults, puppeteers, and therapists think that if they are using the puppet to say something negative to the child it will not be as threatening as if they said it themselves. The truth is that it may have an even greater impact since the child may have felt much safer with the puppet and opened up to the personality of the puppet. This is a serious clinical error I have seen made in work with children. Do not make this error. You can only hurt children (or adults) using such an approach.

CHAPTER 8

Dreams and Storytelling

DREAMS

Dreams are wonderful tools for working with children, adolescents and adults. With children, dreams become enchanting storytelling tools. Adolescents love the mystery and mystique that appear to surround dreams. Adults find the dreamworld to be a fascinating path to discovering secrets and treasure about themselves. Through the dream, we can enter the inner world of the person who comes to us. Now there is much dogmatic mumbo-jumbo about dreams out there, especially from the Jung cult and Freud cult, but that should not negate the importance of dreams.

Whether the dream itself actually means something or not is another whole issue, one that is irrelevant to the concept of working with a child's dreams. Frankly, who cares? The truth is that I don't even care if a child really had a dream. If a certain child hadn't, I might say: "Suppose you had a dream. What would it have been?" Is this dreamwork or storytelling? Probably a little of each.

Through the exploration of a dream we can find out about a person's wishes, hopes, dreams, and fears. Never should we sit and interpret the dream of another. If dreams are ever to be interpreted, the interpretation should come from the dreamer, not from someone on the outside imposing an external symbolic framework. Many believe that a dream is a self-portrait, a reflection of the dreamer and his or her own inner world. Whether this is true or not, I do know that the interpretation of a dream is a reflection of the interpreter. For that reason, dreamers should interpret their own dreams. Some of the most up-to-date research on dreams seems to be pointing to the fact that the deep symbolic meaning of dreams "is constructed by our waking minds after the dream, not by some dreaming unconscious beforehand" (*Psychology Today Staff*, 1995, p. 62). Even Freud noted that "Sometimes a cigar is just a cigar," giving rise to the thought that perhaps he was much wiser than many of his dogmatic followers.

Suppose dreams turn out to be nothing more than psychic farts, to paraphrase Stephen King: then what? Do we abandon all dreamwork whatsoever? No, I think these things called dreams serve many purposes. Whether they are reflections of the unconscious or simply conscious recounting of psychic discharges does not matter. They still provide catalytic material which can be a tool for greater personal understanding in waking life. If they are nothing more than simple fodder for storytelling, we must remember that there are few more valuable tools than storytelling.

The notion of interpreting or analyzing someone else's unconscious or creative material is very dangerous. As healers, therapists and other professionals, we can at best be guides to others on a search for meaning.

In working with dreams I prefer to look on it as a form of play—we are playing with sleeping images. I realize the description used throughout the literature is "dreamwork," but somehow "dreamplay" seems more descriptive. I realize that there are those who think play is not serious and involves no commitment. However, those who think that in fact know nothing of play, or children, or the child inside each of us. Play is a very intense way of experiencing things which might otherwise be too overwhelming or too frightening.

In dreamwork, do not take any one dream out of context from overall trends. The importance of any particular dream (or sandbox scene, drawing, and so on) should not be blown out of proportion. Themes and messages emerge over time. Our disposable, consumer oriented culture—and many therapists reflect the culture—is in too much of a hurry for a quick answer and a quick fix. But healing doesn't come in a quick fix. The unconscious doesn't respond to our desires for quick answers. We are not computers and we cannot upgrade our computer 386 hard-drive soul for a 486 hard-drive soul to make things churn out faster.

We need to observe, and participate in, the process of our dreams over time to gain greater personal wisdom and access to inner resources. On any given night, messages and themes emerge from our dreams (or our conscious interpretation of dreams), should we take time to listen to them. As mentioned earlier in reference to symbolism and metaphor, I do not believe in a cutesy "dictionary" of symbols. Given my earlier suggestion to avoid reliance on a preconceived set of symbolic meanings, it may come as a surprise to find that I do rely on my interpretations of the work of others. However, in examining the inner material of those with whom we work, it is important to keep as open a mind as possible. Gain as wide a knowledge base as possible from many cultures concerning their symbols and sacred meanings. There will come times in exploring dreams and the symbolic representations of others with whom you work when the person will not appear able to connect with any personal symbolic meanings. At that point only, I may offer some ideas on possible meanings behind some of the symbols. This will be based on information from many sources of symbolism: fairy tales; other cultures besides my own Canadian and Irish background; traditional folk tales and stories, and; sacred documents.

Here is one example of drawing on other cultures in helping to understand a dream. A woman with whom I was working on her dreams in therapy had a horrific background of past abuse by her father as well as present self inflicted abuse. She was ultra-critical of herself and physically self-abusive. She would punish herself by beating her legs with a hammer to the point of severe bruising and bleeding. She had a dream that made absolutely no sense to her. In her waking life, she was amidst a process involving giving up old pieces of her life, symbolically burying them, and beginning anew a life involving self-respect and self-care and care for others. The immediate world around her, especially family, still treated her as she was in the past. Despite her immediate environment not recognizing the changes, she was already a new person, a reborn person. The dream she had was almost an exact parallel translation of a certain portion of the *Egyptian Book of the Dead*. To simplify it, the dream outlined the process of her own life, how part of her had died, had gone to the underworld with the assistance of Anubis, the guide, and been transformed and reborn. After we discussed the dream I talked to her about the text of the *Egyptian Book of the Dead* which seemed to parallel her dream. She was amazed with the accuracy[1] of comparison between the two. It enabled her to see that, despite comments from those around her in her immediate family, she was on the right path and really had begun a new life.

I'm not suggesting everyone should have a copy of every sacred document of the world, or that everyone go out and read the *Egyptian Book of the Dead*. What I am saying is that the more you can tap knowledge from other cultures, the greater your understanding of symbolism and metaphors that arise from the unconscious of others.

I have suggested that having checklists of symbols and dreams and the like is downright dangerous, if not outrightly abusive to the person with whom you are working. I am referring here to the kinds of books and checklists such as those found in many bookshops and having titles such as *Your Dreams Interpreted*, *1000 Dreams Interpreted*, *10,000 Dreams Interpreted*, *The Meaning of Symbols*, and so on. There is nothing wrong with those books as fun, fictional items. The problem comes if someone treats them as more than just something with which you can have fun at a party and perhaps to tease your friends with. If we start altering our lives based on the interpretations of others, then great danger and damage awaits. If you are interested in the meanings of symbols throughout the ages and in many cultures there are two good resources to refer to. Both are books by Barbara Walker, who approaches this area with great respect and openness. The two texts are called *The Woman's Encyclopedia of Myths and Secrets* and *A Woman's Dictionary of Symbols*. Drawing from a wealth of knowledge from the fields of archaeology, theology and anthropology, in these extensive documents Walker looks at customs, legends, word origins, superstitions and symbols from many cultures. Each book is a highly recommended, well-researched reference that would be a positive addition to any library collection. My main critique of these documents are the titles, which seem to imply that men have no right to or interest in this kind of information.

The method of writing down one's dreams works only with the literate. If a child (or adult) is unable to write, then this method is obviously of no use. I have used this method with adults and adolescents, but never with children. It does seem to help adolescents or adults remember the basic flow of the dream and it also maintains their interest. It has been argued that it is very important to write down dreams since we begin to filter and change the content immediately. In other words, if the dream is not written down, the dream told to a therapist several hours or days later may be different from the "actual" dream. This is simple enough to prove. Simply write down your dream upon waking, and then recall it again several hours or days later and again write it down. When the two are compared you will often find very different stories. I have a sense, however, that writing down the dream and locking it into an inanimate form potentially kills the process. "Writing down the dream takes the heart, the guts, the emotions out of the dream, and renders it a distant intellectual product" (Langs, 1988, p. 101). The many layers of exploration of the dream become lost in a superficial, cognitive, exact recounting. It is like the difference between telling a story and reading a story. You will have to decide for yourself how you wish to handle dreams. What I have found is that sometimes it can be useful for the person with whom I have worked to write down the dream, especially early in the therapeutic process, when having something to do in the form of writing helps to relieve the very anxiety about being "in therapy." Other times it is more useful to tell a story later based on what is remembered from the dream. It is unwise to have rigid rules about how to process dreams. The only rule is no rules.

In general, I would much prefer a person's recollection in the present over a cognitive referencing to a past notated diary. What I have found over the years is that therapy can very quickly turn into a content session with the client or patient bringing in a duly and self-indulgently recorded dream that we jointly "explore." But the exploring can all too often be somewhat distant. It's like we are sitting aloof of this dream, looking at it from a distance, poking it, prodding it, safely not feeling anything because it's over there somewhere. It's recalled in our head and not felt in the heart and soul. It becomes an externalized thing being analyzed.

A woman with whom I worked had a very scary dream of a light bulb chasing her. I asked her to reexperience the light.... I asked her to close her eyes, enter a sacred place inside herself and let the dream image appear. The light came and she did indeed look slightly distressed. She reported seeing the light and it did cause her anxiety.

I asked her to approach the light. As she approached it, the light turned to a raging fire. She said she saw herself lying down and being healed by the intensity of the fire. She was quiet for some time and then slowly opened her eyes and said, "I think I've been scared of my own raging creative energy inside, which I have been ignoring and trying to pretend isn't there, making it insignificant, kind of like turning a fire into a light bulb. But the thing was so terribly frightening because a light bulb is not supposed to have that much energy."

It is important in the processing of any dream images to remember that simple awareness is merely an exercise in indulgence and without action can only lead to frustration. The wisdom we gain from our inner healer must be applied to our day to day life.

The dream I was talking about above was explored further with Alexandra.... Once Alex returned to the symbolic image, I had her focus on it and I asked her to nod when she felt she knew the fire and had a relationship with it.... I then said "Alex, allow yourself to see the fire. See yourself having a relationship with that energy... where does that energy wish to go, what would it like to do?...now come back and let's see how you can be true to yourself on that path ...." The integration of Alex's symbolic dream messages needed to be applied to her daily life or simply be lost in a process of increasing frustration. I worked with her on a process of "how can you allow the fire to exist today, tomorrow? How can you nurture it?" "Is there a part of you or anyone the fire would like to make warm?" Questions along these lines maintain the integrity of the owner's symbol. This kind of processing cuts down the possibility of it being the therapist's "stuff" that is being dealt with rather than the person who has entered the therapeutic relationship with the notion of being "helped." The dreamer is never told what his or her symbol means. How can anyone but the dreamer know its meaning? To pretend to understand what symbols mean for someone else is a very degrading approach. I cannot know what fire in the dream above means for the dreamer. I know what fire means for me. Fire is healing, soothing, mesmerizing. I have spent many long hours in front of a fireplace as part of a healing and renewal process. If I am feeling at my wit's end, completely exhausted physically, emotionally or spiritually, I know that lighting the fireplace and lying in front of it, staring at it, will bring me perspective, it will allow me to feel a calmness. Now suppose I imposed this view on everyone. Suppose I started to assume that fire meant the same thing for everyone. How much help am I going to be to the little boy whose house burned down around him and both his parents died in a fire when he was 6 years old? We need to find out from those who enter the therapy process with us what the nature of their symbolic communication means by exploring it with them, not interpreting it or analyzing it.

In this particular session above, Alex was not asked to become the fire. That is a Gestalt approach and can be quite useful, but it was not the approach used. You may choose to take that approach in exercises that follow or in your work. I asked Alex to see the fire, to feel it. She did have the option on her own to become the fire, but was not directed that way. This was a new kind of dream for her and I did not wish to tell her how to experience her own unconscious but I was guiding her in the development of a relationship with it. Although I am using an example here of an adult woman with whom I worked, the same approach works very well with any age group.

This dreamwork approach is also different from visualization in that the images which arise from within the client are used, rather than images given. It is a different—not better or worse—just a different, approach. It can be very useful if a client tends to always look to you for answers. A guide does not provide answers but simply points out key pathways, markers and possibilities.

As a healer, the best I can give to someone is a question, not an answer. I can point to doors, I cannot walk through them for the person. I can only make suggestions. In the example with Alex, I could suggest that it might be useful for her to look at where she feels fire in her life and where she feels a lack. In making suggestions it is important to follow the dreamer's lead as much as possible and "go with the energy." If individuals go on at great length with much animation positively or negatively about some part of their dreams, or pictures, or sandboxes, it is probably worth exploring that aspect with them.

In the integration to daily life we apply some gift from the unconscious to our life and personality. We acknowledge a message from ourselves to ourselves. To do this we can create small, awe inspiring ceremonies to recognize the things we have learned through our inner world exploration. We can also use our inspiration from the unconscious to bring us closer to those we love.

STORYTELLING

Storytelling is one of the most caring tools to be used with a child. Just sitting and reading a story to child says "I care enough about you to spend this time with you."

Therapeutic use of stories is a wide open arena, restricted only by your own creativity. There are many ways to use stories. If children are really sad, with poor self-images and feel there is no positive future for them, then perhaps you could read *The Ugly Duckling* to them. This story is a very appropriate metaphor for such a child. *The Velveteen Rabbit* is another beautiful story for any child or adult. It also serves as a metaphor for "realness" and integrity.

Or, you may be running a group which seems "stuck" or caught on an endless plateau. You could unlock the next door for them through a "Once Upon A Time" playful method involving storytelling. I like to end some training programs with this method for certain reasons. First, using a method such as this often leads to considerable laughter from within the group. Laughter, in and of itself, is healing. Humour has very beneficial physiological and psychological effects. Second, the guidelines for this method create a scenario where, when it is an individual's turn, he or she has a great deal of power and can control the course of history for the story. However, it is also reality oriented, for there are some imposed rules which mean one does not have total control over the world. Here's how it goes. I start the story with "Once upon a time there was a seed...." The group continues the story. One person from the group is needed as a note taker to record the story which evolves. After I say the "Once upon a time," then the recorder adds a sentence. Each person in the group continues to add a sentence, going clockwise around the circle. There is no editing allowed. Group members can be as kind and gentle, or as crude and rude as they would like. They have full control of the story each time it is their turn to add a sentence. However—and this is the reality orientation part—the story does not end until there is some kind of negotiated and agreed upon ending. The story could last fifteen minutes, or it may last for two or three sessions.

Whenever beginning storytelling with children and they don't seem to know how to get started, all you have to do is to remember the five "w"s of stories: who, where, when, what, why. You usually only need the first two or three. A session (I say session, but many of these methods can be used anywhere by anyone, not just a therapist with a child—it could be your own child) could begin by you saying: "Why don't you tell me a story today?" The child may go off with some great science fiction saga. On the other hand, he or she may not have a clue where to begin. This is where the five "w"s can be useful. The following is a real example of how this can evolve. The session picks up here after Billy has said he doesn't like making up stories because he never knows where to begin and doesn't know how to tell stories:

Therapist: Well Billy, if you were going to have a story, who would you like to have in it?

Billy: My dog, Spot, would be in it. So would the green monster from the tv show and so would my Grampa who died at Christmas.

Therapist: Where would you like this story to take place?

Billy: In a cave on the side of a hill near the ocean.

Therapist: Billy, now it sounds like a very interesting story is beginning to grow. When would the story happen? What time of year, what kind of weather, day or night? Tell me these kinds of things about your story.

Billy: Well, it's a story that happens in the summer. It's a really nice day and the sun is shining. I go up the cliff with my grampa. It's really hard to climb, so he carries me part of the part that is the steepest. When we get there, he is going to tell me all kinds of things about hidden treasures he found when he was a little boy himself.

Obviously, now the story is already under way. There has been only minimal prompting by the therapist using the five "w"s of storytelling. Using this approach also means the story is left in the child's own space. The therapist has imposed none of the elements of the story, so it truly is the child's story and therefore reflects the child's life. In Billy's real life situation his grandfather had died. Billy had been very fond of his grandfather and had started to have nightmares since the death. After this particular session, which went into extensive discussion (indirectly through the means of the story) about grampa, the nightmares ended. The therapist had never directly imposed the issue of grampa's death, nor directed the child as to what needed to be raised with regard to the loss of grampa. The method of storytelling was directed. However, the issues which arose were non-directive. It allowed the child to proceed at his own pace, as play therapy should, and did not impose issues on the child with which an outsider may have thought Billy should be dealing.

Winnicott (1971) and Gardner (1971) use a technique of drawing and storytelling involving a "squiggle." This can be a valuable approach when total ambiguity is desired. The child is literally given nothing in terms of issues. Thus, what is revealed is more likely the child's own material.

I have tended to use a modification of this and use "a seed," since seeds are ambiguous in their own way. From seeds come growth and seeds are a beginning. Thus, they symbolically represent hope. This can be quite useful in group work, especially a group which has become bogged down or has plateaued. The "once upon a time there was a seed..." story can provide great benefit. There are interesting dynamics at play. First, in the instructions for the story there are guidelines that lead to empowerment. The story is begun by the therapist starting the story and directing the group to take turns. They are told:

> I'm going to start the story and then I want you to go clockwise and each person gets to add a sentence. When it is your turn the story is entirely yours. You can be as kind and gentle or crude and rude as you want. There is no editing someone else's work. I want you to keep going around until you have an agreed upon ending. The story begins with: once upon a time there was a seed.... Now you continue it.

This method builds in an empowerment for each individual because when it is anyone's turn, he or she can completely change the course of the story's history. The technique is also healing and refreshing, for often there will quickly be laughter. Finally, there is a reality orientation, as the story is not to end until there is a negotiated ending.

Traditionally, storytelling filled the air during the passing of winter months. Envision the dark night, wood crackling, the smell of wood burning and apple cider in the air. I think it would be wonderful if every therapy room were to have a fireplace (I know, I know, I'm being an idealist). These stories link us to the past. Use your entire being in storytelling. Your voice, your eyes, your face, hands, body. Bring in props...blankets, boxes, colour your stage with crayons. When you are passionate about your stories, love them and believe in them: you will become a magnet to the child's psyche.

Footnotes

[1] Not my accuracy, the accuracy of coincidence.

CHAPTER 9

ART AND DRAWINGS

Hope and Memory have one daughter
and her name is Art,
and she has built her dwelling
far from the desperate field where
men hang out their garments upon forked boughs
to be banners of battle.
O beloved daughter of Hope and Memory,
be with me for a little.

—William Butler Yeats, 1893

FEELINGS AS COLOURS
YOUR FAMILY
YOUR FAMILY AS ANIMALS
YOUR FAMILY AS A GARDEN
AN ABUSED CHILD
HOW YOU THINK THE WORLD SEES YOU/
HOW YOU SEE YOURSELF/
HOW YOU WOULD LIKE TO BE SEEN
(WHO YOU WOULD REALLY LIKE TO BE?)
YOURSELF AND YOUR BEST FRIEND

There is an almost infinite number of art methods for use in the emotional healing process with people of all ages. A few of my favourites are included in this chapter. These can be both fun and productive in your work with children. Be cautioned that there are a number of art therapists and creative arts therapists who see their work as some mystified and grandiose Divine calling and who see any work with art as both deeply powerful and dangerous. They caution the professional world about the dangers of delving into this material without adequate training. Ignore them. They have a pickle up their butt and take themselves far too seriously. If it's that dangerous, some of the screwed up people I have met who identified themselves as art therapists or creative arts therapists should not even be allowed in the room with a person desiring healing process work. This brings to mind the movie *Crazy People*. There is a scene where it is time for "art therapy." One of the patients is whining "No, not art therapy. I hate art therapy." I think they must have been subjected to one of those art therapists who takes themselves too seriously. Some of these people seem to need to analyze everything because they fear feeling anything. As Szasz notes:

> Humorless persons make poor patients: humorless therapists make pathetic analysts. Beware of the psychoanalyst who analyzes jokes rather than laughs at them (1990, p. 193).

I read many journals and other periodicals. I often see journals with a Jungian or Freudian slant and they are typically filled with articles on the meaning of Peter Rabbit, Goldilocks, The Lion King, and every other children's fantasy on the face of the earth. Like the religious fanatics obsessed with finding hidden sexual and evil meanings in Disney cartoons or discovering backwards subliminal messages (the legitimacy of forward subliminal messages is not proven, never mind backwards!) in some modern song, these are also people with too much time on their hands, too little meaning in their lives, and too few brain cells in their heads.

Really, this stuff is lots of fun. Play with it. Have fun. Don't get all caught up in analytic interpretations. Explore art, don't interpret it. Don't analyze it. Just be with it. Feel it.

FEELINGS AS COLOURS

This is an adaptation of a method called the *Colour Emotional Chart* that I learned from Betty Bedard-Bidwell, who is the President of the Canadian Association for Child and Play Therapy, as well as a play therapist and art therapist in Southern Ontario. I have changed it considerably, but I give Betty full credit for the inspiration behind my design.

With this method, the first thing I do is have individuals draw a picture of themselves. They are given fairly open instructions:

> Draw a picture of yourself however you define this. You can be true to life or abstract. Use whatever colours you wish, and put them anywhere in the picture to express yourself.

In the next step I choose some scene for the person to draw. Some examples of things I have used include:

> Draw a picture of yourself having fun.
>
> Draw a picture of yourself in a safe place.
>
> Draw a picture of yourself being nurtured/nurturing.

The final piece of this exercise is to give the person a list of emotions, feelings, and processes for them to associate colours with. Some of the common ones I have used are:

Love	Rejection
Hate	Comfort
Happy	Sex
Sad	Joy/Birth/Beginnings
Angry	Grief/Endings
Fear	Frustration
Guilt	Escape/Running Away
Lonely	Others of Your Choice.

Older kids, adolescents and adults are usually asked to do each of the above columns on a separate piece of paper. For children under about the age of 9, I would probably have them do only the ones listed on the left side and do only one per page so the exercise does not become confusing or overwhelming. Feel free to change the kinds and number of emotions used. This is a very adaptable exercise. For younger children, you can sometimes use pictures instead of words. For a child with limited or no sight, you can use textures instead of colours. For example, when visually impaired children are told the word "sad," they can feel in a box for just the right texture to describe the feeling. In the box can be a number objects with differing tactile sensations: different kinds of sand, pebbles, flour, marbles, cotton balls, wood chips, grass, sunflower seeds, rubber, many different materials and textiles, clay, soybeans (uncooked), goopy stuff, rose petals, chamomile flowers, spearmint leaves, and so on.

I then give instructions:

> I would like you to imagine each of these feelings or issues and see what is the first colour that comes to mind. Put that colour beside the emotion. You can use the same colour more than once and you can use more than one colour for any particular emotion. While you are doing that, think of a time when you felt that way and try and get in touch with how you acted when you felt that way and what you needed when you felt that way.

After they are finished the exercise, I then look at a couple of aspects of their drawings and colouring. The first thing I like to do is have them see if any of the colours are the same or similar—which of their colours are aligned. For example, have they used the same colour for sex and fear, for love and happiness, for love and sex, for sad and grief, and so on. Which of these colours are similar? This is possibly the way they actually associate such emotions.

Next, I like to compare their colour chart with the pictures they have drawn. Do certain colours show up anywhere significant in their scenes or on their body? Is this perhaps the area of the body where they hold these feelings? Although this, at present, is not a valid researched psychometric tool, I believe it is an interesting therapeutic process door opener. It has proved at times to be an invaluable tool in the therapeutic process.

It is an exercise done "below jaw level." The processing of words is not involved and, thus, some valuable unconscious material can arise without cognitive obstruction. Of utmost importance in the processing of this exercise is not to interpret the meaning of any of the colours for people doing the colouring. That is the value of this exercise. We can find out from the creator of the colours what they mean. This is so much better than metaphorically raping people by telling them what their art and colours mean, as so many therapists are prone to do.

YOUR FAMILY

Drawing a picture of one's own family may be quite revealing. However, it may be a very threatening exercise and give no real details other than what the individual considers to be an idealized family.

Sometimes there is much to be learned from such simple pictures. One young girl with whom I worked, when asked to draw a picture of her family, drew mummy and daddy and her, all holding hands and smiling. This was an interesting picture since her parents were, at least in theory, separated. There was a reality base to the picture, though. Every Sunday afternoon, the parents got together and went on outings with the child. They maintained that they didn't want her to feel bad about the separation. This is an impossibility. If you don't want children to feel bad about a separation, don't separate. If you do separate, allow children to grieve, feel their pain and work it through. As well, whenever either mum or dad would have a spat with their new partner, they would run back to each other and sleep together. Thus, the child was given a contradictory picture of the world. Mummy and daddy are separated but mummy and daddy aren't separated. The child was acting quite bizarre in her behavior at times—major tantrums out of the blue on a fairly regular basis, and she appeared to be confusing fantasy and reality. There was some concern about her stability. In hindsight, the child was quite stable. She was, however, reacting to a very bizarre, confusing and unstable environment. The parents needed to separate themselves and they needed to allow the child to mourn. Making the situation even worse was a very rigid family therapist who believed that, because of her working (actually it didn't work at all) model, she was only willing to see the whole family together or no one at all. I'm not sure where she was coming from. This was no longer an intact family, yet this therapist wanted to see everyone together. This only served to further confuse the child. Obviously there was work to be done to enlighten this family therapist as well. Knock knock. Anybody home? Hey, this couple is no longer together. Why are you insisting on seeing mum, dad and child together?

YOUR FAMILY AS ANIMALS

"A very effective exercise is to have children draw their families as symbols or animals" (Oaklander, 1978, p. 26). Children who come from homes where there is violence may not reveal much about family dynamics in direct drawings. Children whose mothers are regularly beaten may only show a stereotypical or idealized family in their drawings. However, asking them to draw a picture of their families as animals may indicate all the dynamics of violence. Dominance, submission, violence, protection, nurturing, hiding—all of these may come out in the drawing. You may find the violent perpetrator portrayed as a very aggressive animal, an abused mum as a submissive animal. You can often see children's alliances in such pictures—who sides with dad, who sides with mum. I have seen many children who only did highly idealized pictures of their families when asked to draw a picture of their family. These same children, often in the same session, drew very different, and much more accurate, representations of their families when asked to draw members as animals. It doesn't feel as direct to draw an abusive dad as an attacking animal as it does to draw him as an attacking person. That is the benefit of this kind of exercise.

YOUR FAMILY AS A GARDEN

Asking a child to draw a picture of his or her family as a garden is at times even more revealing than the family as animals method. Using a garden gives an even greater sense of distance. In a sense, we are all of the animal kingdom. None of us, though, is a species directly related to plants.

Initially, look at the overall condition of the garden. Is it well tended? It doesn't have to be neat and tidy, just well watered and somewhat weeded. I would be interested and even concerned about the perfectly neat, orderly, symmetrical and tended garden. Those kinds of gardens are simply an obsession rather than a passionate endeavour of fun with the Earth.

It is interesting to see who is the most colourful member(s) of the family in this exercise. Is there someone who is a glowing sunflower providing joy to the rest?

Are there weeds? Are they just a natural part of the overall scheme as in reality, or have they taken over?

Is there a lawn? Is it vibrant and green, or dormant and brown?

Are there any trees? What kind of trees? What meaning do they have for the person drawing them? Do they provide shade and comfort, or do they rob the garden of needed light? What is growing under or near the trees?

What time of year is it in the garden—summer, autumn, winter, spring? Is this a time of increase, abundance, decrease, or hibernation?

What flowers are close to each other? Is there any building or dwelling? Are there animals...birds, rabbits, raccoons, foxes, butterflies, insects, worms? What are they doing?

What is the weather like in the garden? What has it been like recently, and what does the future hold? Is the garden getting the water it needs to be nurtured? Is there enough, but not too much, sunshine?

All of these things may, in some small way, reflect the life of the person drawing. Each area can be explored. For example, ten year old Danielle drew a picture of a blue jay constantly harassing a small sparrow. There seemed nowhere the sparrow could go to find peace. Danielle said the blue jay was her younger sister and the sparrow was herself. All the sparrow wanted was a little bird house to go to and play alone at times or to have some friends in. This house had to be one where no blue jays were allowed.

Danielle went on at great length about her relationship with her sister as we meandered through this exercise. Previously, she had always been reluctant to talk in any way about anyone else in her family. Many of the family dynamics were becoming clear quickly through this exercise.

AN ABUSED CHILD

When working with children who have been abused, it may be overwhelming and far too threatening for them to draw a picture of themselves. You may find them immobilized by such an exercise. They just sit there and there is nothing they can do. On the other hand, you may only get a "cutesy" picture of an idealized image.

It can be helpful to have such children, instead of drawing themselves, to draw a picture of an abused child. Suddenly, you may find all the internal dynamics of the child with whom you are working exposed.

HOW YOU THINK THE WORLD SEES YOU/HOW YOU SEE YOURSELF/HOW YOU WOULD LIKE TO BE SEEN (WHO YOU WOULD REALLY LIKE TO BE)

Like much artwork, this can be very revealing. How do children see themselves with respect to how they think the world sees them? These drawings may be wonderfully integrated and similar. On the other hand, there may be a wide chasm of difference between the two pictures. It may be helpful to add a third picture of how children would like to be seen. If there are differences between any of these pictures, what are they? One ten year old girl with whom I worked on one side of the page drew a smiley, carefree picture with lots of colour and a full environment to show how she thought the world saw her. Beside it, she drew another picture, one that showed how she saw herself. It was close to empty. The outline of the girl was the same, but all colour had vanished. It was only the barest of pictures. Even the environment was gone. In this second picture there was no sky, no grass, no trees, no sun—only emptiness. She felt this way about herself. She was a very sad young girl but presented a happy-go-lucky image to the world. In effect, she was protecting her parents from her deep sad feelings about their separation. In so doing, she was gradually dying inside. She lacked the caregiver support and encouragement to express herself. It was important in counselling work with her to also involve each of the parents in gaining the support each needed, as well as in providing them communication and parenting skills to help their daughter.

YOURSELF AND YOUR BEST FRIEND

As with the picture of an abused child, children drawing a picture of themselves and their best friends may provide a wealth of information. You can learn a lot by asking children how they are like their best friends, and how are they different. Would they like to be more, or less, like this friend?

You may find that children draw pictures of themselves and you. This gives you much material to explore with them (remember, don't interpret it, explore it with them to find out their own meaning). I worry that children drawing me as their best friend may not actually have a best friend in their lives. Maybe, to them, I really am their best friend. There is a great sadness to this. On the one hand, it is nice that they see me as their best friend. On the other, it is sad that there are no peers who fulfil this role. Children need peers as friends and adults as caregivers.

Children drawing you as their best friend may be trying to please you and make you feel good. This, too, is a sad statement that they feel that they must do things to make you feel good. They have become the supporter, or feel they must be the supporter and flatterer in order to win your approval. This may have nothing to do with you or anything you have done. It may be that some children feel this way with regard to anyone in authority in their life. Perhaps they fear conflict and try and avoid any conflict with you by portraying you as this best friend.

All art work needs to be taken as an opportunity to learn something from and about children. If you sit and interpret what children do for you, you may as well be an analyst of computer systems and not work with living things. We cannot know from the outside the meaning of an other individual's creation.

If we are willing to follow the path with others leading the way, we can learn much from those we follow. If we insist on leading the way—by analyzing, interpreting and inflicting our meaning—there is no offer of hope or help. It is only a statement of disrespect and implies that other people do not possibly have the wisdom or resources to find their own meanings.

CHAPTER **10**

Nature I...
Working with the Earth

Sandbox Play

CROSS CULTURAL BACKGROUND
ONE WOMAN'S STORY
THERAPEUTIC HISTORY
THE PROCESS OF SANDPLAY: GUIDELINES
A HEALING STUDY
IN SUMMARY

The young woman's hands touched the sand and a transformation began. She was sixteen and frightened. Her beautiful appearance hid her shyness and fear. She had trouble maintaining eye contact and stuttered significantly. Her life was a miserable tale that none should have to face. Neglect and rejection, physical and emotional beatings, rape: her history explained her fear of life's experiences. She entered therapy on the advice of a high school friend. In therapy she was working very hard on building a new life and facing her fears in the hope of growing beyond and despite the inner turmoil and pain. One day she began her therapy session saying she felt helpless like a young child. I suggested she allow herself to accept the inner child and prompted her to allow the child out. I sat on the floor by the sandbox, touched the sand with my hands and said

"Why don't you just make up a story in the sandbox." She never did make a sand scene, but she did sit directly across from me and she, too, touched the sand, picking it up, letting it fall through her fingers. It was like she connected with Mother Earth and felt her healing presence. Interestingly, she maintained eye contact throughout the entire session and did not stutter once. She maintained this in therapy from that point on. We then worked on her allowing herself the same ability in the world at large. Initially this involved her creating a mental image of sitting in the sand and touching it while feeling stable and calm. She would use this mental picture whenever she felt insecure, threatened or lacking in confidence. She also put some of the sand from the sand tray into a little gold locket she usually carried with her. It was as if that simple process of touching the sand in one therapy session opened a very important door.

When people participate in the process of sandbox play they enter a realm of healing that operates on a very deep and primitive[1] level of the psyche. Sandbox play, referred to as sandplay by most mental health professionals, is a process involving the use of a small sandbox about half the size of a desk top, and numerous small figurines to create imaginary stories and scenes. Through this experience, which actually reflects the person's inner emotional world, the person faces many conflicts and problems and learns to resolve issues which had previously blocked his or her growth and development. I believe that sandplay is one of the most important tools in the healing arts and sciences.

CROSS CULTURAL BACKGROUND

It is unfortunate that civilization and so-called progress are usually synonymous with losing touch with Mother Nature and the Earth, for it is precisely there, in the Earth, that many healing qualities are found.

Many primitive[1] cultures have used sand for its healing qualities. The Navajo Indian religion, with its great emphasis on magic, includes a healing process that involves purification. An "object" that plays a vital role in Navajo healing is the sandpainting.

> The sandpainting is an altar, but an altar composed of the representations of divinity, which becomes sacred in its setting

> after it is placed according to divine tradition. When a person sits on the sandpainting and is treated by the medicine man who applies the sacred-bundle paraphernalia with the correct songs and prayers, he becomes the god and shares in all its miraculous power.... There has never been a time in the history of mankind when medicine or curing was divorced from magic or religion (Reichard, 1977, pp. ix, 14).

The folk magic of many cultures and "old ways" have existed throughout the ages. The ancient religions have an almost infinite variation of sects and labels. Many use very similar methods when it comes to healing and sand. A sacred circle and sand are important in many ceremonies. Both sand and circles are highly significant in the psychotherapeutic process of sandplay.

There are even ancient texts of magic which include rituals that directly parallel the image of modern sandplay. These are prescribed for the purpose of healing psychic trauma and wounds and for simple relaxation and recharging of personal energy. One such document, a *Celtic Book of Shadows*, reveals the use of what we today would clinically label as sandplay, and it says that in times of personal difficulty/illness people should play with a tiny sandbox using whatever tools or toys are necessary to create an imaginary world. Then they should change that into an image of the world as they would prefer it to be and imagine that their own worlds are able to change as well. This certainly sounds like modern day sandplay and possibly even the process of active imagination. The same ancient document suggest that people may, weather and locale permitting, sit on a beach or another sandy location, and draw a circle around themselves in the sand and meditate quietly, allowing the sand to absorb and diffuse any negativity away from the their bodies. We could all learn a great deal from this ancient wisdom.

ONE WOMAN'S STORY

In a variation of this second method noted, I was once treating a wonderful woman in therapy who travelled a great distance to my office on a regular basis. Because of the distance, she was only able to come for scheduled weekly or bi-weekly appointments. She was under great stress. She had left an emotionally abusive marriage and was trying to live a new independent life while raising two teenage children and also developing her own life. She was also a physician, which meant that her career involved a great deal of giving of herself in what was quite often a highly pressured and stressful environment.

One morning she called my office in considerable stress. Some might like to use the word crisis[2] to describe her situation. She was feeling beyond her emotional limit and could take no more pain. I considered this a sign that the healing crisis, a great opportunity for growth, had set in. She was terrified because she recognized suicidal feelings in herself which had previously been quite foreign to her. She felt at somewhat of a loss to be at such a distance from her therapist. I reminded her that I was truly only an outward symbol of her own inner healing process and I suggested—this was a shot in the dark but I've used it several times since—as she lived in a town at the edge of one of the Canadian Great Lakes, that she go and sit in a secluded area of a beach and draw a circle around herself in the sand. Then she was to visualize herself emotionally healing. She was to allow her negative feelings to be absorbed by the sand and then she was to imagine purifying, healing white energy surrounding her and enabling her to step beyond what she was perceiving as the present unbearable pain.

She rather sceptically noted that at this point that, although this was rather foreign to any of her medical training, there was nothing to lose and she would try it. But the tone of her words definitely connoted the feeling, "you've got to be nuts."

I let her know where she could call to locate me over the following seventy-two hours. Four hours later she again called me, this time obviously relieved. She was somewhat reluctant, yet obviously pleased, to tell me that she had just experienced a deeply transformative process. After following all the instructions, she witnessed an energy "leave her body" and enter the sand and simultaneously felt great relief and awareness that she would be okay. She would get through her present difficulties. Although this example does not encompass the depths of the sandplay process, I tell it to illustrate the power of simple contact with sand in and of itself. It also illustrates one of many uses of the healing power of nature in a clinically therapeutic process.

THERAPEUTIC HISTORY

There are, today, many practitioners who utilize sandplay as a tool of therapy. Three key pioneers to recognize the value of sandplay were the European psychoanalysts Margaret Lowenfeld, Dora Kalff and Estelle Weinrib.

Margaret Lowenfeld herself credits H. G. Well's 1911 book *Floor Games* as inspiring her own involvement with sandplay. In 1935 Lowenfeld published a text entitled *World Techniques: Play in Childhood*. The world she described was the sandbox, often called the sand tray[3]. With its recommended miniature size of approximately 57 x 72 x 7 cm., it is quite easy for the tray to become the child's entire world visually and thus it is an ideal projective device on to which the psyche can emerge.

In 1956 at a Swiss psychiatric conference, Dora Kalff, a Jungian therapist, observed the work of Dr. Lowenfeld. Following this, with encouragement from C. G. Jung, Kalff travelled to London to study this technique in depth. Upon returning to Zurich she applied the method within the highly symbolic and experiential Jungian model and found that "an autonomous process was occurring with little or no verbal comment or explanation being given to the child.... Kalff then began doing sandplay therapy with adults and discovered that the same developmental process occurred as in children" (Weinrib, 1983, p. 8).

Estelle Weinrib published *Images of the Self* in 1983 and presented one of the first theoretical and practical studies in the use of sandplay. Although slanted entirely from a Jungian perspective, it was a pioneering effort in this valuable and innovative psychotherapeutic method.

Today, in the 1990s, we are still in the infancy stages of learning to use this technique called sandplay. A 1988 graduate research study by Mary McIntyre noted that "comparatively little has been written on the therapeutic use of sandplay. Much of what is available has been contributed by therapists trained in the Jungian tradition. An in-depth review of the literature reveals that very few actual studies exist on the topic" (McIntyre, 1988, p. 8).

I remind you, however, that although I am giving certain modern day persons credit for developing this as a healing technique, it is obvious that it is nothing new to the world of healing. The credit the modern clinical pioneers have earned is due to the fact that they have adapted and applied old healing techniques to modern practice. All that we are doing today is expanding the variations on ancient practices of "sand healing."

THE PROCESS OF SANDPLAY: GUIDELINES

1) *Ideally, play therapy itself provides what Kalff calls a "free and sheltered space" catalytic to the healing process* (1980, p. 29). This idea that free and protected space is therapeutically important has been well explained by Weinrib (1983). The freedom involves the decisions to use whichever figures and create whatever adventure, picture or story one desires. The protection lies in both the limiting size of the sand tray and in the presence of a therapist. However,

> it would be an unfortunate misunderstanding to believe all one needs is a tray with some sand, a collection of small objects and a dictionary of symbols. Just companioning a patient while he makes pictures will not accomplish much, nor will interpreting pictures as though they were dreams.... Critical is the ability of the therapist to assimilate the feelings and atmosphere of the process and the individual pictures. In an emotional sense the therapist "enters" the sand tray with the patient and participates empathically in the act of creation, thus establishing a profound and wordless rapport. The silent capacity to enter into creation of his world with the patient can, in itself, help repair the feeling of isolation with which so many people are afflicted (Weinrib, 1983, pp. 29, 30).

2) *As the sandplay process develops and deepens and old repressed issues are confronted, a great deal of energy which had previously been utilized in repressing thoughts and painful issues will be released.* The result will be quite a childlike sense of wonder and a feeling of "I can do anything I want," especially in adults. The wise therapist will work with patients in encouraging them to channel this energy into physical activities in their daily lives such as dance, woodworking, creative exercise, martial arts, theatre—any creative activity involving the hands or body. Otherwise the patient, who is psychologically around the age of two, may act this out in some manner that may be detrimental to him or herself.

3) *Sandplay is not a complete therapeutic package, although sometimes it may be a large piece*. Also in our therapy rooms are numerous other tools: creativity supplies, construction paper, face paints, crayons (one of the finest play therapy tools ever invented), clay, glue, pipe cleaners, puppets, musical instruments, doctor kit, handcuffs, toy kitchen, story books, chalk boards, mirrors, and so on. Play therapy is not done to the exclusion of parental guidance, family therapy or marital therapy.

4) *Size and Location of the sand tray.* The generally accepted size for a sand tray is **approximately** 57 x 72 x 7 cm., slightly smaller than a desktop. This size allows it to become an ideal projective device as it takes in the entire visual world of the child (and the child inside the adult), and yet does not go beyond it.

Don't worry if the sandbox is not that exact size. I know there are some rigid programs where it is dogmatically proclaimed that the sandbox *must* be that size. There is no reason for this except the fact that some therapists are insecure and cling rigidly to these numbers. When asked, they have no real reason other than hocus-pocus nonsense. The reason for the size, as already mentioned, is for the box to fit in the person's field of view. If we took the dogmatic "it must be this way" approach, one would need a huge number of sandtrays to fit the fields of view of many clients. Don't worry about it. Just have one small sandbox of any size. If someone gives you a hard time about it, visualize that person having farted out loud in the library and everybody turning to look at him or her for such silliness.

I like to have the sand tray at floor level on casters for easy movement. At this level we are symbolically grounded and closer to the Earth, the true natural healer. It is also where most children do their playing. However, I have also worked on the floor in sandplay with many adults. Once again, keep in mind there is no scientific rationale for the sandbox being on the floor. I maintain that, for me, when I am on the floor I am symbolically closer to the Earth. However, suppose you work on the twenty-first floor of a building. Does thirty-six inches closer to ground level really make any difference? Obviously not.

5) *I prefer to have the bottom of the tray painted blue prior to first adding sand.* This allows the representation of the presence of water, whether or not water is actually available. Keep in mind that children won't necessarily care at all what colour the bottom is painted. If the bottom of the sandbox is purple and yellow stripes and children want it to be water, they will tell you "this is the water."

6) *The sand should ideally be safe or in some way purified or sterilized.* An easy way to obtain this is to purchase it through a teachers' supply store, hardware store or building supplies store. I give this recommendation for very practical reasons. The process of sandplay is an esoteric and fascinating approach. It can also be very enchanting and the healers involved may deeply enter the process on their own time and go off and dig up their own sand. This has happened many times with people I have trained. On some day off they go out into the woods and dig up their own sand as part of their own process of learning this method and making their own sandbox. There have been a couple of unfortunate incidents. Two examples: some of the sand one intern collected had poison oak in it and on several other occasions there were creepy crawlies that ended up all over the office. Please, just obtain sterile sand at a reputable supply store.

7) *Recommended objects to have on hand are obviously those which can reflect psychological growth and development, conflicts, cooperation.* For example, a good collection would include wooden, metal, plastic, clay or natural fibre replicas of:

a) Vegetation. Various trees, plants, flowers, grass. The best place I have found to get vegetation is in model train shops and similar hobby shops. You may live somewhere that does not have such a shop. Many of these companies do have mail order programs. Or, even in most smaller locations, there is once a year a model train fair where you can obtain all kinds of supplies that are useful for your sandbox. It really is a lot of fun hunting for these kind of supplies. One of my favourite finds over the years was a rather large tree, about twelve inches high with leaves and branches that are removable. I was thrilled with this, for finally I had a big tree that was cyclical. It could represent winter, spring, summer or autumn.

b) Primitive animals and beings such as prehistoric creatures, dinosaurs, snakes, crocodiles and spiders.

c) Wild animals. Lions, tigers, wolves, horses, jungle animals. Independent toy stores and zoo shops are great locations to find these.

d) Domestic farm type animals. This is one kind of item that is fairly easy to find.

e) Farm and country people, tools, implements.

f) Boundaries. Fences, tunnels, gateways, walls, bridges. Once again, model train and hobby shops seem to have the most abundant and realistic looking items in this category.

g) Marbles, especially the clear glass variety. These can be used variously as magic crystals, path stones, water, bombs.

h) Crystals and stones. Don't worry about a huge budget for the high cost of crystals these days. Just collect stones by the beach or side of the road. Or, if you are really into rock hunting, get geological maps and guidebooks and go out and search for your own. I am very lucky to live where I do in Eastern Ontario in Canada. We live at the edge of what was a prehistoric ocean and the Canadian Shield, so there is a wealth of mineral deposits within a short travelling distance. We can go out in the woods and find quartz crystals in abundance and many other wonderful gifts from the Earth. But if you don't happen to live in such a location, all you need is a gravel road, a quarry, a beach or a highway roadcut to find some stones for your sandbox.[4]

i) Buildings. Houses, schools, spiritual centres, pyramids, healing centres, energy sources (gas station, hydro poles), castles. Tubes from paper towel rolls, small cardboard boxes, plastic boxes that berries come in from the grocery store are all put to great use in the sandbox.

j) Fantasy figures. Dragons, unicorns, fairies, knights, kings, queens, monsters, vampires, skeletons, coffins.

k) Spiritual beings. Buddha, Christ, angels, gods, goddesses, Santa Claus, wizards, witches, magicians and so on. Many of these and the previous fantasy figures can be found in Christmas stores which are open year round. Other items can be found in "new age" shops and games stores which carry supplies for fantasy role play games.

l) Machines and equipment. The list here is endless but should include tiny hospital equipment and other medical supplies.

m) Vehicles. Cars, trucks, aeroplanes, boats, buses, police cars, construction equipment, fire trucks, ambulances.

n) Conflict figures. Army toys, weapons, pirates, armed figures. I like to shy away from the addition of "cowboys and Indians" because of the harmful stereotypes this could promote. I also like to avoid toys with preconceived images and hero images. It is harder for the child to project onto something which comes with an idea attached to it.

o) People. Many nationalities, primitive, modern, male, female, babies of various sizes, children, parent and grandparent figures, good and evil looking people, clergy, wise looking people, nurturing looking people, cooperative looking people, battling people. Some of the best collections of people (as well as some other unique and interesting items) have come from cake decorating supply stores.

p) Miscellaneous. Those little plastic baskets that berries come in, empty paper towel rolls, pens and crayons and construction paper for making anything that might be missing.

As there are no sandplay stores, you have to build your own sand tray and gradually search for and collect the figures. This search is an important part of sandplay, for it encourages the participation of the therapist in the overall process. It also means the therapist will know exactly what figures are available and what their significance is. Collecting these toys can be an absolute joy and may even become a hobby of sorts. The obvious starting point is the local toy stores. Crafts stores, cake decorating supply stores (these produce some of the best finds such as people of various cultural backgrounds, babies, brides and grooms, pirates ships), gift and specialty shops, religious stores, jewellery, gem or rock shops (for different stones and crystals), school supply shops, model train shops (the best spot for vegetation and realistic looking trees as well as hydro poles and other energy symbols). It will usually take at least a year for the collection to be somewhat complete, because, with each season, new objects become available in stores—Santa Claus, angels, skeletons, ghosts, cupids, leprechauns. But that doesn't mean you should wait this long to begin using the sand tray in therapy. Your collection will always be growing and changing. There is no real endpoint.

As long as you have a sand tray and sand, you have a workable tool. Many children will simply use the sand to draw shapes and make pretend stories with pretend or self constructed figures if none are available. I refer you back to the story of the young woman mentioned at the beginning of this chapter.

Whatever collection you have, do make sure you include construction paper, scissors, and crayons. Many times something will be missing from your collection. It can still be created using these simple arts and crafts supplies. On one occasion, a ten year old girl with whom I was working wanted a graveyard as part of her story. I don't happen to have a set of tombstones as part of my toy collection and doubt if very many people have found such toy items. However, with the construction paper and scissors this young girl created her own. When completed she even took crayons and wrote names and epitaphs on each stone. On another occasion, a forty year old woman with whom I was working wanted a stream and waterfall to lead out of the sandbox onto the floor nearby and into a lake. So she cut out white paper, coloured it blue and created her own stream, waterfall and lake. We truly are only limited by our own creativity.

9) *Record the scenes that the client has made in order to follow progress and changes from week to week.* This can be done in notation form, diagrams, slides or with video equipment. The recording also enables

you to obtain consultation on your work from colleagues, to conduct research and, in hindsight, to check on your previous hunches and intuitions.

10) *I would strongly advise any therapist wishing to develop skills in sandplay to gain as much knowledge as possible of symbols, of mythology, anthropology, and fairy tales from many cultures.* This will greatly enhance the understanding of the sandplay scenes.

> Any symbol can have many meanings. Therefore it is advisable that the therapist have a relatively wide knowledge of symbology from which to choose interpretations. However, the specific interpretation of a particular symbol may be less important than the process itself and the relationship between himself and the patient. It is, of course, imperative that the therapist's ideas about the patient and the pictures are in the right general direction (Weinrib, 1983, p. 16).

11) *A Caution.* A strong word of caution is in order as you discover the sandplay process and are possibly drawn to more and more reading and training on the subject—this is a new area with much philosophy and dogma. Many times something must be done in a certain way simply because "it is written." There are many who treat this new method much like a new religion. Approach this valuable technique with a very critical, open and playful mind.

A HEALING STUDY[5]

Sean was a ten year old boy whose parents had separated and he was caught in the middle. Everyone else's needs seemed to have been addressed before his own were. Each of his biological parents remarried new partners in the same week. This young boy had two processes to complete: 1) coming to terms with the parental separation; and 2) reality construction regarding the fact that perhaps he was actually a full and healthy human being who just happened to exist in a crazy situation.

Thus, his growth involved: 1) grieving the loss of his family as it had previously existed; 2) coming to terms with the lack of control he felt in his parents process; and 3) developing coping and healing strategies that would allow him to exist in his post-parental-divorce situation. The following is a summary of my work with Sean:

His first session involved crayons and huge sheets of paper. When asked to draw how he felt, he drew a devastating storm. There was a tornado and lots of lightning. The roof was off of a house and he was inside screaming for help. Up in the extreme upper left hand corner he put a yellow dot. I asked about the dot and Sean commented "That's the sun, its gotta come out eventually." I told him that it always does, even if we lose sight of it along the way. But even this little yellow dot was quite therapeutically encouraging to me, for I saw it as a sign of hope and symbol of the self just waiting for the storm to quiet in order to reveal itself.

For the next several months Sean gravitated to the sand tray in most of our sessions. There were terrible wars along the mythological path, a journey through life's confusion and conflicts through the eyes of ten year old Sean. The wars were chronic and very nasty. At first there was no apparent meaning, purpose or order to the chaotic battles. Gradually, a sense of order set in. It became obvious who was fighting whom and what their issues were. Following the first scenes of primitive battles that lasted several months, a burial ground appeared and all of the old conflict was buried in a great sand pile. This scene seemed to coincide with the process of coming to terms with the parental separation. Following this, we had new, technologically advanced wars with high-tech planes and weapons. It was as though his other process—coming to terms with the difficult situation in which he was living—was both closer to the surface and more complex.

Then, suddenly, tranquillity, emptiness—beautiful, lonely and conflict-free emptiness—a tree and a lake. In our last session, we experienced a miracle of awareness. We were saying goodbye and talking about what we had each learned through our work together. Sean's scene that day had in the centre a clear marble which he described as a magic crystal. In each corner of the scene there was another marble (magic crystal), plus, in the upper left, a tree with full foliage; in the lower right, a castle with a skeleton overlapping it (death); in the upper right, a "wise old snail" (wisdom); in the lower left, a rabbit who had appeared in many of his scenes associated with chaos. Through the months the wise old snail had often been present to provide guidance, whereas the rabbit had often been in trouble. Sean's words to describe this scene were wisdom from a ten year old:

"There is life and death and in them wisdom and chaos. I know I have no control over life and death but I can choose between wisdom and chaos in my life." Unfortunately, the adults in this child's life did not always share this level of awareness.

IN SUMMARY

Dr. Harold Stone, former President of the C.G. Jung Institute of Los Angeles, in his Prologue to Dora Kalff's *Sandplay* (1980), notes that

> The sandbox is not an instrument of magic. It is a tool, an extremely effective tool, for getting to the imagination and allowing it to become creative. But it is more than a tool. It is also an expression of the therapist, as a creative personality, who relates to patients both personally and symbolically at an extremely deep level (Kalff, 1980, p. 15).

I agree with most of what Dr. Stone says, but I would disagree on his first point and argue that the sandplay process, not specifically the sandbox, is an instrument of magic. Gladys Reichard, who studied Navajo sand paintings in depth, states that

> The worldwide technique which converts the dangerous to the helpful is magic. It often does not include a belief in spiritual beings, but merely the belief that a carefully worked-out procedure will in itself bring about a desired result (Reichard, 1977, p. 17).

To end this chapter I would like to take some magical thoughts from Starhawk, writing in *The Spiral Dance*:

> To work magic is to weave unseen forces into form; to soar beyond sight; to explore the uncharted dream of the hidden reality, to infuse life with colour, motion and strange scents that intoxicate; to leap beyond imagination into that space between the worlds where fantasy becomes real; to be at once animal and god.... The language of the old belief, the language of magic, is expressed in symbols and images. Images bridge the gap between the verbal and non-verbal modes of awareness; they allow the two sides of the brain to communicate, arousing the emotions as well as the intellect... (Starhawk, 1979, pp. 109-110).

This beautifully poetic description of magic is, to me, what sandplay therapy and healing are all about—or should be.

Footnotes

[1] I view this concept of the primitive with great respect. If the world were more primitive today and less civilized, we would not have air, water and soil pollution rampant over the planet.

[2] It is very difficult to convince me that a crisis actually exists. Many people create crises for the rush of adrenalin that goes with the internal perception of crisis. Any staff or intern who has trained with me has been told not to come running to me in a panic with tales of crises. I believe that as long as people are breathing and they are not in danger of bleeding to death, they are not in crisis. I do note, however, that if people are suicidal, they are likely in crisis as they are in danger of stopping breathing or of bleeding to death. And, when I am convinced that a crisis exists, I always try to remember the Oriental interpretation of crisis as being both a danger and an opportunity.

[3] Given its small size, the use of the phrase sand tray, as the Jungians call it, seems quite appropriate.

[4] Anyone visiting Eastern Ontario may feel free to contact the author for information on sites of geological interest in the area.

[5] This section is entitled "A Healing Study". I intentionally use this phrase here as opposed to the typical "case study." There is something degrading and dehumanizing about considering human beings as cases. Beer comes in cases. People come with hearts and souls. It is difficult to conceptualize a process of healing with regard to a "case."

CHAPTER **11**

Nature II...
Working with the Earth:

Plants/Rocks/Animals
In The Healing Process

PLANTS

George Bernard Shaw noted that "Gardening is the only worthwhile endeavour." This statement often rings true. Although I believe there are many worthwhile endeavours, at times gardening may be the only thing which can keep us balanced.

As part of the holistic approach in working with children I believe we need to help them return to consider their place in the natural world. A direct and beneficial method for doing this means involving them with plants and animals. Children need to learn to garden, to become one with the Earth. When we touch the Earth, we become closer to the healing source and closer to our own soul. Symbolically we reach to the depths.

I feel sadness when I realize how many children have never even been in a garden. They spend many hundreds and thousands of hours in front of a television, yet never plant a living seed, wait for a sprout and then watch a plant grow and blossom. The self nurturance of growing such symbolic foods as potatoes, pumpkins, carrots and apples is an experience never known to many children in the world.

Another important aspect of gardening is that when you are out there, digging, planting, you are fully a part of life. You are working below jaw level, not up in your head. You can feel a breeze if it blows, see the wind,[1] hear the birds or crickets and the rustling of leaves in the trees.

I firmly believe that every school should have both outdoor and indoor gardens. Every grade level could become involved in their own way. Once you build this in to a curriculum, the program can easily expand. Next comes composting. Once a composting program is in place, it is only a short step to seeing the need for recycling. It is the ultimate useful science project. It is a living and growing experiment.

The following are a couple of exercises which can be started in the garden. One is called *The Nest*. The other is called *Aloha Nui Loa*. Each of these exercises is created for the older child or adult, but can easily be adapted for younger children.

THE NEST

Every living thing needs a place to nest. A place called home. The nest is the metaphor of the shelter we all need and deserve. It is a very individual space. Like the bird's in the wild, it is a shelter from the storm. It is symbolic of self care and commitment to living in a safe place.

I watch the birds in my garden and the woods out back with joy every spring as they wander through my garden and yard and pick up all kinds of bits and pieces of leaves, hay and grass, tiny twigs, chips of bark and whatever else they can find as they work diligently at building their nests. I know that a little later in the spring I will be seeing nestlings out for their first flights, sitting on a branch looking very nervous between their parents. Each of the parents will take turns feeding the young bird. It is a moment of caring and nurturing from within the garden. We can give ourselves the same kind of nurturing.

To create your own symbolic nest, see yourself collecting bits of natural substances from the outdoors and making your own nest. Perhaps you can bring this into concrete form by making a tiny pillow to place in your bed. You could gather some bits of grass, flower petals from plants which appeal to you, some hair from your dog or cat that comes off as you lovingly run your hand over its back or tummy, bits of paper from a loved one's letter, a favourite stone or mineral, sand from a seashore, herbs, a thread or shred of cloth from your favourite old pair of jeans which may have accompanied you through special and significant moments in your life...the list is endless. Like the purple martin's nest, who knows what wonders can show up in this symbolic nestpillow. Put all these things into your tiny pillow you sew yourself and keep it under your own pillow or mattress. Let it be the symbol of your own safe little nest, the place you can crawl into to renew and be safe.

Turn the sleeping/resting area of your home into a sanctuary. Set aside a weekend or couple of days with no commitment other than to yourself and the purification of your nesting environment. Clean your bedroom. If at all possible, open a window and allow fresh air in. Sweep, scrub, visualize an emotional cleansing as well as the literal physical cleanup. Think to yourself that you are creating a very special place. Perhaps this is a time to change the colour of your room, or put up a new picture or painting.

On some shelf or table place a plant. Cyclamens are considered by many to be protective. Perhaps have a hanging plant as well. Plants help cleanse the air. Have as many as you want, but do have at least one.... Maybe a canary to fill the air with song. (It is a well researched fact that pet owners as a whole have better recovery rates from serious illness—and probably minor illnesses too, but I am not aware of research in this area.) On your shelf or table place some twigs, dried petals and other reminders of Nature. If you wish to live a peaceful life, surround yourself with peaceful substances and objects ...a beeswax candle which you place in a candleholder that you find at just the right time and place. Perhaps at some flea market or yard sale one afternoon you stumble across a quaint item at the same moment as you are thinking a nice gentle thought. This is the kind of thing you should be bringing into your nest.

If you have a partner, you may, at times, feel that you do not have a space of your own. You need such a space even within a partnership. Without it, you will start to resent your partner for something that is not even his or her fault. Your nest and nesting thoughts can be entirely contained in your nesting pillow. You can bring this out when you want to nest anywhere in your living environment. When you travel you can take it with you to the homes of others, to a hotel or campground where you may be staying.

Spend a day with no tv on, no radio on, just simple pleasant sounds on a CD player. On another day have no electronic input whatsoever. No tv, no radio, no stereo, nothing. Open your windows and hear any natural sounds...birds, wind, crickets, bees, leaves blowing, geese, frogs, water flowing, a wolf howling...feel the scents of leaves, flowers, autumn, winter, spring or summer in the air.

We often avoid ourselves by keeping our senses overloaded. It is not good for our nest to be too busy or crowded.

As you ready for a nap or bed time, envision yourself like the bird in a tree or an animal on the earth which lives in its burrow. Do what you need to do so that there is no sense of unfinished business when you retire to your nest. Once you are in there you are safe and secure...in your own self-created nurturing environment. As you enter your bed, feel the safety of the nest. Curl up and find the most soothing position.

Lying in bed or on the floor, allow yourself to feel the life force within you, within the universe...touch yourself anywhere throughout your body where you feel discomfort, tension or pain. Use your own healing energy to regenerate yourself.... Let tension go.

If you are in a process of change or simply want to feel renewed...as you enter sleepland see yourself in the nest. Let yourself be inside an egg. Feel the healing presence of Mother Nature surrounding you with warmth and an all present nurturing. As you go to sleep, see yourself in this very protective shell, knowing that as you sleep you are readying to emerge from the egg and approach life from a new beginning. Several minutes or hours later when you awaken, sense yourself as emerging from an egg and beginning life anew. See things as if you had never seen them before. Take a new perspective. Give thanks for this new beginning.

THE MAKING OF A LEI–ALOHA NUI LOA

Lei in Hawaiian means garland, laurel or wreath. The phrase aloha nui loa translates to "much love." The making of a lei can be a fun and wonderful gesture of love. The lei is the beautiful garland of flowers worn around the neck, head, wrist or ankle in Hawaii. They are often given to loved ones as a gesture of affection, or they may be worn as a natural addition to the day's clothing. There is little that can be as refreshing as such a gift.

Everywhere you go in Hawaii you will see leis being worn. When we run our training programs in the Hawaiian Islands we find people arriving wearing their leis. They are always made of fresh flowers (you can buy tacky plastic ones in souvenir shops but that certainly seems counterproductive) and literally surround you with a refreshing scent.

Hawaii is one of my favourite places to work (and play). I remember some long plane rides from Kingston to Hawaii with over 10 hours on a plane, 6 time zone changes and very stiff legs in need of a stretch. Even under the best of conditions provided by Canadian Airlines, it is still a long flight, being cooped up for that many hours. I usually leave the plane exhausted.... I remember one trip I spent the last two hours fantasizing about crawling into a nice cosy bed...we disembarked from the plane, eventually got through Customs and Immigration and were ready to exit the airport, only to be very pleasantly surprised and greeted by my dear friend Stuart and his wife Sue, who were there waiting with loving greetings and leis to put around our necks. There were also some much welcomed hugs. It is difficult to describe how cared for and how refreshed it feels to suddenly be breathing not stuffy airplane cabin air but the fresh tropical air of Hawaii, intensely scented with the presence of carnations, orchids and many other flowers placed in a long strand over the shoulders. The scents fill the mind with feelings of being refreshed rather than exhausted. This wonderful Pacific custom transforms even the most worn out traveller. It seemed only natural to take this custom and apply it to a healing ceremony.

The making of a lei can be a fun and wonderful gesture of love. The process can also be part of a healing ceremony for an individual. I first used it while working in a healing process with a young woman who had been severely abused as a child. My first call was from an agency working with this young woman who knew of my work and was looking for consultation for ideas to help her. I was at somewhat of a loss for a number of reasons. First, I had never met her in person, which can make it more difficult to get a picture of what exactly is going on. At the time of initial contact, I was running a professional training program in Hawaii and Katie was on the Northeast coast of North America. Being many zones apart we were literally separated by both time and space. The cultures we were each in at the time were very different. I was within a world in the Pacific which did not know cold or snow or the harshness of winters of the northeast, a culture which does not, in fact, have a word meaning weather. Fortunately, the first contact I had with Katie was in the month of July, during the summer in the Northeast, so this helped with what I suggested. (However, I have since realized that this could be used anytime, anywhere.)

Katie was experiencing serious emotional distress and feeling very unsafe and haunted by her past. Fire was a negative symbol for her as she had apparently been burned as part of her abuse. I spoke with both Katie and some professional staff from the institution where she was living and there was a real concern about Katie's emotional health. There was also the feeling that she needed to do something that represented, in a powerfully symbolic way, self care and protection. I was feeling disoriented in attempting to make recommendations. I was too far away and far too relaxed...yet as I looked around I noticed the leis that some men and women were wearing and felt so inspired by the vision—of course, the perfect symbol and the perfect ceremony. I recommended that Katie and a person she was closest to take all the time needed and make a lei that Katie could wear. I gave them the simple instructions that follow for the making of the lei and asked that after it was completed, they go to the nearby ocean and visualize the thought and image of fire which was tormenting Katie being rendered harmless and painless by the water of the ocean. While doing this, Katie would be wearing the lei. In discussions later, it was clear that this process had been very beneficial for Katie.

The healing process involved in the making of a lei is simple. Take a number of your favourite flowers and herbs. Choose scents which you find soothing and refreshing. If you are in a season when things are not in bloom, you may choose to obtain your source of plants from a local farmers' market, florist or even grocery store. Obtain a sewing needle and some thread or cotton string.

Take your string and a needle and thread through the centre of each flower and form a necklace of flowers, leaves, herbs. With each flower you add, think a positive healing thought. Send this thought into the flower and into the growing lei. Thread all the good thoughts together as you form the lei.

When you have finished the lei you have a very powerful and wonderful symbol of healing and protection (the circular form of the lei). This can then be worn within your own healing process or given to someone else. You can give it to someone for use as part of his or her healing process or as a symbol of your love.

One last very important point: the healing energies and spirituality of Hawaii are very potent and vibrant. Huna healing methods of the Pacific are ranked with many traditional healing methods in their depth and meaning. Cautions from within Hawaiian wisdom should be taken very seriously. One such piece of advice is that it is considered unlucky to throw away a lei which has been given to you and you have accepted. Always keep it in a safe manner and treat it with respect. Hang it in your house or on the car's interior rear view mirror. Or place it outside in a location of honour such as on a wishing well handle.

HERBS

We have grown too far from our connections to the Earth and have lost contact with the beauty and healing powers of plants. Strictly speaking, herbs are any plants, part or parts of which are used for healing. The term is more commonly used for any plant which is used for medicinal purposes, flavouring of food or scent. The flavouring and scent capacities can certainly be healing as well, but such properties do expand the true meaning of herb in common thought.

Personally, I owe my very life to plants—and the physicians, oncologists and medical researchers who, through painstaking and extensive research, learned how to harness the healing powers within them. Fifteen years ago I was diagnosed with Hodgkin's Disease. I went through traditional medical treatment, supplemented by a holistic approach to healing. One of the vital elements of my physical healing involved the administration of a drug called vincristine. This drug, used as one of several in a chemotherapy regime, is made from the periwinkle (vinca) plant. The use of such drugs has brought about drastic remissions in many children and adults suffering from leukaemia and Hodgkin's disease. To date, no synthetics have been found to replace the raw leaves which are used to produce some of these pharmaceuticals. Other plants such as mayapple and Maytenus are also among many used to produce drugs which are saving many lives through cancer treatment.

In fact, herbs have been the primary source of medical help throughout time and over most of the world. Even in the present day, according to the World Health Organization

> 80 percent of the world's population depend on plants to treat many common ailments. In addition, 30 percent of modern conventional drugs are derived from a plant source (Murray, 1995, p. xi).

This usage is not restricted to so-called undeveloped countries. Although there are practitioners in Canada and the United States who do understand the value of herbal medicine, the real credit for an increasing understanding of this approach goes to Germany and Asia. In Germany, many physicians[2] have herbal preparations as their primary medicines. Research over the past two decades in some "developed" countries has resulted in "an explosion of scientific information concerning plants, crude plant extracts, and various substances from plants as medicinal agents" (Murray, 1995, p. 2).

It is often asked, if they are so effective and widely used, why aren't they more popular and more widely used? There really is a rather simple explanation for this, yet a highly complicated solution. You cannot patent a plant. This immediately cuts down, by millions of dollars, the profit that can be made after researching the effectiveness. Thus, the pharmaceutical companies have little or no interest in herbs. It is also interesting that pharmaceutical companies have and do isolate constituents of plants in attempts to develop pharmaceuticals (the "active constituents" can be patented). Unfortunately for profits, the crude herb has often been found to be more active (and often far less toxic) as a gestalt than when components are isolated. There is also government influence. It is estimated that, "in the United States FDA approval of a plant-based drug typically takes 10 to 18 years at a total cost of roughly $230 million dollars" (Murray, 1995, p. 3). In the United States and Canada, "herbal remedies" (even the phrase makes them sound like something sumbuddy wud take for roomatiz), are sold as food supplements and no therapeutic claims can be made with regard to such products. In Germany, the legal requirements for the use of plants as pharmaceutical drugs necessitate that they are both safe and effective. These are the same standards applied to all drugs in Germany. Availability over the counter is based entirely on application and safety and herbal products sold by prescription are reimbursable by insurance if prescribed by a physician (Murray, 1995).

The consuming public somehow has come to feel protected by our North American all-encompassing and overseeing political structures. We believe that anything the government will allow is fully understood, good and safe. This is an illusion. Aspirin is a prime example. This has been on the market for much longer than its action has been understood. The main mechanism of action responsible for aspirin's anti-inflammatory effect was not even understood until the early 1970s, and its mechanism of action for pain relief, as of 1995, had yet to be fully understood (Murray, 1995). If we were to assess aspirin on the same basis as herbs, it would have to be labelled as possessing no pharmacological activity.

It is quite safe to say that herbal medicines are usually far less toxic and have fewer side effects than modern synthetic pharmaceuticals. The modern "drugs" are quite often designed to alleviate the symptom rather than the underlying cause. Take aspirin, again, as an example. If people have a fever, they may take aspirin to make themselves feel more comfortable. This may be wise to do if a fever is too high for too long. But the action of taking the aspirin[3]—if this is the only treatment undertaken—to reduce the fever does absolutely nothing to deal with the underlying condition which has caused the fever. If no other action is taken—such as rest and sleep and whatever else is medically advisable for the specific cause—then taking the aspirin is identical to hearing a fire alarm and throwing water on the fire alarm to stop the alarm mechanism, rather than dealing with the fire which has resulted in the activation of the alarm.

Where does this all fit in along a healing path with children? Yes, always have the best medical advice and treatment available for our children. But let's also expand our vision of healing. What a different world it would be if, instead of watching television, being inactive, becoming ill, and taking drugs to deal with the symptom... children were able to grow up spending time being outdoors with a caregiver, planting potatoes, planting a new chestnut tree, digging the earth, listening to the Canada geese fly overhead going south for the winter, holding a worm and talking about what worms do for the garden, smelling the lavender growing, planting herbs in the garden, watching those plants grow, harvesting them during the waxing moon...and using them in teas and tinctures to self-heal. Kind of makes Saturday morning in front of the television start to appear absolutely gruesome, if not downright evil.

ROCK COLLECTING

I would classify rock collecting as a form of gardening. It may seem like an odd comparison, but it is a form of harvesting that makes many children tingle with excitement.

There is something basically good about being out in the woods or along a rock wall looking for crystals or some treasured stone. I think the younger the child, the less "real" or sparkly a stone has to be to be perceived as absolutely magical.

A fun approach to using rocks and crystals in the counselling process designed by Viki Takacs (1993) is called *Talking With Rocks*. Her process follows:

> Julia walked past the play therapist into the play therapy room. She turned, looked at the therapist and shrugged her shoulders. Julia, who was eleven years old and had been abused when younger, was not interested in playing with anything in the room. Julia did not like to play in the sandbox because she was afraid of getting "dirty." She claimed she disliked playing with the puppets because she could never think of what to say. Drawing on paper was out since she did not consider herself creative enough.
>
> Sound familiar?
>
> Every therapist has worked with at least one Julia who refuses to do anything. However, this difficult moment can give the therapist some opportunities to consider other options. One would be to

wait it out. Another option is to introduce the child to something which appears to be completely new and different, but something the child probably has some previous experience with. That is, the therapist's "Rock and Crystal Collection," put together especially for children in play therapy.

Some professionals' reaction to this rock and crystal idea is scepticism. They have the "prove to me that it works" look on their faces. Some people catch on right away and realize what a useful tool this could be for them to use. Come people question, "why a rock collection?"

Rocks and crystals come naturally from the earth. They can be raw, tumbled, polished, faceted, etc. Their colours are natural and beautiful. In ancient times they were worshipped. Nowadays, people still worship gems, especially in jewellery stores. In daily life, crystals are indispensable. For example, in electronics, crystals are used in timing devices, radios, electronic communications and in computers. Crystals are also used in telephone systems, hearing aids, spark plugs, lasers, souring powder and in the porcelain of toilets. Incredible.

But a rock and crystal collection for kids in play therapy? Recall yourself as a child walking along the beach looking for pretty pebbles. Perhaps collecting a pailful to look at. Remember how smooth they felt between your fingers? Remember the pretty sparkling steaks of different colours? Did you find flat stones that you skipped over the water, trying for the "world record" of 27 times? Did you ever find a fossil? Collecting pebbles/stones was a relaxing experience, finding a neat one was pretty exciting. The best part was quietly looking them over, meditating as to which one was the prettiest or best. Perhaps, what is most interesting to note is that, as an adult, you probably still like to go to the beach and find a nice looking pebble. Try it. That could be the start of your "Rock and Crystal Collection."

People like to look at and touch rocks and crystals. They like the colours, how they look and feel. They like to know where they came from and wonder why some are so smooth and shiny and others so jagged and sharp. The same goes without saying with kids who are in play therapy.

Imagine this: when children walk into the therapy room they notice a closed wooden box lying on the table or floor. Curiously, they approach the box and open it as if there is a treasure to be discovered on the inside. "Ooh, aah, look at all the rocks!" They are encouraged to pick them out, touch them (lick them if they must) and ask as many questions as they want. What the therapist does not know can be answered (hopefully) by the next session. Next, the therapist can ask children if they have ever collected rocks before, or, even more basic, have they ever seen some neat rocks before. Ta dah! A safe topic that they do not mind talking about. Notice as they talk they are touching and playing with the rocks more than ever. They may also begin to talk more animatedly and look directly into the therapist's eyes. Aren't rocks fun to look at?

Notice that the child is beginning to talk more about personal experiences from the past. Starting with rock collecting, nature, places they have been to and where they may have seen neat rocks (*i.e.*, a rock cut on a highway or a boulder by the school). Perhaps they may have experienced a "rock unit" in school and, thus, have a greater appreciation and knowledge base about rocks and crystals. Whatever happens, you will notice that the handling of the stones seems to open up the child's vocal cords. Pretty rocks and crystals can be very exciting, especially if the therapist makes them special.

A rock and crystal collection is useful to start a good trusting relationship between a therapist and child. Stones are solid, natural, innate. They do not break like plastic toys. They can be used creatively. Also, in good weather, time can be spent outdoors looking for special rocks. These rocks can turn out to be invaluable to kids in so many different ways.

For the therapist, to collect rocks need not be expensive. Rocks can be found anywhere: by the roadside, by lakes, in nearby quarries or at old mining sites. Inexpensive small stones can be bought in rock stores. Children's favourites tend to be any kind of quartz (eg. smoky, rose, rutilated, amethyst, tiger's eye), Herkimer diamonds, fluorite, malachite, halite (salt) in different colours, labradorite, sodalite, and mica. Some rocks and crystals may be found lying around in your own home area. However, if you wish to hunt for you own, it is important to dress accordingly, have a pail/knapsack, geological hammer, safety glasses, work boots, first-aid kit and plenty of mosquito repellent. Information on rocks and crystals can be found in any library. Just take the time to look and find a book that is right for you.

The results with children can be astounding. As they open up the box, faces light up. Oh, the beauty of rocks and crystals! Quiet children begin to chat. Loud children quiet down as they hold the stones and earnestly tell the therapist of their experiences. All energy is spent on touching, feeling and talking. Overwhelmed kids (be prepared) will not talk at first. Relax. They may be meditating on which stones they like the best. As soon as they find just the right ones they will also tell stories to the therapist. If they stay silent, there are many children's stories about rocks that can be told to help open the children up.

Questions that the therapist can ask are: Which stone do you like the best? Do the smooth/rough stones want you to tell me a story? What colours do you like the best? What feeling goes with that colour stone?

Stones are good to play with, as they are hard to break. If one does break, it is always be easy to replace. Since they are replaceable, they become vital when it comes time to say good-bye to children. What better gift to give but the rock/crystal they liked the most? It would be small enough to fit in a pocket and can be kept as an "emergency" rock for the children. For example, when they are going through a rough time they can pull out the rock from a pocket or from under a pillow to hold and touch as they hopefully recall play therapy sessions where it was safe and where coping skills were learned. Rocks and crystals may help the child to survive in the big world. It will be almost as if the particular stone was acting like a symbol of what the child had conquered or as an amulet to ward off "evil spirits."

For Julia, the "Rocks and Crystals Collection" opened up a new door. She loved to hold them and play with them. Clear quartz was her favourite. She shared many stories with her therapist which opened up parts of her younger life. It was a good start. After several months of intensive sessions it was time for Julia to

> leave for good. As she crossed over and through the play therapy door, she wore a new necklace with a quartz crystal as a keepsake and reminder of her healing time in the play therapy room.

A bonus to this is that it can bring a great joy for a therapist to collect rocks on their own, just for the fun of it.

WORKING WITH ANIMALS IN THE HEALING PROCESS

Animals are a link to our primitive roots. They take us to the past while grounding us in the present. This is an area where there is an abundance of research with regard to positive benefits. For example, it has been found that "a dog is able to exercise a calming influence in a situation that generates fear or stress" (Bergler, 1988, p. 47).

These benefits apply to children and adults. Further, it is a mutually beneficial relationship. It has been found that pulse rate and blood pressure in dogs and horses both show a significant fall as these animals are stroked by humans (Anderson & Gantt, 1966; Lynch & McCarthy, 1969, 1977; Lynch, Fregin, MacKie, & Monroe, 1974).

Certain uses of animals in therapy and rehabilitation have been around for some time. These include the use of dogs for the blind and deaf and horse-back riding for the disabled. But animals have a much broader working track record than even these.

Animals and pets can be very good for children. When a child is given responsibility for the care of an animal, there is the need to develop a routine and consistency. The child can also see how hard it may be for a pet to learn a trick and thus, metaphorically, identify with the animal. However, when a pet does learn some new trick or task, this serves to boost the self-esteem of the child. This will assist the child in dealing with other difficulties in life.

It is important to note that what a child learns through pet ownership will not automatically be generalized into social skills in human interactions.

> Love and sympathy displayed by a child for a pet are not always transferred automatically to the sphere of human relations. In other words, a pet can "teach" a child to love it, to identify and associate with it, but this does not necessarily mean that the child

> is able to identify with and understand other human beings. Here the parents must step in and supplement the educational process, encouraging the child to transfer his experiences with the animal to the interpersonal domain (Bergler, 1988, p. 54).

Animals may be beneficial in helping a child understand the life cycle. Through births and deaths of pets—most of which have significantly shorter life cycles than humans—the child can come to learn about life, death, memories, mourning, planning for the future, the different needs at different stages of a life cycle. Please note that this does not imply that you should run out and breed your cat or dog in order for your child to witness the birth process. There are far too many uncared for dogs and cats in the world already and, unless you are a breeder in the first place, I strongly recommend against taking this on as a task. It is far more work than the uninitiated can imagine and, unless you are a professional breeder, you may well add significant stress and resentment to your life rather than giving your child a positive experience. The inexperienced breeder who is simply dabbling will quite possibly cause harm to the animals as well.

One of the most important aspects of pet ownership is the loving touch that is part of a nurturing relationship with a domestic animal. Animals allow safe, non-exploitive touch. There are many studies that have definitively proved this benefit.

Pets have such positive potential. They are close to essential when we are mourning, alone, isolated. The elderly, disabled, and children all benefit from having a pet. As Dr. Leo Bustad, co-founder of the Delta Society—a non-profit organization dedicated to the study and application of the human/animal bond—has found that "when we care for others, we feel as if we are cared for. The pet gives the bereaved person a reason for going on—as well as a comforting, constant friend" (Pearce, 1991, p. 20).

Bergler (1988, p. 63) has described a number of benefits of pet ownership. These include:

- Tactile contact which has no sexual connotations and therefore carries no taboo. As George (1988) notes: animals "help children in a society that seems to frown upon excessive emotional expression. Hugging, fondling, petting, and kissing animals is usually accepted" (p. 403);

- Empathy, i.e. the feeling of being understood and loved by one's pet;

- A sense of one's own importance;

- The experience of loving and being loved;

- Feelings of closeness to nature;

- Security—the pet is always there, never judging, never rejecting. "Stressful events in the life of a child, such as the birth of a sibling or the illness or death of a family member, may be eased by an animal" (George, 1988, p. 403);

- The inculcation of socially desirable characteristics;

- Opportunities for play—Mummy or Daddy may be too tired, or too busy, or just absent, but Rover is always ready and willing to be a playmate;

- Enforced adoption of a regular daily routine. Although this is a general benefit, there are possible drawbacks. The kind of pet really needs to be geared to a child's developmental level. Likewise, the amount of the children's caregiver involvement in the pet's care must be modified depending on the child's age and developmental skills;

- Feelings of being needed.

What Kind of Animal (and where to find it)

Obviously, a child's age needs to be taken into account when considering the type of pet for a child. When obtaining any animal as a pet, a trip to the library or book store is a necessary first stop. Learn about the kind of pet you are thinking of obtaining. What kind of care does it need? How much attention, space, exercise, and so on does it need? Read through the books about this animal. Get some technical books about the species as well as some more child oriented books so your child will understand the needs of the animal. If the pet is intended for an office setting, keep a number of books in your office about the animal so everyone can have access to information. Whatever animal is used, it "must be nonaggressive at all times, tolerant of children, and quick to respond to the commands of therapist and child" (George, 1988, pp. 408-409).

Birds:

Birds, not exactly cuddly, have certain wonderful qualities. Some, like canaries, sing the most beautiful melodies. Be aware that pet store owners tend to charge more for male canaries because of their song qualities. First, this is somewhat of a scam. I have owned many canaries over the years. Darned if both males and females don't sing. Granted, the males sing a lot more, but females often do have quite a beautiful song. (And, yes, I am certain they were female—they both laid eggs, nested, and hatched the eggs and nurtured the young.) Next, pet stores like to charge more by calling a canary a male because of its reported singing qualities. Canaries are very hard to sex and it is unlikely the store really knows what sex the bird is. So the store guarantees that the bird is a male. If it doesn't sing amply in a certain number of days (usually 60 to 90), they guarantee you can return it for another "male." But really, who is going to own this little creature for three months, become attached to it, and then return it because it appears to be a female. Well, maybe misogynistic Freudians, but the average person is going to love it and want to keep it. The pet stores are in a no-lose position on this one. The best place to obtain your canary is from a specialty breeder or a store that is obviously knowledgeable and specializes in birds.

Budgies and cockatiels can make good pets and turn into very chatty companions and playmates. Prior to obtaining one of these birds, a child's caregiver should be aware that they can be more than just a little "chatty." They can screech for attention, scream when ignored, and be a royal bother with their demanding vocal and flapping antics. As with most pets, they need and deserve a great deal of attention and care in order to become positive companions. Both of these kinds of birds have a great deal of character, and each can be a real clown. They are in need of minimal physical care, but you should be prepared to give them time and attention.

Rodents:

These are minimal care creatures that can be a treat to watch. However, many of them are nocturnal and can be very grating as they burrow and dig, gnaw and bounce, and spin their little wheels at 3 a.m. This can also mean a lack of sleep for a child. Although these little animals involve minimal care, they do need to be fed daily and cleaned regularly. Failure to do this will mean a diminished quality of life, or an end of life, for the little animal. They are more useful in teaching the need for consistency and quality of care than they are as companions. An exception to this may be guinea pigs, which can become more sociable than the average rodent.

Fish:

Although fish have been shown to decrease anxiety and promote a calm and relaxed attitude, they obviously lack the cuddliness of a dog or cat. You can't even touch, hold or stroke them like you might be able to with a bird or rodent. Like rodents, they tend to be more useful in helping the child develop a care routine than in providing companionship or a playmate.

Their best use is for kids with severe allergies who may not be able to own furred or feathered creatures. They are also of great use in medical care settings. Their presence in medical and dental offices and waiting rooms has been shown to decrease the anxiety level of patients.

Exotic Animals:

Under no conditions whatsoever are these appropriate animals as pets for children. A major problem in the trade of exotic pets is the incredible rate of destruction involved in the capture, storage, and shipping of these animals. Their commercial trade is nothing short of a tragedy. Their domestic upkeep has an extremely high rate of mortality. Their life expectancy and/or quality is drastically reduced from their life in the wild.

Exotic animals tend to come from, and need, exotic environments. They should be left in their home environment. Avoid them as domestic pets. These kind of animals only serve to reinforce the ego of the person who desires to own them. Such people tend to have rather weak personalities and feel worthless and invisible. They believe that, if they own this very unique animal, they must be a unique and noticeable person. These people should get a life of meaning and not exploit animals. If you know people like this, they should be encouraged to find meaning in life by giving to others rather than by being noticed. If they want to feel unique and meaningful, let them volunteer several hours a week in a nursing home or at a local Humane Society.

Dogs:

Dogs are the animals most often used in pet-facilitated therapy. The reason for this is

> their constant willingness to give affection and tactile contact at all times and in all situations, together with that "innocent, child-like" trust which dogs unfailingly display towards humans. This reliance on the part of dogs elicits a reciprocal response from humans, who are prepared to put their trust in a dog (Bergler, 1988, p. 39).

Dogs can be held, they respond to love and affection and they really show appreciation for the relationship you have with them. Finally, they are potentially highly trainable. I will try and stay away from breed types here, but will need to mention a few with regard to research that has been conducted. Almost all dog (and cat) owners think the breed they own is the most intelligent and best there is on the face of the earth. This is good for the individual pet, but not a good reference in terms of choosing the best kind of pet for a child or a professional's office.

Although dog-owners may not like to admit it, some breeds are much smarter than others. Some, like a well bred German Shepherd, are both intelligent and cooperative. Some breeds are both stubborn and stupid, a very bad combination. Coren (1994) has ranked dogs on the basis of obedience and working intelligence and found that the highest ratings are obtained with the Border Collie, Poodle, German Shepherd and Golden Retriever. For use in the therapy process, we also need to consider nurturing qualities of the animal. George (1988) recommends German Shepherds and Newfoundlands as ideal types to be used in pet-facilitated therapy.

Although the German Shepherd is almost an ideal dog in many ways, this does not mean you should run out and get one. They are highly intelligent and loyal creatures and there is probably no better dog on the face of the earth than a well-trained German Shepherd. On the other hand, there is nothing worse than a poorly trained German Shepherd and there are far too many of these poorly trained creatures around.

Obtaining a dog is an issue that can raise emotions. Two of the most popular places to get a dog are pet stores and Humane Societies. I would avoid pet stores at all costs. I know folks who feel that you should only obtain a dog from the local Humane Society. By doing this you save a dog's life. I agree in principle, but in principle only. If I want a dog that is going to be used professionally around children or will live with children, a Humane Society is not going to be my first site to search. I am going to go to a reputable breeder. The Humane Society is a location where unwanted animals end up. They may be victims of abuse, neglect, or lack of care. We know that there is a certain kind and amount of socialization needed for ideal companion dogs. The Humane Society is not the best location to find properly socialized animals. However, they are certainly far above pet stores and puppy mills as good sources of pets. The professionals who work there are not in a profit making business and they do tend to care deeply for the creatures they take in. They do, in fact, have the best interests of the animal as their mandate. Approach the Humane Society with caution. Do not obtain a pet there on a whim or because it had "such sad eyes." Check out any dog obtained there with great caution. Take it outside on a leash to play. Watch how it relates to you. Does it cower in response to any particular kind of movement—or worse, growl and show a defensive response? As cute as this animal might be, as sad as its eyes might seem, avoid this timid or aggressive animal for a child.

Cats:

Well, cats are cats. This is the ultimate existential animal. "I purr, therefore I am. I am here, therefore I am worthy." In selecting a cat, like a dog, try and find a well socialized animal, ideally, one who has "stayed with his mother and litter mates for the first three to four months of his life" (Kilcommons and Wilson, 1995, p. 31). It is such a tragedy to find kittens as young as seven or eight weeks old in pet stores. That is far too young. If they are being sold at eight weeks, at what age was the poor thing taken away from its mother and littermates? No doubt the pet store owner will rationalize that they only "need" to be with their mother for the first four to six weeks. Physically, maybe, but even that cannot be justified. Kittens have physical and emotional needs. These are not met by early removal. If you are looking for a kitten at the Humane Society, choose the one

> who reaches out a soft paw through the bars, makes eye contact, is close to the front of the cage, and is basically trying in every way possible to interact with you (Kilcommons and Wilson, 1995, p. 27).

If you are getting a cat or dog for companionship, remember the animal needs companionship too. If you are away for many hours a day and are never there to provide company for the creature you hope will keep you company, better to get a fish or canary. Or get two cats—many people will argue against two cats but, if you obtain two at the same time, possibly littermates, they can be wonderful companions and playmates for each other. I happen to live with two cats (no one really owns a cat). They are sister Bengal leopards[4] and I have never for a second regretted living with the two of them. I am home a great deal of the time, yet, when I don't have the energy or time to play with one or the other, they find each other to play with.

Other Animals:

A number of other domestic animals have been used in therapeutic processes. For example, therapeutic riding programs involving horses are some of the oldest and most well developed of all animal facilitated programs in many areas of North America. The effectiveness of these programs has long since been shown to be of great benefit to children and adults with many kinds of handicaps—physical, emotional, mental. Early efforts in the late eighteenth century in animal-facilitated therapy involved the caring for farm animals by mental patients. Wildlife programs have been integrated into treatment programs. I have even recently been introduced to a program in Florida involving dolphins. Swimming with dolphins has even been used for chronic pain.

The Animal's Background

I will focus here on the use of the dog in pet-facilitated therapy, as this is the basis for most of the research to date. There is an optimum upbringing in the early development of the dog. The Monks of New Skete (1991) offer excellent developmental guidelines in the raising of puppies. Between four and six weeks of age, interaction within the litter is crucial to a pup's development. Under no circumstances should a pup be removed from the litter at this early stage.

> The sixth week (35-42 days) is pivotal in puppy development. The main emphasis of socialization begins to shift from mother and littermates toward human beings and the world beyond the nest (p. 51).

It is important in early contact with puppies to encourage and foster non-threatening eye contact, as this will lay a foundation for training and the development of a long term dog-human relationship. The puppy then needs to become accustomed to a number of humans, different ages of people, and the many sounds of the average home.

> From the fifth to the seventh week it is imperative that each pup be handled individually by different people, both men and women, every day (p. 59).

Obviously, all such socialization is going to be denied in puppy mills and cramped commercial environments. Optimum development and socialization—especially over the first three to four months—of the pup takes a great deal of time, energy, and care. As you can see, there is more to it than just buying a dog. Early socialization is only the basic beginning. The dog "should be well trained if it is to be used in the playroom or therapist's office" (George, 1988, p. 408). Such training takes a great deal of time and patience.

Research

There are positive physical and emotional results from including animals in treatment programs. It has been found that both angina and heart attack patients have a "400% better chance of survival if they owned a pet" (Bergler, 1988, p. 48). What was significant about this particular study was that the same result was found even when dog-owners were not included in the study. It was felt that there might be skewed results because of better physical fitness resulting from the need to walk a dog. It became clear that a decisive factor "is the anti-stress effect which the pet has on its owner" (Bergler, 1988, p. 48).

Pearce (1991) reported on a number of research efforts and found that: pet owners are more self-sufficient, independent, and optimistic; pet-owning children tend to be less aggressive with other kids; children with pets do better in social interaction and social integration; pet owners consistently score higher than non-owners in feelings of life satisfaction, self-esteem and overall well-being, and; pet owners are more responsible, more dependable, less egotistical and less self-centred.

Likewise, George (1988) has reported on numerous research studies pointing to positive aspects of the use of animals in therapeutic processes: studies of kindergarten children found that animals help children develop imagination; an animal in an unfamiliar room with a stranger present has a calming effect on children (based on systolic and diastolic blood pressure being lowered); animals play and bring children back into the reality of the relationship; children who develop sympathy for animals tend to be less destructive and more careful of other animate and inanimate objects; stressful events in the life of a child may be eased by an animal; animals can be particularly important for a child who is physically ill, helping the child maintain a fairly normal psychosocial development; children may be able to discuss many more problems and issues when an animal is present; an animal can help a child regress; animals are recommended with the young, nonverbal child, the withdrawn and socially disadvantaged child, and; pet-owning children score higher in being able to ask for needed help. They are also given a higher status by their peers; animals help children develop self-esteem, a sense of achievement, socialization, cooperation, and nurturance.

Using Animals in Work with Children

There are many techniques and methods for the use of animals in working with children. "The practicalities of using animals—pets as well as farm animals—are as limitless as the creativity of the therapist" (George, 1988, p. 416). Abby, the Dalmatian I mentioned earlier in the book, has, at times, been in a deep sleep during a session with a child. The child and I may have been playing or talking and suddenly Abby groans and almost sounds like a cow. The child asks "I wonder what Abby is dreaming." Obviously, I have an immediate entry to the child's world if I ask "I'm not sure. What do you think Abby might be dreaming?" Now the dog has become the object of the child's projection.

The child can be asked questions through the animal and this significantly increases a sense of safety and comfort for the child. For example: "Suzie, Abby wonders how you're feeling today" is much more likely to engage children in a discussion of their feelings than if they simply entered the room and were asked questions directly by an adult. This can work very well with even younger children.

I have had children comment about my canaries: "I wonder what they are singing." My reply would be something like: "I wonder that too. What do you think they are singing. Can you tell me the words to their song?"

Sometimes words become irrelevant.

> When an animal is used in psychotherapy, the need for language is reduced. While it is often easier for the child to express himself through acting out with the animal, the therapist must depend more on the posture, tone of voice, and facial expression of the child in interpreting what the child is trying to communicate. This means that the therapist must be trained in the dynamics of body language—as should any good play therapist (George, 1988, p. 409).

The animal does not criticize or judge. It doesn't degrade children by telling them how they are feeling or interpreting their art. Finally, and the most important issue of all, the animal accepts children without question. If the animal in the room happens to be a dog or a sociable cat, the cat can sit on the floor with the therapist and touch the animal while talking, drawing or playing. With a larger animal, like Abby the Dalmatian, kids can lie on them, lean on them and use them for pillows. This is a nurturing nest that serves as an ideal place to heal.

Footnotes

[1] All children know that you can see the wind. Many thousands of times they have been subjected to nagging lectures from teachers who try to emphasize that "you cannot see the wind, you can only see the effects of the wind." But kids know that you CAN see the wind. Too bad if teachers have never seen it.

[2] An estimated 40% of physicians in Germany have herbal preparations as their primary medicines.

[3] This is not meant to slam aspirin. It may, at times, be a very useful drug and of great benefit to many people's health. I am using it here as an example because it is well known and extensively used. I have used aspirin. I have used many modern drugs in their time and place. And I try to exercise, sleep, grow as much of my own food and herbs as possible, as many of my own medicines as possible. I get vaccinations. I make sure my children's vaccinations are up to date. I do not want anyone to get the impression that I think we should abandon decades of research and knowledge and return to the dark ages and operate on belief systems rather than facts and the experimental method.

[4] These are essentially domestic cats. They are one-eighth leopard. Not long ago, the Asian leopard was on the verge of becoming extinct, as it was a favourite prey of fur trappers. This wild cat was bred with certain domestic cats, such as the Egyptian Mau and Abyssinian, in order to preserve (not for the fur industry) the beautiful spotted and silk-like pelt while obtaining a domestic cat's personality. The result was definitely a beautiful animal, as well as a highly intelligent (keeping in ming my earlier comment that every dog owner thinks their dog's specific breed is the smartest on the face of the earth—by this point you can probably see that this also applies to cat owners), confident, and dependable pet. They, like any specialized breed, have their quirks and idiosyncrasies. They tend to love water and can be prone to joining you in the tub

or shower, in certain play they are known to growl rather than mew, and they have quite an affinity for climbing and viewing the world from the highest vantage point, and I mean highest vantage point—hey, what's that on the ceiling fan? Oh, it's just the cat. Or, where's the cat—check the ceiling.

CHAPTER **12**

Nature III... Working with Air...Fire...Water

AIR

I have written elsewhere in this book on the importance of breathing exercises for children. What I will deal with here are some of the more playful aspects of air.

Picking dandelions or milkweed as they have gone to seed and blowing the seeds to the wind.... Imagine that the seeds are actually fairy wings and make up stories about the world of the fairies. The scent of flowers fills the air. Flowers bring all the elements together: they dwell in the earth, yet reach to the air. They need both water and the energy of the sun to live and grow. Children can learn to treat flowers with protective respect.

Kites can promote family togetherness and teach children of the power of air. The family can build kites together and then sail them in a field. Watch the wind and air currents take the kite on soaring journeys. Look around and talk about what you each see around you on the ground. Then imagine what the kite can see from way up high in the sky.

Blowing bubbles can be an all around giggly activity. They float, they pop, they squirt. They can be followed into wondrous fairy lands. In northern climates where winter can be terribly cold, try blowing bubbles in the coldest weather and watch them freeze in mid-air.

Balloons bring mixed emotions. They can be fun for kids as well as tragic. They tend to symbolize parties and playtime. Tragically, children have died from choking on balloons while attempting to blow them up. Many young children have been frightened by a bursting balloon. Ecologically, despite their prettiness at the party, and even when disposed of properly in the garbage, balloons can spell doom for many species of birds who ingest them at the landfill site and either choke or have their digestive tracts blocked.

THE SOUNDS WE ABSORB

Sounds and music are nothing more than energy transformations that occur in air. Atoms and molecules vibrate and reach our ears and we perceive sound. The vibrations that we perceive as sound influence our thoughts and actions. They can tranquillize us and they can invigorate us. The mind of any human being, upon hearing sounds, sends energy through the nervous system.

> Traditionally, tribal peoples have employed power songs and group chanting for healing. In devotional and monastic traditions, mantras, invocations, and sung prayers have for centuries been considered to have healing powers.... Sound, in the form of tone, music, or chanting, works on the right hemisphere of the brain.... Healers who use sound have been discovering that it is a powerful instrument for releasing and balancing energies in the right and left hemispheres (Laughingbird, 1978, p. 276).

Music can create good times and bad times. Music can bring back memories of a childhood Christmas or a day at the local exhibition or fair. Sounds can tranquillize or terrify us. The gentle drops of a summer's rain or the soothing sounds of a bubbling stream flowing over rocks will have a very different influence on our mood than a powerful and intense waterfall or the howling rage of a hurricane slashing at our home.

Music soothes, relaxes, energizes us. Music can make a hectic moment tranquil, but it can also make a tranquil moment unbearable. Music has the ability to touch the soul.

Sounds of Nature

I live in an area where the sky is not obliterated by the lights of civilization. Standing outside my house late at night I can seen millions of stars glowing in the heavens. I hear frogs croaking, crickets chirping, loons "laughing" and nighthawks screeching. When I step outside late at night I feel nurtured by nature's sights and sounds. Or perhaps some sunny afternoon I am out on a country road in a country field and I hear the wind. The tall corn or wheat rustles with the breeze and I take a deep breath and smell the grains and wildflowers bursting everywhere. Listening to the breezes and bugs and birds is healing. It sends energy rushes through my spine and I feel my shoulders pull back.

When we are in civilized space too long, headaches creep in, shoulders curl inward, muscles tighten, car horns sound, tires squeal, sirens, the constant hummmmm of engines, air conditioners, streetlights.... All these send tension into our psyches.

This is not to imply that civilization is, in itself, bad. We can use its advances to our benefit. Being able to hear the music of Enya played on a CD in your living room is the end product of years of invention, discovery and extensive research. The machine which plays this music is a wonder of science.

SCENTS

The scents that enter our sensory awareness can have an effect on our emotional and physical well-being. Scents, perfumes, odours and the smells of nature, the earth and cities can influence moods, trigger old memories and even alter our way of perceiving the moment we are in the middle of experiencing. Ancient Egyptians are the first known culture to combine scents with bathing, adding perfumes and oils to their baths for the purposes of healing the body and soul.

Aromatherapy involves the use of natural aromatic substances to metaphorically help heal the soul. There is a literal aspect to this healing as well. We know that aromas and scents can influence the brain (Worwood, 1995, p. 25). Many scents can be used to create an ambience of nurturing and healing in the office or home environment. An excellent guide to the use of scents and aromas is Worwood (1995).

NATURE MEDITATIONS – FIRE

Only recently have we begun to reawaken to the power of positive thinking, of prayer, of making wishes and of healing words. Each of these can have beneficial effects on the world. We are beginning to realize that perhaps there is something more dynamic to these processes than simply self-fulfilling prophecy or "wishful thinking."

For this exercise you will need a safe place to light a fire. This may be a woodstove, a fireplace indoors, perhaps a copper kettle or some bricks surrounding some earth outdoors. A campfire would do nicely.

The assumption behind the exercise is that if we think it and imagine it, then what we wish for can come true.

> If there is something of great importance for you, something you would like changed in your life or a wish you would like to come true, a healing you would like to see fulfilled...focus on what it is you would like to see happen...create and enter your sacred space...take all the time you need to get a very clear image of the situation being changed....
>
> In making your wish do not make wishes that directly alter the behavior or views of others. It would not be right to try to control others without their permission, even though you may think what you are wishing for may be well intentioned. An exception to this may be a healing request for someone in a crisis situation from whom you are not able to get approval. For example, several years ago a dear friend had entered a medical crisis situation quite suddenly and was in the intensive care unit of a local hospital. There was no way to physically be in touch with him. Some friends and I decided to gather and participate in a healing ceremony dedicated to his well-

being. The decision was actively made to participate in this event in which we all offered our prayers and wishes for a healthy recovery even though we had not asked his permission or even spoken with him. With regard to prayer for others without their consent, Larry Dossey, in *Healing Words*, notes that "I would maintain that as long as our efforts are filled with compassion, caring, and love, there is little reason to fear that our prayers for others without their consent are somehow unethical."[1]

Please note there is a definite difference between wishing for the well-being of others and wishing someone, other than yourself, would change or do something you would like. Always focus on the well-being of everyone.

Close your eyes and think, sense, feel and see what you want to happen. See it happening. Watch the results of this change. What are the repercussions of such a change? Is this really what you want? When you are clear about the matter and when you can get an image of both what it is you want changed and the implications that such change will have on the world, you are ready for the next step in this exercise....

Write your wish on a small piece of paper...use virgin parchment paper such as that used for calligraphy...write it out in red ink...red is the colour of the life force that flows through our bodies....if you can, use a calligraphy pen or some other pen that is refillable with ink—or best of all, a quill pen that is only used in very special moments for writing of intense significance to you...make your own ink using natural dye from flowers, herbs in your garden (go to a library to find methods of doing this. This could be a whole new journey for you. Libraries can be wonderful places with offerings of so many new things to learn)...do not be ambiguous or vague in your writing. Do not go on at length. Simply and clearly write out what you would like to see exactly as you would like to see it. After you have finished writing, continue to sit with an image in your mind of the situation being changed, your

> desired wish fulfilled.... See the process happening and then see the results after it has occurred. Know that this can happen.
>
> When you feel this phase of the exercise is whole and complete, hold onto your paper. Feel the importance of it. Next, light the paper and set it on fire. Let the energy from the fire enter the world with your message...put the burning paper in the campfire or fireplace or container you have set aside for exercises such as this.... See the smoke from the fire entering the world.... The energy of thoughts and images you have so carefully applied to this process goes off into the very real being of the world, influences it and the desired change begins. See this happening. Know it can happen.

Getting Rid of Negatives

Like the exercise above for sending your wishes out into the universe, we can also rid ourselves of negatives in the same way. What we wish to rid ourselves of should be written or drawn on a piece of paper. Set the paper afire and allow the negative to be changed into only ashes which are returned, harmless, to the earth.

For some further readings in this area, refer to two works of Larry Dossey, M.D.: *Healing Words: The Power of Prayer and the Practice of Medicine* (1993) and *Space, Time and Medicine* (1982).

NATURE MEDITATIONS – WATER

Children have a natural affinity for the elements and water is no exception. A catalyst to endless hours of a child's play can be puddles and streams on a neighbourhood street. Splashing, building, damming, rerouting...the creation of whole new worlds. Puddles have brought more joy and growth to the lives of children than the billions of dollars spent on the many consumer products of the corporate child exploiters.

What wonderful creations develop when the elements of water and earth are combined! Mud, sand castles, dirt worlds are all intensely sensuous. Touch and tactile stimulation are healing. Playing with mud and water and the earth are healing. "We're going to play in the mud" is a life affirming statement of joy from children. Pity any child who is scared to play in the mud for fear of getting dirty.

"The creek," if a child is lucky enough to live near one, is often the most fascinating place in a child's life. I was fortunate to live near such a creek. Many long hours were spent racing sticks with friends, imagining just where the fairies lived and hid (twilight was an enchanting time in the fields, woods and creek near my childhood home), picking raspberries in the huge fields of wild berry bushes that grew near the creek, skipping stones across the water.

> Water is very mysterious for the young child: how quickly the icicle melts which only a little while ago was hanging from the roof glistening in the sunshine. the child's small hand scoops up water, but the water does not stay there: it runs out through her fingers. And how mysterious it is to look down into water. The depths are so very dark, while the heavens are reflected on the surface, and the child discovers her own reflection there. Or the experience of rain: how quickly it can change the child's world! The rain creates puddles, those miniature lakes in the street and on the pavements.... There is an old German country saw which describes the rain as a friend to children:
>
> Rain in May brings joy to earth
> So if on us it showers,
> We too will gladly grow
> Like grass and flower (Ingeborg, 1987, p. 55).

In watching any natural flow of water the child can also experience the seasonal flow of life. The life flow is at its fullest in the summer when bees buzz, birds sing, insects chirp and buzz, water bubbles over stones, and flowers send their enchanting scent for all the world to enjoy. Then comes autumn with its gradual decrease in temperatures, changes in vegetation. For those who live in cooler climates, there will be the falling of leaves. These leaves flow along streams, filling the yard. What romping fun to pile leaves and jump in them all day long. With winter in cooler climates comes a freezing. Ice forms beautiful patterns on the surface. What shapes and stories form in these shapes. Finally, with spring the joy of rebirth. The melt, the increased flow, a great increase in activity.

For children who are not fortunate enough to live near a clean and safe natural water source, they need not be deprived. Regular trips to the river or the lake or seashore with a caregiver can bring much joy. A child of the inner city can enjoy nurturing playtime using simply a bucket and water or two little pots and something to dip in the pots like a spoon or spatula.

Water is essential to life...without enough water in our lives—literally and symbolically—we become harsh, shrivel and eventually die, spiritually and physically.... I remember once living in a city with no real water source—there was no river, lake or ocean nearby.... It always felt symbolically hot in that place.... It was not a good place for me to be and eventually it was necessary for me to leave for spiritual and emotional survival...living beings need water.

Water is also important to our spiritual lives. Water is where our soul reaches its depth.... If you are feeling a lack of nurturing in your life—maybe you feel the need to be nurtured more or to give to others and nurture more...you are in a healing process...you wish to pass through a rite of purification...or perhaps you wish a new career or job, or for good things to happen in your life in general....

Throughout the ages, water has been considered healing and cleansing[1]—symbolically and literally purifying. Thousand of years into the past, the Egyptians and other ancient cultures used water and bathing as a way of healing the spiritual and mental aspects of one's life.

The following exercise can be used to be in touch with water on the physical, emotional and spiritual levels:

> You can go to a lake or stream or the ocean...or you can pour water in your own tub...sit by the water and see an image of your desired goal in the water...when you really feel you can see and sense the goal being reached, let yourself enter the water...allow yourself unlimited time to exist within the water...as you are covered by the water...sense the goal envisioned in the water being fully absorbed into every cell of your being...deep into your heart and soul.
>
> You are opening yourself up to your own potential for change in this process. Through this bathing process you are opening

the door and giving permission for new things to happen in your life.

When you leave the tub or outdoor water, stand naked and sense the water which has intertwined with your body. As the remaining water on your body evaporates, feel it taking your desire out into the universe where it will come to be.

A nice addition for this exercise is to add some herbs or flowers to the water as you are preparing to enter it. Pick something that will amplify your desired wish or heighten the desired feeling.

Many herbs which can be used in this way are easy to grow or obtain. For a real sense of wholeness and completion of a journey, use as many herbs as possible that you or a friend have grown.

Some recommendations:

Chamomile. If you wish to be calmed put some chamomile stalks and flowers into your bath water. Its scent is very soothing. This can be used in a calming ceremony to promote restfulness or to help rid yourself of stress after a difficult period of life or a hard day at work. As it is a rather easy herb to grow, you could grow it yourself. You could take some herbal tea bags and open up one or two to let the chamomile spill into your bath water. You may find it at the side of a road or in a field. It is easily recognized by its flowers and scent.

Peppermint. For healing or purification. Use in your bath water during a phase in the healing cycle when you are wishing to feel stimulated or inspired. Like chamomile, pure peppermint tea is readily available. You could open up a tea bag and let the contents fall into the tub water. If you are able to grow or find fresh peppermint, just before entering the water, rub some peppermint leaves on your forehead or temples and feel the power of the peppermint going to work instantly. If you do decide to grow your own peppermint, be cautioned. It would be best to grow it in a pot or an old oak barrel or somehow contain it. Peppermint tends to spread easily and take over other parts of the garden.

Clover. For a sense of protection or for a feeling of youthfulness. You can put some in your bath or carry some with you. If you are including clover in the tub and wish to feel protected, put several stalks of clover in the water before getting into the tub. Lie in the tub and focus on the clover. Hold the flower up and breathe in. Notice the kind of protective scent it exudes. As it floats around in the tub see the beautiful and gentle colours of the clover flowers. Allow yourself to absorb the feeling you sense coming from the clover.

Lavender. As part of a purification process. This is one where we only recommend fresh lavender leaves and flowers be used. There is a world of difference between fresh lavender and lavender that has been dried and stored and used in sachets and potpourris. The latter can be intrusive and overwhelming. On the other hand, fresh lavender scent feels respectful, magical, cleansing and inviting. A mild scent of lavender oil has actually been shown in clinical tests to aid in sleep in the elderly with insomnia.

Periwinkle. To aid in thoughts of protection or renewal and symbolic rebirth. Periwinkle is another hardy and stable little plant that grows under some adverse conditions. Float a number of periwinkle flowers in the tub water around you and lie there focused on this natural beauty. See yourself as safe and sheltered. Life begins anew.

Rose. Love, love, love. Its shape, colour, and scent. What better method to promote a feeling of love. To give yourself the best of love luck, scatter and toss fresh rose petals in the bedroom on your honeymoon. When you are working to increase a sense of love in your life (and remember the best way to get love is to show and give love and kindness to others), include some fresh rose petals in your bath. You may add some rose water. Real rose water is available at many bath and scent shops these days.

Sandalwood. For a powerful sense of healing, protection or purification, add some sandalwood oil to your bath water. Since it is unlikely you have grown your own sandalwood, you can obtain sandalwood oil from bath and scent shops, or you could simply burn some sandalwood incense in the bathing area prior to your bath.

Oak/Thyme. Strength, stability, endurance. You may have a long run tomorrow or a swimming championship coming up. Perhaps you are entering the hospital soon for surgery. To symbolize your desire to be healthy and strong, take a meditative bath and put three or four oak leaves in the tub to focus on. Perhaps put some thyme in as well. Crush some of the thyme in your fingers before you put it in the tub. Inhale the scent and feel renewed, refreshed and ready to take on this upcoming task.

Cedar. To purify and heal. Take some fresh cedar and crush it in your fingers. Inhale the scent and let it flow through your entire body. Allow it to enter every cell in your body and fill your whole being and soul.[2]

Learn about herbs, wildflowers and trees from naturalist field guides such as Audubon or Peterson guides. Take a workshop on cooking with herbs or herbal gardening. Go to the library to discover and explore some books on herbalism. Herbs have been used in many ways throughout history and by different cultures. Enjoy the benefit of what you learn. Share the benefits of your new knowledge and skill with others. Have a friend or friends over for a dinner you have prepared using herbs you have grown yourself. As an offering, give them a little herbal collection that they can use in their own bath water.

Footnotes

[1] An exception to this occurred during the times of the fourteenth and fifteenth century when anything beautiful was considered a work of the devil. Even bathing was considered evil. It was thought by certain church writers that any exposure of the naked body, including during washing or bathing, was sinful. This was taken quite seriously. Apparently, upon the death of Thomas a Becket, his body clothing and linen simply fell to pieces when there was an attempt to remove it. It was rotted and caked with filth and lice.

[2] Please do not take this discussion to imply that if you have a cut, you should put cedar on it to heal. Nor does clover, by itself, protect you, and so on. Each of these plants is metaphoric of a process.

CHAPTER **13**

Nature IV... The Wheel of The Year Cycles of Life

INTRODUCTION

I am often asked what I consider to be the greatest problem facing the world today—is it crime, poverty, lack of government funding for social programs, bleah, bleah, bleah. No, really, I think the greatest problem on the face of the earth today is an alienation from nature and our own spirituality. As a result of this alienation, we have an unwise use of resources. A big threat to the natural balance is overpopulation. People and pollution: these are our greatest problems. The greatest loss we have suffered as we have become "civilized" is our fading awareness of our dependence on nature and of our relationship with the spiritual. Of the many changes that modern technology has delivered,

> perhaps the deepest and least understood is [our] loss of the land, of weather, of growing things, and of the knowledge of [our bodies] that these things give (Reich, 1971, p. 188).

We have refrigerators to keep our food cold, ovens to create our fires, furnaces for our warmth in winter, air conditioners to eliminate the sensation of heat in the summer, offices with permanently sealed environments, and so on.

There was a time not so many decades ago when tribes spent lifetimes in the same location. In a similar environment for generations, individuals learned to read the signs of nature, signs of change, signs of stability. There were cultural ceremonies celebrating the changes of the year. We have lost much of this in our modern urban environment. Such a loss, such trends

> cannot be counteracted merely by providing public playgrounds, or by organized walks, for nature speaks much more spontaneously and intimately than this to the young child. [There is a] despair which can come over children when the experience of nature is taken from them little by little—as happens in the cities when one natural playground after the other is built upon (Haller, 1991, p. 85).

In the natural flow of life, there is an interconnectedness of all. The very word ecology

> means the relationship of organisms to each other and to their environment. The word ecology is derived from the Greek, oikos, meaning household, and in this instance, the household is the whole earth (Sisson, 1987, p. 160).

The tide ebbs and flows. Life ebbs and flows. The sun and moon each rise and set. The moon has cycles of its own—the dark of new moon gradually turns to the light of full moon, followed by a decrease. The cycle is repeated throughout time. Even a child in an inner city core who has never seen a horse or a field can come to gain an awareness of natural cycles simply by following the sun and moon.

BRIDGES AND PASSAGEWAYS

The Cycles of Life

Life is cyclical. What we plant in the autumn gives us beautiful flowers in the spring. Life arises and life disappears.

In each of our lives, we travel from place to place, both literally and symbolically. We also travel from one phase of life to another. A child is born...the child is welcomed to its family and culture...the child begins school...graduates...finds a partner and mate...marriage...divorce...death...funerals...there is life, there is death, there is rebirth. We leave one thing behind and begin another. We need rites of passage for our changes and transitions in life. These serve as bridges from one place or stage to the next. There is a sad lack of ritual and ceremony in the modern world. This lack leaves many clinging to obsessive rituals, rigid manners, and superstitious beliefs. There are times and places for rites of passage. We need methods for crossing from place to place. In our emotional and spiritual lives we also need such processes. Any time you are entering a new phase of life or a new psychological process, you can visualize a bridge moving into this new area of life.

An example of a symbolic ceremonial act to acknowledge an important moment in life is the Celtic habit of planting a tree to honour the birth of a child.

We need such symbolic passageways throughout our many changes in life. These bridges and ceremonies acknowledge and honour the changes and growth. They also allow us to grieve and leave old ways behind. Therapists need to build bridges into their work with children. Parents need to build ceremonies and rituals into the ongoing life of the family.

TRANSITIONS

Our culture does not help its young move into adulthood. We act as if we resent or even hate our teenagers and offer them no means of symbolically reaching and entering adulthood on the other side. We seem to just sit back and hope they make it without getting killed by drugs, an automobile fatality, or a drive-by shooting. The transition to adulthood takes several years. The rite of passage is a beginning. Today's rites of passage include many self-destructive rituals and activities like gang involvement. There are some positive rites of passage. One of these is the leaving of home to go to university. But most children do not get to go to university. Only some get the opportunity. The rite of passage needs to be the catalyst for entry into adulthood. Transitions begin with separations. The transition ends with a party—such as the graduation celebration. Things worth doing are certainly worth celebrating.

The entering of the new phase can be acknowledged with "You are now old enough...."

With new rights come new responsibilities. Children should be expected to have a part time job, to contribute a small percentage to their family and to save a percentage toward their education or to have increasing responsibility for some household duties.

With beginnings come endings. One cannot exist without the other. We need to acknowledge endings, divorces, death. Ceremonies are needed for endings. After a year and a day (which allows a full year to pass), a party could be held to end the period of mourning.

If you are working with a child in therapy, the time of an ending needs to be acknowledged. It will be important to draw in the caregivers as well so the acknowledgement is not just something abstract that happens in therapy.

CYCLES

As we journey through life we need a familiar place around which to orient ourselves, a reference point. In our life journey such a reference point brings us safety and security. A meaningful place to begin to centre ourselves would be to follow natural cycles: the changing seasons, day and night, lunar processions. We each have to find our own symbols of our place of sanctuary on the Earth. In the modern corporate state, many people are cut off from life, from the natural cycles of life.

To understand life and nature and cycles we need to be in touch with ourselves and our own rhythms. We breathe. Our hearts beat. We sleep and wake. Members of our species and other species live and die and are reborn. We see the sun and the moon rise and set. The seasons come and go. As we actively participate in our own lives and the life of our planet we become more connected. "Since ancient times Nature's rhythms have been signals for celebration, helping people to deal with their fear of Nature's powers and to express their gratitude for her generosity.... Festivals raise us above the daily grind, revitalize us, and strengthen communities" (Oldfield, 1994. p. 242).

In some ways, our culture does mark cycles since we do tend to celebrate birthdays. We need many other remembrances as well. Reminders of the ancient ones, our ancestors. We need to remember those who have died. A celebration of life on the date of death of a loved one. A celebration of new life on the date of death of a relationship. We celebrate wedding anniversaries but not divorce. We need to celebrate the endings as well. They open doors to new worlds we have entered. They offer new opportunities, beginnings.

Celtic Cycles

From the perspective of my own Celtic background there is a solid emphasis on lunar cycles. This is not entirely what many might consider superstitious, since we know that even tides are influenced by lunar cycles. Following lunar cycles can help a child learn about rebirth, about hope. Indeed, as sure as the moon wanes and becomes smaller for two weeks, after the darkness there comes an increase until again there is fullness.

"For people dependent on the seasonal rhythms of the earth, the movements of the sun and moon were vital" (Sharkey, 1979, p. 75). The cycles and rhythms of the year are clearly marked in the Celtic calendar. This tool of measuring where we are in the year was agriculturally based. Unfortunately, much "new age" and "occult" gobbledegook has been placed on the Celtic calendar, but such fads pass and the depth of Celtic beliefs remains as always. In the Celtic framework the day and the month are each divided into two halves depending on available light. In each day there is light, daytime, and there is darkness, night time. Similarly, in the Celtic month, there are two halves, each of which correspond to a lunar phase. The cycle of light involves the waxing moon. This is the time from new moon to full moon. The cycle of darkness, during the waning moon, stretches from full moon to new moon.

The actual Celtic annual cycle was agriculturally based, not solar or lunar based, for very practical reasons. It was

> adapted to the husbandry of an agricultural population whose livelihood depended on corn-growing, stock-raising and dairy produce, with ploughing in the early spring, calving and abundance of milk in the early summer, harvest in early autumn and storage in early winter: that was their annual cycle of work (Danaher, 1981, p. 223).

There is none of the new age hocus pocus on any of these festivals that many modern esoterics try to create. These festivals were equidistant in time and were celebrated based on solar equinoxes (they took place 45 or 46 days after a solstice or equinox). The actual solar solstice and equinox did not seem to have been the days of celebration that they would become later, with more modern Celtic observance.

Thus, Samhain, the Gaelic word for the month of November, marked the end of one year and the beginning of a new year. Since inclement weather would be coming soon, it was expected that all crops be in by this point in time:

> all provision of food, fodder and fuel should be stored away. Cattle were put in byres and sheep were folded. No more fruits, domestic or wild, were picked. Fishermen drew up their boats and repaired and stored their gear.... Many fairs were held.... These, too, were occasions for general family outings for a day's enjoyment in the local market town.... In some areas great bonfires were lit. Every household had a festive supper at which young and old feasted on rustic goodies and took part in marriage divination games. Groups of young people in disguise or fancy dress went about collecting minor tribute from the householders and often playing tricks upon the ungenerous (Danaher, 1981, p. 219).

Obviously, we have here the origins of what would become known in North America as Hallowe'en. It has certainly changed in meaning over the years.

The other great festivals of the Celtic year were Imbolc, Bealtaine and Lúnasa. Imbolc, on February 1, is considered to be the first day of spring, since the weather was improving and ploughing could soon begin and fishermen prepared to go to sea. It was a time to seek blessings. St. Brigit's crosses were put up in both house and stable. Again, masked children went from house to house.

Fortunately, North American commercial marketing strategists have not yet picked up on this one! In this case, the masking tended to represent something about the Saint, and her blessings were called down upon the houses visited (Danaher, 1981).

The first day of summer was known as Bealtaine and occurred on May 1.

> Summer was welcomed by strewing of flowers, by setting up green or flowering branches or decorated May bushes. Bands of young people, bearing bushes, garlands and other emblems of May and singing songs to welcome the summer, went from house to house, receiving small gifts from the householders (Danaher, 1981, p. 218).

Bealtaine celebrates the end of winter, the returning flowers and warmer days, which are the harbingers of the fertile summer. It is a time to sleep outdoors overnight, make love, arise to drink water from a well before dawn, and return to the village with flowers and leaves twined through the hair. At Bealtaine, the ordinary laws of morality are suspended. It is a time for sexual license. It is a time to ignore restrictions and previous commitments, and in the exuberant transition into summer, fall in love. For centuries May was considered an unlucky month in which to get married; it was the month for illicit romance, not marriage, and couples who wished to marry waited until June, thus making that month the traditional wedding month. However, any child conceived at Bealtaine was considered sacred, the offspring of the God of Fertility and the Goddess of Spring.

The first day of autumn arrives on August 1, Lúnasa. This is also the beginning of the first harvest. It is a time to reap the harvest of our year's actions. As a harvest time, it is a festival of bread. It is also a time of baking with all the fresh crops providing berries and other yummy fillings for pies. Another playful harvest celebration activity involves the making of corn dollies, originally created from

> the last sheaf of reaped wheat. The stems were braided together to make a roughly human shape – the personification of the Mother Goddess of the harvest. Such a treasure remained in the lucky house for a year, guarding it, until the dolly was destroyed and a new one fashioned (Cunningham & Harrington, 1988, p. 142).

Each festival in traditional Celtic culture is the first day of a Celtic season, each was regarded as bringing a change in weather conditions, each marked an important change in the daily work of the farmer or fisherman, all had ceremonies and invocations to ensure protection and blessing during the summer season. Each was a time for fairs, payment of debts, divination of the future (once again—betwixt and between being times when entry to the Otherworld is closer), festive ceremonies were observed, groups of youngsters took part in masks and processions, and supernatural forces and beings were considered to be very active (Danaher, 1981). Later in history, the solar cycles would come to be included in Celtic ceremonies and the equinoxes and solstice would be acknowledged.

Many earth oriented cultures celebrate similar festivals and cycles. A child does not have to live on a farm or out in the woods to be taught about, to appreciate, and to enjoy these cycles. In fact, the further one is removed from nature, the more important it becomes to connect with nature by honouring such cycles and festivals.

Daily Rhythms: Each day we both fall asleep and we awaken. The sun rises and sets as does the moon. There are many cycles and rhythms we cannot see. We may not even directly be aware of them or feel them. Physiologically, our entire body is on a cycle over a given day. For example, levels of melatonin rise and fall in our body depending of time of day, amount of sun and other factors. Our body naturally prepares us for sleep by releasing melatonin, providing it is not blocked by certain factors such as medications and stress. We are active and we rest over the course of any twenty-four hour period.

Weekly Cycles: As there are few apparent "natural" weekly rhythms, these tend to be acquired through repeated activity. However, Dr. Michaela Glockler (1994) does note that there is a certain

> inherent seven-day biological rhythm which is evident in the healing process of many infectious diseases [like pneumonia, measles, and typhus] (p. 282).

In the past the week had predictable activities. There was a wash day, a cleaning day, a Sunday-go-to-meeting day. We need to build in predictable weekly activities. The Sunday dinner, a lost tradition in many homes, should be reclaimed. In my Irish Catholic home, we always had fish and chips on Friday, since it was the day to fast from meat. I still love to eat fish and chips on Friday. It brings back loving memories of life at home and sitting on a couch in the living room window of our second storey flat, watching Dad cross the street to the fish and chips store and then seeing him come back out with the fish and chips wrapped in a newspaper. Our Friday dinner was fun, playful. My dad had the next 2 days off work and I knew the whole family would have some playtime together and that Dad would be a part of it all. What a wonderful feeling with which to end the week. Oldfield (1994) notes that "with a little thought we can establish routines to fit with our own lifestyles. For example, if there is only one day in the week when there is time for a leisurely family breakfast, we can make it a special occasion by, perhaps, serving food that the family does not have during the rest of the week. These special family rhythms are welcomed by the child" (p. 241).

Monthly Cycles: There are many monthly cycles. These actually approximate lunar monthly cycles rather than calendar months. Every 28 days the moon is full, every 28 days it is dark. There is a time in the month for planting (when the moon is waxing) and a time for harvesting (when the moon is waning). The closer a culture is to the earth and the flowing cycles of nature, the more likely its activities relate to such lunar cycles.

Lifetime Rhythms

All living things are born, grow, reach maturity, deteriorate and die. We need rites of passage for entering each new phase.

Birth. In many cultures, upon the birth of a child, a tree is planted. This was part of my own Celtic upbringing. I was amazed to learn over the years how many cultures practice this wonderful ritual. "From Switzerland and Sweden to Java and Africa, trees are planted as a way of commemorating the introduction of the child into society" (Dunham *et al.*, 1991, p. 156).

Past, Present, and Future. We can find our place in the natural flow of life by honouring our past, living in the present and having hope for thc futurc.

Family photo albums are one of the very best ways of remembering and honouring the past. Different members of the family should be involved in putting these together. Family evenings or afternoons can be spent deciding which pictures to put in, what notable quotes to include and what little memorabilia to place in a cherished spot in the family album. Things like leaves collected on the trip through the Berkshire Mountains, the ticket from the plane ride to Texas, a little plastic bag with sand from the beach on the coast of Prince Edward Island, a bill or the menu from the favourite little restaurant you stopped at in downtown Kingston,[1] the flyer about whale watching from Bay Bulls in Newfoundland. Each of these treasures can be included in the family album. Although these family photo albums are usually associated with one's family of origin, I think they have great use for many children in foster care. Each new family the child lives in becomes a part of that child's history. Too often the impact of these families is devalued and too often children are just supposed to forget the past family and get on with the new. This is a cruel injustice to both children and the families with whom they shared a part of their lives.

Annual Cycles:

A New Year

Every January 1 (Or November 1—Celtic, or February—Chinese, or another date depending on the culture) is a new year. It is a time for rebirth. A time to wipe the slate clean and start over. Once a year there are birthdays, anniversaries of marriages, deaths and other events, and remembrances of things past.

Winter Festivals

In many religions and cultures throughout the world there is a tradition of honouring the birth of God, the Son of God, or the Sun God that is held at the darkest time of the year. This is "an ancient belief based on the returning power of the sun and the lighting of candles and fires is an important ritual" (Oldfield, 1994, p. 255). For the Jew there is Hanukkah, a festival of lights that features the lighting of candles. For the Christian it is the time of Christmas. Since no one really knows the date or place of birth of Jesus, in the year 435, the church voted to celebrate the birth of Christ on December 25, the time of the ancient Roman celebration of Saturnalia when candles were lit to ward off evil spirits. With German influences, homes started to honour the birth of Christ with the Christmas tree, a symbol of life, adorned with candles. Today, millions of homes feature a modern adaptation of this with the use of tiny electric lights replacing candles.

Spring Festivals

This is the time of rebirth. Winter is conquered. The days lengthen and by the spring equinox in March the length of sunlight grows greater than the length of darkness. Christians celebrate rebirth through the festival of Easter. This is a celebration taken from the ancients. Even the name reflects ancient fertility rites. The date for the celebration of Easter likewise reflects ancient cultural practises predating the birth of Christ. Easter is celebrated every year on the first Sunday following the first full moon after the spring equinox. The Chinese, Hindus, Jews, and Buddhists all similarly celebrate some great festival of rebirth or of victory of good over evil at this time.

This is a time of great awakening. Caregivers should be spending time outdoors with their children showing them the many little sprouts which are poking up through the ground – the bulbs and seeds planted with the child during the previous autumn. It is also a time when many seeds can be planted. For a young child, fast sprouting plants like radishes and carrots can bring observable results in just a few days. Even the youngest children can help dig the tiny furrows necessary for radishes and carrots. They can help water the plants on a regular basis and they can help pick their harvest in just a few weeks. From there, the harvest can go to the kitchen for the preparation of a salad and the children will have accomplished a great feat of helping to supply nourishment for their families. These are the tools of true self-esteem building. Children who are nurtured and have learned to nurture in this way will not need sappy and misguided self-esteem exercises. Nor will they need the behaviourist's gold stars or charts. A deeply loved child of the earth will never need a therapist. As mentioned earlier in this book, therapy is for people who don't have friends or inner resources – without friends, faith and hope, a desperation results. With loving caregivers, a garden and real quality time, self esteem emerges naturally.

Summer Festivals

Summer is the season of fullness and of growth. Muslims honour the prophet Muhammad and celebrate his birthday in the summer. This is the time when the sun has reached its fullest. It is a time for rejoicing and playing, a time to passionately embrace nature at its fullest.

Autumn Festivals

The classic modern day autumn festival in North America is Thanksgiving, held in October in Canada and November in the United States. This is a joyous and wonderful festival both celebrating the harvest and giving thanks for rebirth in a new land. This is a time in many cultures for celebration of the harvest and a time to mark the end of gathering and preparing for winter.

CELEBRATE

In your own family it is important to honour your past. Develop family festivals to honour your own culture. You may have many cultures in your family tree. Take aspects of each and turn them into family ceremonies. If you are working with children, learn about their cultural backgrounds and help them celebrate the festivals of cycles from their own culture. This is more important for some cultures than others. For example, Iranian children of Persian descent will likely have great pride in their culture. "Iranians are nostalgically tied to the past. For an Iranian, loss of Persian identity is shameful" (Behjati-Sabet, 1990, p. 96). Laotian and Cambodian children are likely to have celebrated the Buddhist New Year in their family histories. This takes place in April. It is actually celebrated at a time marking the end of the dry season in Laos. Thus, with rain, comes renewed growth. To Christian children, Christmas and Easter are the most important celebrations. They mark the birth, death and resurrection of Christ.

You are doing no one a favour if you try and help children acknowledge the cycles of life and wheel of the year in a way that is not culturally and spiritually appropriate to them. Take the time to learn about the cultural background of people with whom you work, the celebrations of the culture, the religion of the family. Celebrate their uniqueness. Experience the beauty of their festivals and discover the strength they find from their religion.

Footnotes

[1] For those of you ever lucky enough to visit "Canada's best kept secret," otherwise known as Kingston, Ontario, don't miss Chez Piggy, Kirkpatricks, or the Toucan. Each is joyfuly quirky in its own way.

CHAPTER **14**

Special Issues

LOSS – THE GRIEVING CHILD

There are many losses in any child's life. Some of these are natural and wonderful. Some are tragic. When children begin to speak they have lost their preverbal exclusive nonverbal communication. When they go to school for the first time they lose a part of their childhood. Many of these processes are important and desirable. But they are also endings that can lead to grief and we may forget to acknowledge the pain of growth. We think that all developmental change is wonderful and without emotional pain. Children going off to high school have made great steps, but they are also leaving a part of their childhood self behind. They may be very scared and insecure about taking this very big next step.

Death and endings come to the lives of many children. A parent may die. A friend may drown. A best friend may be gunned down in a drive-by shooting. Their beloved dog or cat might die.

These are tragedies in the life of a child. It must be recognized that healing occurs after such wounds and that healing can take a long time. It is important to be aware that beginning to grieve and intense grieving can easily take a full year in a child's life. We need to build in ceremonies and rituals to acknowledge the grief and mourning and to allow the child to move beyond the grief.

Several months after the death of a loved one, children may suddenly act behaviorally disturbed, they may become very depressed, grades may plummet, they may become aggressive in the school yard. This is quite possibly the grief emerging. If it had happened in the first two weeks following the death, it would have been accepted as a function of their loss. Coming several months later, it may be seen as inappropriate by authority figures around them. After some initial brief grief and shock, it is not unusual for children to then sit on their grief for an extended period of time with no visible signs of upset. That doesn't mean we should actively try to make children grieve. It means that when it finally emerges, it should be accepted and the child understood and assisted. I think many of the difficulties in accepting a child's grief derive from our culture's lack of ceremonies and rituals in general, from a specific fear of goodbyes and death, and a lack of passion and intensity for life that permeates the Western world.

CHILDREN OF SEPARATION AND DIVORCE

This is a rather unique kind of loss due to the confusion of knowing that mum and dad are both still there but they're not together. It is quite a difficult process for children. On the one hand, both caregivers are still alive. On the other hand, something more abstract, a relationship, has died. With the end of the parental relationship there are a vast number of secondary losses. There is the loss of the intact biological family unit, the loss of dual financial resources, the loss of family events with both parents hand in hand. There are many other potential changes for children following parental separation. These may include changes in schools, clubs, the local grocery store they visit, sports teams with which they participate, the usual route to school, neighbourhood friends, all because of change in residence location.

In the recent past there has been a mental health myth that

if the parents do okay, the kids will do okay. This is definitely not true. If the parents deal with and begin to resolve their own issues it really helps the children work through their difficulties, but it is not an automatic process. Children likely need much help in getting through the pain. Just when children are in need the most, their parents have their own loss and pain to deal with and have the least to give. Children and parents need as much outside support as they can get through this difficult time.

Another modern myth with regard to children is that divorce is not necessarily bad for children. "In this myth, changes in the American family, especially divorce and remarriage, are viewed as good for children and adolescents. The expectation is that every historical period gets the family form it needs and deserves. Thus, the obvious outcome of a more technological and complicated world is a more diverse and stratified family form. Recent research has demonstrated amply that this myth has developed because it is difficult for us to tolerate the notion that the interests of children and of adults may be diametrically opposed. But children and adolescents are truly conservative by nature. The more stable and predictable their world, the happier they are. Changes in family structure are seldom as beneficial to the involved children as adults would like them to be, and are often associated closely with emotional problems and violence of all kinds" (Straus, 1994, p. xvi-xvii).

Mendell notes that

> children in all age groups reacted to parental divorce with rage, sadness, self-blame, evidence of narcissistic injury, fears of abandonment and rejection, and a shaken sense of security and identity...[that] may overtax the young child's emotional and cognitive abilities (1983, p. 321).

One of the most painful issues I have seen for children with whom I have worked over the years involves fears of being abandoned. Children are vulnerable, do not have adult resources to survive, do not have control over the situation and feel at a complete loss as to how to gain some personal control. The younger the child, the greater the helplessness and vulnerability. Children are at the mercy of others and need their caregivers. They see mummy and daddy abandoning each other and fear they could be next. The initial need is as consistent an environment as possible, with repeated reassurances.

Another painful situation for children involves idiotic parents who put children in the middle of their petty battles. I have worked with many children who have been far more mature than their parents. Putting down the other parent in front of the child is nothing less than outright abuse. If you weren't able to maintain a relationship in the first place, don't worsen the situation by putting your children in the middle of your post-separation battles. I worked with one family group where the father had actually taped his wife on the phone with her lover. This father claimed that when his son was old enough (he was 6 at the time), he would show the boy "what a slut his mother was and why the marriage broke up." Mature guy. If the kid's lucky, the old man will kick off before he inflicts this damage.

Another father with whom I worked quit his well paying executive job and returned to live with his own parents so he wouldn't have to pay any child support or alimony. Grow up, bud, and take some responsibility for your stupid actions. Somebody sterilize that guy before he reproduces any further and has more children he can wound.

This is not to say that it's only fathers who can be idiots following separation. I worked with another family where the mother, actually a very loving woman who was trying very hard to be a good mum, made some key parenting errors in the area of discretion. One weekend she and her son went up to the family cottage. Mum drew dad's face on blocks of wood and then chopped the wood in half. Unbeknownst to her, the child was watching. The 12 year old child was suicidal within 36 hours. Mum had not intended to do this in front of the child, but they were both at the cottage. Mum's indiscretion caused major emotional problems for this child.

Typical Responses

All children experiencing the divorce of their parents will experience distress. Each child may show it or hide it differently. However, there are some general responses you may see in certain age groups. Some of these responses are listed below (adapted from Freeman, 1985). Keep in mind as you review this list that just because a response is listed under one age group doesn't mean you won't see it at a different age. The listings simply include the most common responses for this age group. For example, in the 6 to 9 year old group, reconciliation fantasies are listed. I have known 30 year old adults whose parents have divorced. These 30 year olds have had the same reconciliation fantasies as the 7 year old. With that in mind, the following are typical responses[1] in each age group:

Preschoolers

- *Aggressive behaviour.* This may be obvious at the day care, the preschool, or even at the supper table between siblings. The anger and frustration inside are symbolically *boiling over.* In an attempt to reclaim a world that is out of control, the child becomes the aggressor. Every attempt must be made to understand the confusion and sadness that are underneath the aggression. At the same time, the aggression needs immediate negative consequences.

- *Regressive behaviour.* We really see this kind of response in any child under stress. It is more noticeable in the preschooler since regressive behaviour in a preschooler often means difficulty in previously well-developed toilet habits. They may start needing diapers again. Thus, it is much harder to ignore than the 10 year old who starts acting like an 8 year old.

- *Anxious behaviour.* The preschooler often becomes remarkably clingy and whiny, with a number of seemingly unrealistic heightened fears.

Early School Years (Ages 6 to 9)

- *Reconciliation Fantasies.* Children spend a considerable amount of idle time thinking and daydreaming about life with mum and dad back together. It is a prime wish in life.

- *Nightmares are reported to be common for this group.* However, I am not convinced that this is related in any way to the divorce situation. We know that the most common age range for nightmares, regardless of home situation, is in the 7 to 10 year old (Garfield, 1984).

◗ *An increased demand for objects.* A child feeling neglected, sad, and lonely may push for material objects from a parent in order to gain an indication of love. At the same time, the parent, out of guilt, may be only too willing to provide material objects. This is sometimes referred to as the Santa Claus Syndrome. In reality, what the child needs is as much attention and natural fun time and playtime as possible with each parent.

◗ *Intense expressions of sadness.* You may see physical mourning reactions of extreme grief. These may even include children curling up in fetal position as a result of an overall feeling of physical unwellness from the overwhelming events that they perceive happening to them.

◗ *Guilty feelings.* In an attempt to gain control of a situation that feels beyond control, children feel guilty. Feelings of "I caused it" are an attempt to bring some sanity to the insane world around them.

◗ *An intense longing for the absent parent.* This can border on obsession at times. It again is an attempt to return the world to a predictable form.

Later School Years (9 - 12 years)

◗ *School and/or peer difficulties.* This is also a warning sign of the need for immediate intervention. At this age range, children's peer groups have taken on significance. If they are having trouble with peers and alienating themselves, they may be eliminating a major source of support that they badly need at this time.

◗ *An intense expression of anger.* This may be very direct and aimed at one of the parents, or it may be indirect and take the form of a general bitter attitude or be directed toward some outside source—a friend, a teacher, the world.

◗ *Blaming of a parent.* One of the parents may take the brunt of the blame for the divorce. In younger children it is often the person requesting the separation, regardless of cause. For example, the badly abused woman who gathers the strength to leave the abusive relationship may be blamed by a young child for the entire end of the intact family of origin. On the other hand, older children may not be so predictable in the direction of their anger.

◗ *Support for a parent.* The child may become a shoulder for a parent. Filling the vacuum of the parent's missing partner, a child in this age range is often able to show compassion for a troubled parent. This is unfortunate for all involved. If it went no further than a child showing compassion, there would be no major issue. However, with the parent in a position of great neediness, he or she may start to use the child as support in an unfortunate exchange of appropriate roles. This is far too much weight on any child.

Adolescence

◗ *Expression of pain and anger over the loss.* Like other ages, the adolescent may have intense feelings such as sadness and anger directed inward or outward regarding the divorce.

◗ *Inappropriate adult-like behaviour.* This may include pseudomaturity in any number of areas. I have worked with many adults over the years and, in meetings with the family, it has felt like the adolescent was a full adult partner in financial, custody, property and child-rearing of younger siblings. This is a terrible and inappropriate load for an adolescent to be carrying.

◗ *Acting out behaviour.* I mention this response, as it is noted in the research. However, much acting out behaviour is typically adolescent anyway. To view this as a "symptom" of something specifically related to divorce may be stretching a point.

Fortunately, research (Freeman, 1985) has shown that children experiencing the separation and divorce of their parents can be helped significantly in a very brief period of time. A six week group program that focuses on issues of divorce has been found to be particularly effective. Indications of effectiveness include a dramatic decline in frequency of reconciliation fantasies (wishing mum and dad would get back together) by the children participating in the group; children in a control group who did not participate actually had an increase in reconciliation fantasies.

Travelling throughout North America and the Pacific, it seems that these days there are children's separation and divorce groups by the dozen in most cities in North America. The fact that such groups are needed is a sad reflection on the state of the modern family. However, children need these groups badly and their involvement in such groups should be fully supported. Most of the groups run on fairly similar psychoeducational formats and run between 6 to 12 weeks. If your child or a child with whom you are working is in need of one of these groups, you can check with local professionals to see where one is run near you. A local minister, lawyer, family physician or school guidance counsellor will likely be able to direct you to someone who runs one.

One last recommendation for children who have parents who are in the process of separating or divorcing is that someone be available for the child. This is a time of great stress for parents. They may not have the resources required to care for their child at the emotional level the child needs.

CHILDHOOD DEPRESSION AND SUICIDE

People of all ages become depressed. Some of them commit suicide. Many people do not consider children as candidates for depression or suicide. Not long ago the idea of a young child committing suicide was not taken seriously. We now know that even young children are capable of becoming depressed and committing suicide.

What is Depression: Clinical depression is described within the *DSM IV*[2] (American Psychiatric Association, 1994) as a mood disturbance and can include either

> depressed mood or the loss of interest or pleasure in nearly all activities. In children and adolescents, the mood may be irritable rather than sad (*DSM IV*, 1994, p. 320).

A bleakness or desolation is felt in one's core. To classify as clinical depression there must also be several additional symptoms such as changes in appetite or weight, sleep, and psychomotor activity (this does not appear to be as common in children as it is in adults); decreased energy and complaints of tiredness and fatigue with no apparent reason preceding such complaints; feelings of worthlessness or guilt; difficulty thinking, concentrating or making decisions; or, recurrent thoughts of death or suicidal ideation, plans, or attempts (*DSM IV*, 1994, p. 320)

Other indicators of childhood depression include frequent irritability, weepiness—or periods of feeling like crying—in younger children, and numerous physical complaints such as tummyaches, headaches, and leg pains, all without any physical causes (Poznanski, 1982).

Unhappiness in a child is usually fleeting and temporary. A typical child is able to have fun. It is an important part of a child's life to play and have fun. Fun is not a part of a depressed child's life. The unhappiness of a depressed child is not fleeting or momentary. It typically is long lasting (more than a week). The most reliable sources of observation of a depressed child are teachers.

> In a good school system, with a sensitive teacher, the teacher is often the best observer of the child's affect. The parents are somewhat less reliable for several reasons. It is as hard for parents to be objective about depression as about any other psychological problem the child may manifest. Parents often gloss over the child's pathology because it makes them feel guilty, or their relationship to the troubled child frequently is so strained or attenuated they cannot observe objectively. In addition, a high percentage of the parents appear clinically depressed themselves (Poznanski, 1982, p. 309).

In depressed children there is often an apparent loss of interest in normal, everyday activities and a change in cognitive self-perception. Their affect may be depressed and reflect sadness, pessimism, anxiety, fear, worthlessness and hopelessness. Behaviorally, you may find them withdrawing from peers and social activities and other normally pleasurable pursuits such as their favourite sports, games and other recreational activities. There may be a general fatigue, eating disorders, headaches, heightened distractibility, abdominal pains of unknown origin and other general physical complaints. Depressed children may have a negative worldview and self image, no hope for the future, and be critical of themselves (Poznanski, 1982). When suicidal ideation or suicidal gestures are clearly present, no interpretation should be required. The message is clear.

Children may display their depression inwardly by withdrawing, becoming less verbal or completely non-verbal, or isolating themselves. Children appear quite sad, but the sadness is generalized and cannot be related to any clear issue. Suicidal children begin to make hidden or indirect statements about their intentions. Alternately, children may act out their depression through their contact with the outside world by becoming physically or verbally aggressive, more impulsive. Acting out children may act quite angry, but this anger is generalized and it is not clear what the anger relates to.

There are a number of myths about suicide. These include things like: people who talk about suicide don't do it, they are just asking for attention; suicide strikes more often among certain cultural or socioeconomic groups; suicide happens without warning; once things start to improve after a threat or attempt it means the risk is over, and; the suicidal person is fully intent on dying.

Suicidal people, children or adults, have a desire to get away from their pain – emotional, psychological, spiritual, physical. They are experiencing hopelessness and helplessness to resolve their difficulties. In this hopeless and helpless view they may perceive death as the only escape. Suicidal people clearly want to be out of the painful situation. It in no way means they want to be dead.

Childhood suicide can differ considerably from adult suicide in a number of areas ranging from time of day/year attempted, to methods used.

Attempts at suicide by children often involve guns, hanging, drugs, carbon monoxide or jumps. Children's suicide attempts may occur anytime, but afternoons seem popular. This may partly be because a depressed and suicidal child returning home from school to an empty house is being given a key opportunity to act out any suicidal intent which may be present.

There are different levels of involvement with children who are suicidal. You may be having a conversation with a child and you realize he or she is talking about suicide. You may be having your first meeting with a child following an uncompleted suicide attempt. If children have attempted suicide you may be dealing with different levels of seriousness. You may be seeing a child who attempted suicide but left clues and hoped to be found before dying. On the other hand you may be working with a child who survived the suicide attempt only by chance.

In working with suicidal children, confidentiality is waived. A human life is at stake and that takes all priority over the issue of confidentiality. You need to be direct in your questioning and you need answers to questions like "have you ever tried to do something to hurt yourself before?" If the response is affirmative, "How did you try to do it?" The exploration is an attempt to find out what kind of immediate danger this person is in. If the child, at present, is in the same emotional state, has a plan to commit suicide, has attempted in the past and has the same method available to now, then this is an indication of an immediate crisis situation.

Signals

There are a number of signals to watch for in the depressed child. Is there a general preoccupation with themes of death obvious through conversations, musical interests, artistic or other creative output? Has there been a general withdrawal and notable change in motivation from what is typical of this particular child?

Some of the most common signals of increasing depression with a potential for suicide involve changes from the individual child's own baseline behaviour. These may involve physical changes in activity level, amount of sleep, affective and cognitive issues.

A profound sense of personal failure that appears to reach deep into the soul may be evident. Do not assume you will see the reasons for this sense of failure. It is an internal perception of failure. The outside world may view the child as accomplished and successful. Perhaps the "A+" student receives a "B" on a test. The average individual is not going to perceive this as a meaningful failure. The depressed child might.

In addition to this sense of failure may be combined a social inadequacy. We know that involving others in our lives can bring joy and rewards. On the other hand, a sense of aloneness and isolation through perceiving yourself as socially inadequate or a misfit can bring depression.

Assessing Suicidal Potential

In assessing the seriousness of suicidal children, it is important to know if they have attempted suicide in the past. What happened then and how were they feeling at the time? Do they have a perceived method available to them now and is this method part of their suicidal plan? For example, if they plan on overdosing on drugs and their medicine chest is full of potentially dangerous substances at home or if they plan on using a gun and there is a gun in the house, then they are in great danger.

How much planning has gone into their suicidal plan? Have they or will they isolate themselves? Have they written a note? Do they have any supports? Do they anticipate death as a result of their plan of action? Have they given away some favourite possession (one of the most serious warnings that some children give of imminent suicide)? Each of the previous items is a serious warning. If the person with suicidal ideation is asked "Do you think you will carry this through?" and they answer no, it is vital to find out why not. They may simply be trying to throw you off.

Is there alcohol and/or substance abuse? These can be related to suicide

> because they tend to reduce anxiety and psychological pain. There is a reduction of inhibitions, which allows the adolescent to express his or her anger and unhappiness more easily through suicidal behavior. Alcohol and drugs also allow suicidal impulses to be magnified, thus increasing the risk (Shamoo & Patros, 1990, p. 7).

A child does not necessarily have to have an alcohol or drug problem. We know that approximately one-third of young people who commit suicide do so while under drug or alcohol influences. Such substances, when the person is already thinking of suicide, can distort judgment enough to make that person more willing to take chances (Nelson & Galas, 1994, p. 44).

In working with a child you suspect may be suicidal, a professional needs to assess and work with the child and/or caregiver. Don't leave this situation to a nice chat with the favourite aunt, your kind and loving minister or family doctor (your minister or family doctor may, in fact, be a highly qualified mental health professional, but if not, make sure to have your child referred to one immediately on an emergency basis). Don't assume that it is just a phase and the problems and issues will go away. The underlying problems leading to the depression and possible suicidal ideation need to be resolved.

Prevention/Treatment

The best treatment for childhood suicide and depression is prevention. The second best treatment is lack of availability of suicidal methods. Children in homes where guns are kept are ten times as likely to commit suicide as children in homes where guns are not kept. This simple fact has far ranging implications for the saving of thousands of little lives.

All children must be viewed as unique and their individual vulnerabilities taken into consideration. The stresses, conflicts and losses in children's lives need to be assessed and explored. Has there been a recent significant loss: the death of a parent, a relative, or even their favourite pet? Young children (and older children, too) may try to join the lost loved one through suicide. With older children, the final and precipitating event prior to a suicide attempt may be a romantic relationship breakup.

Work with suicidal children is initially very directive. Depression involves a withdrawn inward journey, a closing off, and curling up into oneself. Physical positions and body posture often tend to reflect this. Physical activities to counter this are important. Bodywork involving opening is used. For example, breathing exercises that include pulling back the shoulders and opening up the body are taught to children. Neck rolls to the front and back are easy for children to understand and learn.

With depressed children we want to encourage success. New activities with positive results are set up for them. The simpler, the better. For the first four months of treatment the possibility of failure needs to be eliminated. For this reason, a complete team approach that includes the teachers, parents and other external resources is vital. Work with the caregivers—not necessarily family therapy with the entire family together—separate from work with the child is crucial. In addition to the therapeutic work going on, the team has to be fully aware of who is responsible for what in the monitoring plan. You can have the best intentioned plan in the world with wonderful and effective interventions, but if the child is a latch-key child who is isolated and alone after school with no support at home, you are defeating your entire plan by failing to monitor him or her from 3 to 5 in the afternoon.

You need to assess children's abilities to perceive affect in themselves and others. The treatment plan will need to address the identification of affect. Feelings games may not be particularly useful with depressed children. They may be so depressed as to not have access to their own cognitive abilities to process words like sad, frustrated, and so on. You may need to use pictures of individuals with numerous affective expressions.

The impulsivity of children must receive a thorough assessment. You may be working with a very impulsive child and a momentary suicidal tendency could result in his or her death if impulsively acted out.

Activity and social involvement should be included in the treatment plan. Initially, this activity may be as simple as relaxation and breathing exercises. As quickly as possible it should extend to more active and social events. This is another method of "going in the side door." The depressed child is increasingly inactive and socially withdrawn. Here, in addition to dealing with the underlying causes of the depression, you are putting the child in active and social situations—a club, a team, a school event. This may seem quite contradictory. What you are actually trying to do is push the child into positives. It is hard to be depressed when opened up. However, this must be handled carefully and, I realize I am harping on this, with intense monitoring. You don't just tell the little boy to get out to his hockey game. You work with the caregiver to make sure they understand the importance of this and perhaps you set an appointment with the child and one with the caregiver on the Saturday morning following the hockey game.

All of these recommendations raise the issue of stress for the professional involved. To be doing a first class job of treatment means quite a lot of time, effort and personal investment for the professional involved. For this reason, I do not recommend that any professional work as the prime therapist with more than 2 or 3 suicidal children at any given time. The stress is intense. Professionals involved need their own support network when doing this work. They need professional supervision and consultation, as well as personal support. They are truly saints and should be rewarded as such.

In working with suicidal people, you will be with those who feel pain so greatly that they see death as a better opportunity than life for escaping the pain. Psychological work needs to deal with the feelings of helplessness and hopelessness. Anger and sadness inside the person must come to the surface and be worked through. Suicidal people need to regain a sense of control and empowerment in their lives. However, despite saying this, they will need to be monitored intensely when in the suicidal state. This may seem like a contradiction from the view that they need to regain a sense of power and control in their lives. However, if they are not monitored while acutely suicidal and for about the next four months, you may have a dead person rather than a suicidal person. Your initial goal is to keep them alive and to do this with suicidal people means to monitor them intensely. The depression may appear to begin to lift. Maintain the monitoring for about four months after this. They are still at great risk. Often deeply depressed and suicidal people are so depressed that they do not even have the energy to kill themselves. However, after early successful therapeutic intervention or administration of medication, their mood begins to lift. Now they have slightly more energy, perhaps enough to kill themselves. The problem is not the therapeutic intervention or the medication but the lack of monitoring during and following the period of intervention and administration of medication. It has been found that "the most dangerous time for those who might make another suicide attempt is about 80 to 100 days after the first attempt" (Nelson & Galas, 1994, p. 30).

On the other hand, people who have been depressed or suicidal may suddenly appear in perfect spirits and all the old problems seem to have disappeared overnight. Do not be lulled into a false sense of security. What may have happened is that they have come to a plan and resolved to kill themselves. Now they have a way out of their existential suffering and they appear quite happy. Then, there is great shock the next day when they are found dead. Severe depression and the potential to commit suicide do not disappear overnight. Children who are very depressed today but in perfect spirits tomorrow still need the therapeutic monitoring to ensure their safety.

The Very Real World of Suicide

Despite the previous academic discussion about suicide, no words can prepare us for the reality of suicide, when life and death really happen in front of us. I was in Toronto one night in late autumn, taking a break from my day to day activities for some time to refresh. I had just been teaching play therapy at the University of Western Ontario and had come into Toronto at the end of the day-long presentation. I checked into one of my favourite hotels right behind The Eaton Centre in downtown Toronto and then parked in the hotel parking lot. I often prefer to walk than to waste the energy of elevators, so I had walked down several flights of stairs while whistling and was feeling quite content and excited about a couple of days to myself, all alone with nothing to do but write and refresh. Almost no one even knew where I was, so I thought I was not at any risk of being disturbed.

I reached the ground floor and left the parking lot to go into the hotel and I stopped short in my tracks. There was a body on the landing. Part of me immediately tried to find some pleasant explanation. "It must be Toronto street theatre" a part of my brain tried to say for a second or two. Then I thought to myself "no, it's real. It must be someone who's past out for some reason. Maybe they're drunk."... But I felt more power to this scene than that. Then a staff person from the hotel came running up the stairs to the landing and was yelling "They just jumped. You can come around." Come around? The landing was about six feet wide. I would have to literally step over this person, this body.

The horror and tragedy of this was beginning to hit me. This was a real person who had just jumped fifteen storeys from the top of the parking lot. I slowly stepped over her. Time felt frozen. She looked so peaceful, so young, so alive, sleeping. She was on her back with her face up. Wispy and light blond hair hung over her forehead caressing the side of her face. She was angelically dressed all in white, even her running shoes. Her pale colour and her light clothes amplified the tragedy. Her sweater was quickly turning red as blood flowed out from her chest. Blood was pulsing from the side of her head. This was a young woman, about eighteen years old, who had just died in front of me.

I felt so helpless. I wished I could turn back the clock by 10 minutes to park my car on the roof, see her, talk with her, take care of her, let her know that someone in the world would listen. As I stepped over her I watched her face. I wanted her to open her eyes so I could talk with her. I felt so close to her. We had just shared such an intimate act, her suicide. I didn't even know her name. I was shattered thinking, this is someone's daughter, someone's sister, someone's friend. I was even more upset by the fact that perhaps no one cared that she was dead.

In a daze I took an elevator up to my room on the seventeenth floor of the hotel. I wanted to watch the Toronto skyline for a while and just try to collect myself. I opened the curtains in my room and looked down below and realized I overlooked the suicide scene seventeen floors below. I was visually glued and could not take myself away from watching what was happening below. I heard sirens and saw the police and ambulance crew running up to the landing. Someone took a pulse on the young woman's neck. Then they lifted up her sweater and revealed a bare chest covered in a pool of blood between her breasts. Her chest must have opened up from the impact of the fall. She was then covered in a white sheet, toe to head. Dead. Very dead. I wanted to give her something. All I could do was send her an image of an angel to guide her on the next phase of her journey.

Across from me I could see police cars at the top of the parking lot at the site from which she must have jumped. Eventually, Angel (that's what I named her) was taken away on a stretcher in an ambulance. No sirens for the dead. Just a slow drive out of the hotel entrance off to the morgue. I still watched.

Anger filled me when a maintenance staff stood at the death scene with a hose and sprayed away all the blood. Now, not only did the possibility exist that no one cared, but no one would even know that anything had happened here. Yet a life and death scene had just been enacted. I was angry at how it was just being washed away as if it didn't matter. No marker, no memorial, no dignity for this young woman. I withdrew from the world and remained in shock for some days in complete existential crisis. I vowed to be as kind, giving and considerate a person as I humanly could in the hopes that perhaps, through my giving to others, someday I might give some little thought, a smile, a kind gesture to a stranger and, in so doing, prevent his or her suicide.

To honour Angel, I returned to Toronto and went back to the suicide scene two weeks later. I bought a dozen red roses and three white carnations. I scattered them in a circle at the scene where Angel had died. I drew a star at the spot where her heart had been. On the wall beside where she had lain I wrote "Always Care." Something began to feel complete after that ceremony in honour of Angel. There was a joy, a beauty and a loving presence felt for Angel. Yet there was also an eeriness at the site. Still hanging there was a bit of "police scene—do not cross" plastic tape which had been tied to the railing to block off the scene. But now, two weeks later, the lamps and building were highly decorated with ornaments for the Christmas season. It made the situation that much more surreal.

Although deeply sad, I also felt intensely happy about life the next day when I returned to the scene in the daylight to say a goodbye and look at the writing on the wall. The world can be such a wonderful place. I thought that the flowers might be gone or something drastically changed, the memorial somehow gone. But it had been saved and nurtured. I didn't see the flowers at first, but the star I had drawn was there and so were my words "Always Care." Then I saw the flowers. Someone had taken the time and put the effort into collecting the flowers, placing them all together and carefully placed them on the ledge just above the words. So here were these beautiful red and white flowers highlighting the words. I said goodbye to Angel and will return to the memorial scene regularly to leave flowers and say a prayer for this fallen young woman.[3]

In talking with a friend after all of this happened, we both acknowledged how meaningless all of our training can be when forced to feel the pain and witness such tragic events. It is no longer a diagnosis on a page of paper but a real human being suffering to the point of self-annihilation. I am convinced that to be effective with people we must always maintain our capacity to feel. The theories, words, and education are irrelevant if we cannot feel the joy and pain with others. Feeling this deeply can be very trying and stressful.

Always remember that allowing the feelings is a vital part of the healing process.

Recommendations

If you are working with a depressed or suicidal child, always have professional consultation for your work. Outside consultation, expert opinions and supervision are vital. If you are the parent, relative or friend of a depressed or suicidal child, get professional help immediately. Do not risk that person's life by your own inaction. I absolutely recommend always erring on the side of caution, especially with the issues of depression and suicide.

On the other side of this issue, however, are the vested interests of mental health professionals. According to Szasz:

> Overestimating the danger of suicide, and underestimating the danger of psychiatric coercion, serve the economic and professional interests of the psychiatrist, not the existential needs of the (adolescent) patient. That is why I contend that coercive psychiatric interventions are more likely to promote, than prevent suicide (1994, pp. 81-82).

Even if one does believe that psychiatric intervention is necessary,

> even the most ardent supporters of psychiatric coercions admit that the confinement of allegedly suicidal adolescents does not help to prevent their suicide (Szasz, 1994, p. 81).

For this reason, among others, I agree with the view of Szasz that we should be addressing the moral problem of suicide and the practical problems of suicide prevention.

At the risk of harping on the same old issue here, we need to meet children's love and nurturing needs early in life, and help them to make decisions and become responsible and disciplined as they grow. Children with positive parenting are much less likely to commit suicide than children who have grown up amidst a stressful family, without the support they need, and with a lack of meaning in their lives that would promote their full involvement in life and giving to others.

The Survivors Left Behind

> Every suicide intimately affects at least six other people, usually the family and closest friends of the young person who committed suicide. This number grows much higher when you include classmates, team members, neighbours, and extended family—aunts, uncles, cousins (Nelson & Galas, 1994. p. 89).

It is estimated that there are between 4 and 5 million suicide survivors left behind in North America (Nelson & Galas, 1994, p. 89). They are at great risk of depression themselves. In families where there has been a suicide attempt, children are at an increased risk of becoming suicidal themselves. They have been given a model of suicide as a means of dealing with pain.

An excellent model for dealing with suicide inspired grief comes from the work of Nelson and Galas (1994). Their easy-to-read and straightforward text on suicide deserves a great deal of attention. It offers both hope and effective strategies for working in the field dealing with suicide. Although written for teens, it is a valuable addition to any clinician's library. Their model is useful for all ages in dealing with grief following the loss of a loved one through suicide. The model involves the following ways to work through grief:

- Tell yourself that feeling sad is normal;
- Cry when you need to;
- Spend time with family and friends;
- Do things you enjoy;
- Stay active;
- Talk or write about your feelings;
- Find ways to help others;
- Join with others and come up with ideas on how to stop suicide;
- Put your ideas into action (Nelson & Galas, 1994, p. 94).

Following the loss of a client, a friend or loved one through a completed suicide, there is a great deal of confusion and spiritual chaos in the lives of survivors. It is important for survivors to have their own supports, sacred places to heal and to realize that, although the physical lives of their loved ones are over, their own aren't. This can be a new beginning. A time of death holds the opportunity for the time of rebirth.

SEVERE STRESS/TRAUMA

Some children endure such severe stress that they become traumatized. These children have a long journey of healing ahead of them. The process of trauma results from the perception of an overwhelming event with its concurrent feelings of helplessness, powerlessness and hopelessness. It is possible that a child could experience an extremely stressful event and not be traumatized. For example, there may be a natural disaster such as a hurricane or earthquake. During the entire event the child is with a caregiver and is nurtured and protected. This child has supports. Trauma occurs when severe stress is combined with a sense of "there was nobody there for me."

Terr (1983, 1988, 1990, 1991) has been involved in some fascinating studies on the effects of extreme stress and trauma in the lives of children who have suffered validated trauma. Through her work we have learned a great deal about the effects of trauma on children. One such effect is a psychic numbing – this "numbing" serves as a protection from feeling too much, from being overwhelmed during the stress. Tragically, it

> may become a way of life, a debilitating character flaw. The person who lives his life in a place beyond expression, beyond feeling, will present a scary picture indeed. The absent eyes, the blunted responses to another's response, these vacancies frighten anyone who recognizes what they really mean. Who lives behind the empty eyes? Sometimes – too many times – an ordinary child once lived there (Terr, 1990, p. 94).

Another possible effect is a tendency to misperceive. For example, young children who have been molested by strangers may think their perpetrators are nearby and that they see them even if the offender is known to be imprisoned. Children may see the site of the traumatizing event even when far away from it. This misperception may be triggered by smells, tastes, the season of year, by hearing about the event, or any other association. Children often replay the traumatic event during times of calm daydreaming; a destruction in a comfortable trust in the future. Even a sense of the present and future becomes distorted and they become more oriented to the past. The future is no longer safe."Once a seemingly impossible event happens, everything else becomes possible for the traumatized child" (Terr, 1990, p. 163). Furthermore, post traumatic play is common.

Terr's raw material and data are quite valuable contributions. Some of her studies are utterly fascinating. Two of the most extensive studies involved: 1) Chowchilla—children from the town of Chowchilla in California were kidnapped, along with their school bus. They were all buried alive while inside the school bus. Everyone survived with only minimal physical harm; and 2) the Challenger—Terr studied the effects of the Challenger space shuttle explosion on different ages of children and the differences of hearing about the tragedy versus "witnessing" it first hand by watching it at the time of the launch.

Unfortunately, her psychoanalytically influenced beliefs and training seem to lead to some rather strange interpretations and extrapolations of her raw material. Ofshe and Watters comment that "her role as compelling storyteller eclipsed her role as a scientist" (1994, p. 263). For example, Terr notes that "by hearing about the play and by knowing little else about the child, you can postulate a certain traumatic event" (1990, p. 247). Ofshe and Watters note that

> to believe that therapists can have knowledge of an unknown event through an analysis of symptoms is fantasy. Terr's notion that psychiatrists, because of their advanced training, can relate symptoms to a particular event is not accepted within the ranks of scientific psychology or scientific psychiatry. To allow this belief into a courtroom is, to put it mildly, dangerous (1994, p. 270).

Furthermore, Terr is a proponent of the controversial concept of repressed memory. However, her belief is not supported even by her own studies and data. It is interesting that in Terr's own work on both Chowchilla and the Challenger

> each child remembered the event even many years later...[in her work] all of the traumatized children above three years of age who had suffered repeated trauma could remember and talk about it.... That Terr's empirical studies show little evidence to support the idea of the sort of massive memory repression...did not stop Terr from confidently confirming these beliefs (Ofshe & Watters, 1994, pp. 265, 267).

Replaying the Trauma

There are therapists who advocate replaying the trauma or who insist that the child (or adult) verbally deal with it. I do not believe this is required or even necessarily beneficial. Therapists who push children are functioning as voyeurs who risk further hurting them. They are psychic rapists who are meeting their own needs, not the child's. For example, in the area of sexual abuse, what is important is the impact the sexual abuse has had on children, their feelings, their sense of self, their developmental process. If these issues are the focus of therapy, then what is left to be accomplished by knowing exactly what went where? If children wish to talk about the abuse, link it to their feelings and daily life, this is fine. However, knowing the exact details is in no way linked to the success of therapy. In fact, pushing the child to state what happened could serve to retraumatize or further traumatize the child. I like to draw from the kind, gentle and respectful work of Gina O'Connell-Higgins who notes that "You need to realize that, at times, it is simply too physically and psychologically dangerous to *work it out*" (O'Connell-Higgins, 1995, p. 343).

The belief that children must verbally state what happened to them in order to heal is contradictory to the underlying philosophy of play therapy. In play therapy, we are often functioning in the world of symbols, not words. The child may have been abused when they were preverbal. How, then, do words help?

Post-Traumatic Play

Children who have been traumatized through witnessing violence, being abused, being a victim of a car accident, a death and so on, *may* engage in post-traumatic play. Intervention is crucial.

Otherwise feelings of hopelessness and helplessness are only reinforced. Such play is distinctive in its monotonous ritualization and the fact that it may not be openly observed, as it tends to occur in secrecy (Terr, 1983). Even though this play is initiated by the child, it is not necessarily beneficial. In this kind of play the child is repeatedly acting out the trauma rather than processing in a manner leading to any kind of resolution. This is a painful activity and many children who have gone numb and distanced themselves during their abuse may do the same during their replay of the situation.

Post-traumatic play is a distinctive type of play involving a rather rigid repetition, literally or symbolically, of the traumatic scene. If this kind of play includes some kind of resolution or new world view it could be highly beneficial. The problem comes with fixed post-traumatic play, where there is identical negative outcome, no change, no resolution, only a constant repeating of the traumatic event. It is significant in this type of play that there is no resolution to the painful process.

Post-traumatic play involves a joyless scenario, lacking in expressive freedom. This stark picture of play is in contrast to the normal world of childhood play which is free, spontaneous and enchanting. The normal play of children is "is bubbly and light-spirited; whereas the play that follows from trauma is grim and monotonous" (Terr, 1990, p. 238). For the typically non-traumatized child, even when engaged in wars and battles, the everyday play has a spontaneity to it. There is an exuberance and release rather than the obsessive quality that is found in post-traumatic play.

> Play does not stop easily when it is traumatically inspired. And it may not change much over time. As opposed to ordinary child's play, post traumatic play is obsessively repeated. It is grim. Furthermore, it requires a certain set of conditions in order to proceed – a certain place, a certain assortment of dolls, certain playmates, or a certain routine. It may go on for years. It repeats part of the trauma...[it] is able to do very little to relieve anxiety. It can be dangerous, too. The problem is – post-traumatic play may create more terror than was consciously there when the game started (Terr, 1990, p. 239).

Terr (1990) believes that allowing the child to continue long term fixed post traumatic play is counter-productive. Continuation would only serve to reinforce powerlessness and hopelessness. I would maintain that, if it clearly is post traumatic play, there is no rationale for allowing it to continue at all.

Intervention for post traumatic play initially involves helping a child to ground in the safe presence of the here and now. I would recommend using movement exercises and breathing exercises here—anything which allows the child to leave the spacey yet restricted realm of the post-traumatic play scenario and focus on the present. Before talking about any issue, I would suggest asking such children to put their hands together (folded pointing up, as in prayer), and then take a big stretch with their arms reaching around in a big circle until they meet again above their heads, then holding them in the upright together position to slowly bring their hands down until they are in front of their solar plexus, again, as if in prayer. When they reach that point, I would ask them to then take a very slow, deep breath and to imagine they are surrounded by a very calm healing energy and to breath in this energy. I would ask them to roll their neck around to the front in a circle, back and forth a few times, then, to the back, rolling back and forth a few times. Finally, I would ask them to pull their shoulders back as far as they could stretch. My reason for doing this is multi purpose. The physical exercises give the message that they have control over their bodies. It also allows for a symbolic opening up. It is difficult to be depressed or anxious when opened up. Through this process I am trying to give the message that there are alternatives to feeling out of control and at the mercy of others.

After doing this a couple of times, I would recommend being quite directive with the child's play. I would intrude into the play to bring about a new world image. For the child who has repeated some tragic event, I may build in a new ending so the child can see new possibilities. This is very directive—but the children who are involved in fixed post-traumatic play may repeat that play for an indefinite period of time and only continue to feel helpless and vulnerable with no positive hope. You could ask questions about their play such as: "What would happen if we were able to build in some help and a safe place for the [child/victim/person who has been hurt] in the play?" Later, follow with questions like "What does it feel like to see that safe place there?"; "What's different now for you in your life compared to when the abuse was going on?"; "What do we need to do to help you feel safe?" My intention in recommending these kinds of things is to give children an external image of hope on which they can later internally focus. Talking with the child can help if metaphors for hope and change are used. Stories that show very difficult times being overcome are extremely useful.

If you are dealing with a situation where the prime caregivers were traumatized at the same time as the child—for example, in a major accident, crime or natural disaster—it is crucial to build in outside supports. If possible, extended family members, close family friends, or a carefully chosen professional should be accessed. The most important support for children will involve helping them reclaim a safe and protected environment or the rebuilding of such a sanctuary for them. Caregivers should watch for signs of severe stress and, above all, avoid denial. If the caregiver is aware of post-traumatic play or the child is having terrible nightmares or very strange fears, then immediate professional consultation and help is crucial for that child's well-being.

Simply re-experiencing the traumatic situation through play accomplishes nothing. It is vital to process the feelings and dynamics of the experience. We must build in a sense of resolution, safety and protection. Children need to be provided with a long term sense of a world that is safe for them, a world where someone outside of oneself will help during difficult, even overwhelming, times. So when I am talking about intervening in post-traumatic play this *in no way* means that children are not allowed to talk about the trauma or deal with it. They need to play things out. They need to talk about what happened to them. Make very sure that any interventions are not serving the purpose of protecting yourself from feeling overwhelmed. If you can't handle it, how can we ever expect the child to? The most important task is to not become overwhelmed,

> to be able to hear the entire grim tale if your clients are going to heal.... Anything less than bearing witness to the full catastrophe can be silencing, no matter how well intentioned you are or how subtly you convey your fear. If *you* can bear it, they might bear it. Your bravery may lead clients to relinquish their solitary, ashamed anguish. While this puts a tremendous burden on therapists to tolerate far more atrocity than most of us *ever* bargained for, seeing human hope reborn potentially transforms *you* (O'Connell-Higgins, 1995, p. 337)

I think it is also important to realize that, in their pain, some people have reached some equilibrium and cannot safely go further, nor do they need to. I think this is something that many mental health professionals lose sight of as they strive for some theoretical optimal goal of functioning that does not accommodate everyone.

Distancing/Dissociation

Sometimes under great pain, our minds allow us to distance ourselves from the stressful situation or event. Dissociation is a highly mystified word and process. I use the word here only because of its extensive use in the mental health field. All I really mean when referring to dissociation is that people have an ability to distance themselves from extremely painful or horrific situations. They leave the situation behind. They distance themselves by "spacing out." In clinical use, the concept of dissociation is used to mean that the integrative functions of identity, memory or consciousness are in some way disturbed or altered (*DSM IV*, 1994, p. 477).

Many mental health professionals believe that an important indicator of past severe stress/trauma is dissociation and that all dissociative phenomena are, at some level, related to past trauma (Gil, 1991, p. 14). I would like to make clear that this is a belief, not an empirically based scientific fact. Thus, this belief is certainly not beyond dispute. There is, in fact, much disagreement over this issue.

Dissociation can be seen in a process I refer to as compartmentalization. Traumatized victims are able to distance themselves from overwhelmingly painful pieces of their lives and identities to allow themselves the ability to deal with them. Integrating the total psychic (personality) being would be the long term goal of therapy.

Some children's art can clearly be indicative of the compartmentalization process. I am reminded of two girls with whom I was working. One was six, the other fourteen. Both had been sexually abused. They were each asked to draw a picture of themselves. Neither drew a person. Each drew only carefully crafted compartments when asked to draw a picture of herself. Although at first glance, the pictures looked like the typical doodling that anyone may do, upon closer examination, it was clear that there was an extreme attempt to keep the compartments separate, not to get any colours mixed together. They also referred to the compartments with words like "this is the part of me that...." Now despite giving this description, I can only say their drawings were consistent with how I knew they thought about themselves and their abuse. They could not look at everything at once. Each had to break the many painful aspects of their experience into manageable pieces. Isn't this what we all do on some level?

The danger in giving this kind of description is that some professionals like simple, quick and easy solutions to very complex and painful situations. I would not want anyone to think that you can look at someone's piece of art, or any other creative product, and think that we can diagnose, confirm or even assume past trauma, abuse, or whatever by simply looking at the drawing. I am only able to say that the drawings I described above were indicative of the dynamics in each of these girl's lives because I know the dynamics of their lives. This cannot be inferred from drawings. Empirical evidence to support the use of such projective interpretations simply does not exist. However, there are many who believe that this can be done. All such beliefs should be filed in the science fiction section of your mind.

Another example of compartmentalization comes from my own research with female prostitutes. There may come a point in the career of a prostitute where parts of the body actually go "numb." No feeling, good or bad, is experienced physically in certain areas of the body. For example, this may initially be a "numbing" of an area of circumference around the body that occurs in the region of the genitals. The area of reported numbness may initially be but a small perimeter of only about half an inch to an inch. Gradually, with increased time in the profession, this physical numbness may extend so that there is actually no sensation felt in the body in an area that can be as wide as 18 inches. When the "numbing" reaches that large an area, there is often a drastic increase in substance abuse and/or a suicide attempt on the part of the prostitute. This is an example of anatomical compartmentalization. It is more than just emotional feelings that go numb, but physical sensations as well. This should not be taken to imply that the person does not remember the event that was occurring. It simply means she does not have any physical sensations accompanying the event.

There is no doubt that the ability to distance oneself from pain exists. Everyone dissociates at times. Dissociation occurs along a continuum. Sometimes we daydream, sometimes we will drive along a highway and realize we've made turns and passed signs that we heeded but didn't really pay attention to. However, we still remember that we took the trip. It is not as if we suddenly wake up in Washington, having left Philadelphia some time earlier and have no recollection whatsoever of getting from point "A" to point "B." There may even be much more intense levels of dissociation. As a psychological defense against a sense of being overwhelmed by a highly traumatic event, dissociation serves purposes of psychological survival. This is still significantly different from believing that there is no awareness or memory of the event.

Dissociation has gained an ugly reputation and is often viewed very negatively. This is quite unfair because being able to distance oneself from overwhelming pain, be it emotional or physical, is a valuable tool that has saved many psychological lives. People, under severe stress and in deep psychological pain, may learn to do this in order to survive. For example, they may space out and feel nothing when being abused. This is a functional response within a highly dysfunctional situation. Rather than psychologically going "over the edge," they dissociate and leave their identities behind for various lengths of time. Again, I am in no way implying that they do not remember the event. There is a somewhat strong and unsubstantiated view in the mental health field that people can completely "forget" things that happened to them. I have seen little evidence of this except in the extremely rare event of amnesia. A person might have a distorted view of the event or a fragmented memory, but, this is different from absolutely no memory. This is really an area that needs considerable research to obtain some definitive answers.

In "treating" dissociation, first we must come to respect it for the valuable tool it has been in people's lives. Then, rather than try to eliminate it, we need to help them build lives where they *are* safe and protected and *feel* safe and protected. When this has been accomplished, they will no longer need to dissociate. Alternate ways of dealing with affect and painful issues will need to be learned.

In working with someone who is dissociative, we need a common language. We need to have some way to describe and communicate the process. With regard to dissociating, the first step to working with it is to give it a name. Rather than focus on the word dissociate, which I never use except in professional presentations, I would ask the individual what he or she calls it. Many times you will hear dissociation called "spacing out," but there are many other titles that it is given and it is important to know the unique name the child or adult with whom you are working gives it. This allows a description of the process to develop without it being forced. There are many ways of describing the process beyond the typical phrase of "spacing out." I have heard things like "leaving," "disappearing," "ghosting," "watching myself from outside." There are quite a number of names given to this process.

It is also important to understand in what situations, where and when, this distancing is most likely to occur for an individual. This helps to understand the triggers preceding the need to distance. It also allows you to explain the process to the person with whom you are working. I use words similar to those that follow, depending on the age of those with whom I am working to let them know that "sometimes, when under stress or when we are scared or during our own healing, some things may seem too painful emotionally for us to bear. We may try to distance ourselves from what is happening. It's kind of like daydreaming, but, generally, you just don't feel like you're there. It may happen when someone feels certain emotions or certain emotions become too intense. As we look at the emotions that are painful we will be able to start looking at what you need when you feel that particular way and how to help you when you feel that way. You can learn new ways of dealing with pain in the present and for the future."

VIOLENCE AND SUBSTANCE ABUSE

Children living with substance abusers may be terrified, depressed, suicidal, angry, sad, anxious and full of shame.

> Many have experienced repeated abandonment, as well as physical and/or sexual abuse. Others suffer from extreme isolation and silence...many are actually traumatized. (Levy & Ruttman, 1992, p. 167).

Children who live in homes where there is violence, like children of substance abusers and children who are sexually abused, have had their childhood stolen from them. Instead of playful joy, they are given scenes of violence that would scare most adults.

Childhood should be a time of learning through play, a carefree time without adult responsibilities, a time for fun, makebelieve and, above all else, a time for being nurtured and taken care of. When abused, witnessing violence, or abandoned by a "stoned" parent, the sacred act of caregiving by a parent is destroyed. The child in this situation has no childhood. At some point, this childhood will need to be reclaimed, through living it later, or by giving to children when one is an adult. The world of play in childhood is a biological need. Without a time to play and have fun, we are deprived of a full capacity to learn.

Children of violent and/or substance abusing parents will take a long time to learn to trust the therapist. They have already learned that adults are not capable of meeting their needs in a mature and responsible manner. They will have to begin to learn that not all adults are like their prime caregivers. This trust can take a long time to develop. When there are issues of abuse, true and basic trust can easily take six months to even begin to develop. This, along with safety and protection issues, is of prime importance in work with these children.

THE ABUSED CHILD

Issues for Children Who Have Been Abused

Every child must be viewed individually, not as some case to fit our clinical perceptual patterns. This means abandoning theories at the door and allowing ourselves to see the world through children's eyes. Do not assume these children feel angry, sad, betrayed, etc. Rather, explore their worlds with them and discover how they perceive it. It is crucial that we have a grasp on the full worlds of the children—their lives in session with us, at school, at home.

At present there seems to be disagreement in the field on whether every child is traumatized by sexual abuse or whether every child needs therapy following abuse. Eliana Gil wisely notes that

> some victims of child abuse seem to emerge unscathed. Garbarino et al discuss "stress-resistant" children who become prosocial and competent in spite of their harsh, or even hostile, upbringing. he concludes that these children receive "compensatory doses of psychological nurturance and sustenance [that] enable them to

> develop social competence, that fortify self-esteem, and [that] offer a positive social definition of self" (1991, p. 11).

I prefer to take another approach with regard to the "need" for therapy. I would rather emphasize that every child has the *right* to one-to-one intervention. I agree with the view that not every child is traumatized following sexual abuse. However, I would rather not take the risk of missing any that are. For that reason, the opportunity should be available for work with a skilled therapist. This raises another issue. There are many people practising child therapy, especially therapy with abused children, who lack intensive and specific training in the area of child therapy in general, child sexual development, and child sexual abuse (besides the typical "what to look for" workshop training). They are professionals who have taken minimal (hours/weeks rather than years) introductory training in the area of abuse and end up doing a great deal of work in the area, resulting in greater damage rather than healing.

This unfortunately includes a number of family therapists (who usually lack individual child therapy training) who will conduct a family therapy session with the entire family "present" but the therapy consists of the therapist having a conversation with the caregivers while the children (especially young children) play off on their own in some other section of the room, and, for the therapist's peace of mind, hopefully not bothering or disturbing the adults. As Gil (1991) notes:

> Family therapists encourage the presence of all family members in therapy sessions, but they have been considerably lax in demonstrating methods for conducting family sessions with very young children (p. 47).

From what I have seen over the years, family therapists don't understand children, nor do they truly understand systems in the full sense of the word. Viewing family therapy as a biologist, the descriptions such therapists give of "systems" are odd. There is even a school of family therapy known as ecosystemic whose use and understanding of the word ecosystem, taken from the field of biology, is almost sacrilegious to a biologist.

Repetition

Time and again, a child may deal with the same issue. Don't assume because it has been discussed or worked through once, that this will necessarily be the end of it. The same feelings and the same issues may need to be dealt with many times over. The same conversation may need to be held over many months, or even years, until the child really feels a sense of resolve.

Privacy versus secrecy

Protection of the child must override all confidentiality concerns. As mentioned previously in this text, children should be told in the very first session that they have the right to privacy. They also need to hear in this same conversation that their safety is most important and, if you are concerned about their safety and well-being, you will tell whomever you need to in order to make sure they are taken care of. For a more complete discussion on this issue refer to pages 145-147 dealing with confidentiality.

Trust

Trust is a prime issue when there has been past neglect or abuse. Trust can take a very long time to develop between a caring adult and a child who has been abused. It is important not to confuse trust with comfort or with a complete lack of boundaries. Trust takes time and relationship building. For example, when I give public lectures, I may be speaking to a room full of 200 people. I can usually immediately be very comfortable in such a situation. However, and this is no offense to any of the many wonderful people in the room, I don't trust anyone there. It is not a sign of their lack of trustworthiness, nor is it a sign of paranoia on my part. It simply means that a relationship is not present with anyone that would allow trust to have developed.

On the other hand, boundary issues, or a blurring of personal boundaries, may result in individuals having no sense of their own rights to personal time, personal space, safety, and privacy. Five minutes after meeting such a person, be it child or adult, I have already heard from them that they are a "victim" (the fact that they are using such a word implies to me that they are indeed victims, but most likely victims of mental health professionals who have indoctrinated them with a worldview that includes such words), and all kinds of deeply personal information that I believe it is unwise for strangers to share. This is not a sign of trust. It is an indication of a lack of personal boundaries. Such a lack is typical of many children (and adults) of sexual abuse.

To develop trust with someone, we must have integrity and be trustworthy. We need to be consistent and predictable. If I am working with someone I know has been sexually abused, I will make every humanly possible effort to keep my appointment times, to the point of showing up for appointments even when feeling very ill or exhausted. Some may argue that this goes against my view that all mental health professionals need to take care of themselves. There are times for exceptions. My taking care of myself may need to include methods for dealing with this kind of stress on my system.

Consistency

James (1994, pp. 176, 177) reports a useful approach in working with abused children that could facilitate trust. With some children, a week between sessions may be too long, so sessions could be increased to twice a week. In addition, it might be helpful to send a child home with something that is made with the therapist. This object becomes a reminder, helping the child internalize the image of the therapist as a caring, nurturing outsider who continues to exist even when not present.

Acceptance

The immediate therapeutic goal for children who have been abused should be acceptance as full human beings who have the right to express themselves. We far too often relate to children who have been abused, especially those who have been sexually abused, as objects. We do this by seeing them only as victims (objects) and ignore or forget the fact that they are full human beings who happen to have been abused. The abuse may have a huge impact on their functioning lives, but it is not the only influence. They have already been objectified through the abuse process. We should do everything in our power to make sure we are not responsible for a parallel process that could result from our perception of them as objects.

Safety and Protection

Children who have been abused—physically, sexually, emotionally, spiritually—will do many things which may seem bizarre to the outside world.

They may act out sexually or appear to act in ways that are viewed as seductive. This has been argued to result from a number of factors: children's experiences may lead them to expect that needs for loving attention will be satisfied only through sexual encounters, and; to ward off anxiety about being a passive victim children may take an active role in the "seduction," since sexual contact is felt to be inevitable. I don't really believe either of these philosophies. I think, in reality, that the child may be testing the safety of the situation, therapeutic or otherwise, before venturing to discuss sexual experiences.

Another important factor here is that children who have been abused by intimate caregivers have learned the insidious lesson of physical, sexual, emotional, and spiritual abuse

> that "people who love you will hurt you." Neglected children learn that "people who love you abandon you." Either way, intimacy implies threat, and the child who feels reassured or consoled will inevitably feel endangered. Feeling in peril, the abused child may attempt to take flight emotionally, physically, or through some acting-out behavior. Understanding the child's need to flee or need to evoke an abusive response from the clinician provides direction for the clinician's serene and persistent responses (Gil, 1991, p. 56)

Therapy With Children Who Have Been Abused

As noted by Axline (1947), play is the natural medium of expression for a child. Children's experiences may have taught them the lesson that people who love you will hurt you physically, emotionally or spiritually. Play provides emotional space for the repetitive expression of many intense feelings such as sadness or anger (among many others). Play time provides a structure to relearn about one's own power and control, as well as to deal with the memory of feelings without the need to use words. This time with an adult allows reestablishment of the capacity to develop a close relationship with an adult who can protect the child.

Mann and McDermott (1983) report that with long term (more than nine months) play therapy, there are improvements in a number of areas including: self esteem, capacity to experience pleasure, impulse control, cognitive functioning, object relations, behavioral symptom control, social relationships, and school performance. However, they note that "controlled studies are not yet available to compare the outcome of treated and untreated groups of children..." (Mann & McDermott, 1983, p. 305). Thus, despite the glowing indication of improvements, this is really only a belief and not a scientific fact. Unfortunately, this is typical of the field of play therapy. From numerous studies where control groups have been used, it is also quite possible to predict that with no treatment—providing a safe environment is present—there would also be improvements in a number of areas.

The lost childhood

When children have been abused, a part of their childhood has been ripped away from them. Play time or play therapy allows a return to this time of childhood. During this time, the precious aspects of childhood may be re-experienced and reclaimed in a positive way. Simply having time to safely play is a gift for a child who has been abused.

Although abuse of children is very serious, it does not mean that therapy must be very serious at all times. Especially initially, it is important for there to be a fun component so the child is not completely overwhelmed.

As therapy progresses, frame things in relation to the child's day to day experience. Make it *playful.* For example, you may be running a group for victims of sexual abuse and Halloween rolls around. Why not do a trick or treat role-playing exercise (Hindman, 1991, pp. 357-359)? The kids will be in tune with this already and they can have fun. At the same time, they learn some valuable boundaries and street survival skills. In this example, they can become empowered by learning how offenders manipulate. In the exercise the kids can take turns playing the "trick or treater." They approach a door, knock, and are greeted by someone who tells them "You can have your candy treat to take with you if you come in and let me take a picture of you with your costume off." There can be an almost infinite number of variations of role playing.

Kids can begin to learn to treasure themselves by using such exercises as *Finish the Thought Sentence Completions* (Hindman, 1991, pp. 302-303). In these exercises, kids are given cards with sentences on them. They are asked to complete sentences like "Being me is nice because.... I deserve friends because.... I deserve to be taken care of because.... I need to be taken care of because.... I need to be loved because.... I deserve to.... Being me is great because...."

As you work with sexually abused children, it is important to understand their sense of powerlessness which may be a significant theme in their lives. Their young psyches have been intruded upon and they need to be empowered, to learn to have power from within. This is vital in their future development and healing.

Therapy with children who have been sexually abused must remain therapy in their interest and at their pace. For example, if you are expected to be doing the investigation, it is unwise for you to be the long term therapist who will be involved with the child. You are there for the child's needs and these needs may be completely different from the systemic legal needs (which are also important). If you are working as an investigator you will definitely *not* be proceeding at the child's pace.

Useful Methods in Working with An Abused Child (or Adult)

Some general methods specifically useful in dealing with sexual abuse include things like exercises to promote an awareness of personal boundaries, puppets, sandplay, phone, the mail box, masks (paper plates, NOT paper mache), sunglasses, storytelling, feelings games, art, expressive and creative techniques, and movement. Many of these are discussed elsewhere in this text. Some that have not been mentioned include:

Boundaries

The child's personal space has already been intruded upon in the past. Boundary problems result from earlier intrusions. Therapy should counter that process, not repeat it. This does not mean the therapist is inactive. It is important that the therapist be an active observer and participant in the therapeutic process. One can work on boundaries in a very concrete way through modelling behaviours. For example, perhaps you are using crayons and involved in colouring or drawing exercises. The child may be sitting nearby. You could place blocks, sponges or a string all around you in a circle to show the amount of personal space with which you are comfortable. The child could do the same. Then, I would make sure that I had all of the crayons of certain colours within my own space. Whenever the child wanted these colours, he or she would have to ask permission to reach into my space to get one of these crayons. This very concrete activity is a way of representing the right to personal space.

The Phone

Having a phone in your play room can prove both enlightening and beneficial in your work. Children may be able to say things that would have never been said if they pretend someone is on the other end of the phone. Whole conversations may develop and reveal a great deal of information, as well as allowing children to work through some painful issues. They may have an entire conversation with a perpetrator, with a caregiver who wasn't able to protect them, and so on. All kinds of important things that were held close to their hearts may come out through the phone.

Masks/Sunglasses

I think it is quite helpful if there are a number of masks and some sunglasses in the play room. Each of these can function as a safety valve. They allow a certain sense of anonymity and distance in dealing with the real issues at hand. When children put on masks, they are "someone else." They do not feel like they are in the hot seat. The mask relates to the teacher, therapist or other significant adult.

Likewise, when the sunglasses go on, children feel they are hiding, slightly safe. Their souls have become at least slightly camouflaged. I learned this one from a New Jersey State Trooper a number of years ago while doing consultation on child sexual exploitation issues. This one particular officer, having been involved in a lot of child abuse investigations, noted that he found children to be less reluctant to talk with him if he let them put his sunglasses on. Suddenly, he had all kinds of disclosures and information to deal with which had been completely absent prior to the child putting on the sunglasses. This was not a pushy fellow. He would not have pushed and prodded the child for information. He would not give the child words, suggestions or scenarios that may not have occurred. He was prepared to go with no information rather than ask the child any leading questions. But the sunglasses suddenly seemed to work "magic" for him. I was a little sceptical when he first told me about this. However, trying to keep an open mind, I started to have sunglasses clearly available in my play room. Darned if he wasn't right! For more than fifteen years now, I have made this a suggested "toy" to include in playrooms, thanks to this wise police officer.

My recommendation of having masks available for the child to use does not extend to the use of theatrical mask-making with children. In classical mask making, people must lie down with eyes closed, while vaseline, then plastic wrap of some sort is placed on their faces, followed by the application of the mask material which can take 15 or 20 minutes to harden. This is a very dangerous activity to be using with an abused child. It is one I absolutely recommend not using. Too many children have been abused after being told to lie down? How many children are going to space out or feel very vulnerable or threatened in this position? Do not use this creative arts method with children. Use it with great caution with adolescents or adults.

Creative and Expressive Techniques

Children who have been abused have learned under threats and pressure to keep secrets, to hold in expression of their innermost feelings and thoughts, secrets and pain. Any techniques that can work to counter this tendency can help children learn or relearn to express themselves. Many of the creative and drawing methods in this book may be useful in this work. When children are allowed to express themselves through creativity, they are given the message that, "it is okay to feel, to express yourself, and to be a full human being."

Magic Bottle

This is a method that grew out of a method I designed called the Emotional First Aid Kit.[4] With the Magic Bottle, I first take people through a relaxation session as described on pages 89-91. Next, I ask them to

> envision a peaceful setting in nature. Imagine a grove of trees nearby. Let yourself relax as you watch the beautiful brown and green colours of the trees. Sense the texture of the bark on the trees and the rustling of their leaves. As you focus on one of the trees you see a wise and caring person emerge. This being is a healer. This person has come to give you a gift. It is a healing image or message.
>
> Focus on the healing image or message for a moment. I will be quiet and not speak as you sense and feel the impact of this healing gift.

I allow at least 3 or 4 minutes of silence as they focus on this image of message and then continue....

> Now, slowly, it is time to leave. Say goodbye to your wise healer. Thank him or her for this gift you have received. Watch him or her leave, knowing you can go back to this place anytime you wish. See your healer blend back in among the trees. Gradually, begin to let your eyes feel lighter and slowly open. As you return and your eyes are aware of where you are, remember the gift you were given. Without speaking a word, draw the healing image or write the healing message you received. After you are finished, put this healing gift into your bottle. Then, later today, next week, or sometime six months from now when you are feeling very stressed and at your wit's end, go to your magic bottle, take out your gift and focus on it to bring healing.

This exercise allows people to tap their own healing resources at a time in the future when they do not feel they have access to their own inner wisdom. It does not intrude and allows their own healing to emerge without an outsider telling a person what their healing should involve. There is another exercise by this name that is much more complex and designed for use with older children and adults (Revell in Barnes & Revell, 1994, pp. 50-53).

Movement

People who have been sexually abused have learned strange messages about their bodies. Movement exercises, dance, and gymnastics can all be wonderful activities for children to learn how they relate to the world physically. It may be much more appropriate for 7 year olds who have been abused to be in a gymnastics program rather than therapy. They gain physical skills as well as social skills in their interactions with other children. They learn about physical boundaries. That is often more than they gain in therapy.

Yes/No

This technique is meant to allow people a sense of choice, a sense of boundaries, and a feeling for saying no or yes. They do not have to always say either yes or no in their life. A big "Yes" can be written on a giant piece of paper. People lean against it and get to imagine someone telling them to do something against their will. They get to continuously say "No" to this demand. This may be quite foreign to them, especially if they have been abused in the past and always were expected to go along with whatever has been happening. Similarly, so they do not get locked into the position of always saying "No," they are also given the opportunity to say "Yes." A big piece of paper with "No" written on it is taped to the wall. The person gets to lean against it and say "Yes." This exercise is not done for very long, only seconds. It has a great deal of impact in a very short period of time. The exercise has been used in residential treatment programs in England in group situations as a method of promoting catharsis. Not that there is anything wrong with that, per se, but I do prefer to use it in an individual manner as described above.

I have used this method in training programs and am always amazed at how serious this can get in a very short period of time. I have members of the training group stand up and lean against each other. One gets to say "yes" and the other says "no." For the first few seconds there is often a great deal of giggling and laughter at the apparent silliness of it all. But very quickly, the giggles disappear and a deep seriousness sets in. Before long, there could even be aggression. For this reason, as soon as I see pairs move from giggles to serious work, I yell "Stop!" Then they get to reverse roles. In this simple and quick exercise, deep meaning can emerge. I do not let the exercise go for a long period of time in training programs due to the speed with which an intensity of feelings can arise. I want people to get a feel for the exercise, not dive into their personal issues.

Because of apparent power in this process to quickly reach deep feelings, I would never use it in an office setting for an extended period of time. You could be taking someone further than he or she has time to come back from in the period of a short interview. Its use is for experiencing a sense of power and control in one's life. Therein lies the benefit.

Assessing Sexual Abuse

During training programs, I am often asked "How do you know when a child has been abused? How do you go about finding this out? What are some key indicators?"

Obviously sexual abuse is easier to assess if there is physical evidence, multiple incidents and so on. Such evidence is often not available. Assessing abuse is also easier if a child has approached an authority figure and disclosed firsthand. Even this is not a guarantee though. Contrary to the mental health myth of the past few years, children do, in fact, lie.

Many of the typical indicators used in assessing sexual abuse, unfortunately, do not tend to be highly accurate. Some typical indicators that many mental health professionals consider to be indicative of sexual abuse include the following behaviours: acting overly compliant, acting out, pseudomaturity, hints about sexual activity, inappropriate sex play, early at school/late leaving school/few absences, age-inappropriate understanding of sexual behaviour, poor peer relations, lack of trust, lack of participation in extracurricular activities, fear of males, seductive behaviour towards males, running away, sleep problems, regressive behaviours, sudden drop in school performance, withdrawal, depression, suicidal feelings, and school changes (Sgroi, 1982, p. 40). The reality is that this list of "indicators" is not particularly useful because so many of these so-called indicators which are often presented in sexual abuse training programs are either indicative of numerous other issues besides sexual abuse and cannot pinpoint sexual abuse as the issue at all, or they are perfectly normal processes that may occur during any child's development.

Such a list may become useful when you see a cluster of behaviours, some of which seem to contradict each other. For example, the "indicator" of early at school, late leaving school with few absences describes many healthy, well-adjusted children attending excellent teaching institutions. However, if you add another item from this list—lack of participation in extracurricular activities, then you have an unexplained contradiction. Such a contradiction becomes worth noting and exploring.

For children who are victims of incest in the home, that home is not a safe place, so you may find those children always at school early, leaving late and never missing school. The contradiction that will exist here, though, is that these same children do not participate in extracurricular or social activities for, once they are home, they are not allowed out again. One would expect healthy and adjusted children attending an excellent school program to also be involved in a number of extracurricular activities. These kind of contradictions are important to take note of. On the other hand, it still in no way necessarily indicates sexual abuse. It might just indicate that a child lives quite a distance from school and for that reason cannot be involved in extracurricular activities.

Wexler (1990) notes that an examination of commonly available pamphlets on sexual abuse which list behaviours and indicators of sexual abuse

> turned up seventy-one different "behavioral symptoms" of sexual abuse alone.... There is hardly a child in America who has not experienced at least one of the symptoms at one time or another. They include: clinging, anxious, irritable behavior; nightmares, bedwetting, fear of the dark, difficulty falling asleep, or new fears; increase or decrease in appetite; drawings by the child that are scary or use a lot of black and red; poor relationships with friends; difficulty in concentrating at school; low self-esteem; and emotional upset (p. 99).

Wexler is crystal clear when he notes that "sometimes the pamphlets say more about the groups who wrote them than about the problems they purport to address" (1990, p. 100). I would take this view a step further and note that these checklists *always* say more about the groups who write them than about the problems they purport to address. Such lists are useless and, worse, may cause great damage by instilling fear in the hearts of caregivers concerning their own normal and healthy children.

One of the most ridiculous and unscientific methods from the above lists is used extensively by some mental health professionals in their assessments of both children and adults. This approach involves the erroneous assumption that certain colours mean something specific for all people. This method is best left as a party game for Freudian wannabees and not something to be used with children. Colours, like all symbols, mean something different to each individual. I have seen red mean warmth, comfort, and nurturance. I have also seen it mean fear, anger, and loss of control. Black may mean pride in one's culture, mystery, unknown magic, and depth. It may also mean fear, negativity, anger. There are an infinite number of meanings for any colour, depending on the person using it. Avoid checklists of what colours mean like the plague. They are the realm of heartless and soulless automatons stuck up in their heads who need checklists because they do not understand the depth of the healing process. One who does not fear touching passion needs no checklist.

There may be some clues in children's play that could lead to *suspecting* sexual abuse. Mental health professionals do not want to hear this reality, but it is possible in many situations that we may *never* be able to *confirm* it.

One indicator of the stage being set where sexual abuse may have occurred or could more likely occur is seen in blurred personal boundaries. For example, this can be seen in children with no sense of their own or anyone else's right to privacy, their own space and time. They may have no idea of personal space. When they greet you, they are literally offending your personal space and may be standing right "on top of you." Your warning lights should go off as to the possibility that something different has occurred in these children's lives. Tread cautiously. It may only indicate poor social skills.

Children such as these may have been sexually abused. On the other hand, children who had very early, life-saving and necessary medical intervention may present in a manner similar to children who have been sexually abused. Both children had their personal space boundaries intruded on, but for very different reasons. Great caution is needed in assessments. Keep in mind that in our present cultural obsession with sexual abuse we can end up abusing children by putting them through intrusive investigations when nothing has actually occurred.

Parenting styles may be a clue to abuse of children. It has been found that many parents who abuse their children want the children to make up for what has been lacking in their own lives. These parents become disappointed and angry because of unmet expectations. They may engage in inappropriate competitive play, acting like siblings rather than adult caregivers. These parents have a desire to control the child, but have only coercive behaviours—such as pouting, manipulative anger, physical power—available for such control. An example of this desire to control may be seen in non-play processes as well. If children of such parents are asked to clean up, the parents make commands and expect instant compliance. If they did not immediately respond the parent would likely clean up themselves but simultaneously threaten some dire and ridiculous consequence such as "well that's it, you are never going to go outside again." Meanwhile the children go outside to play 2 minutes later (Fagot & Kavanagh, 1991).

Finally, in assessing sexual abuse there are certain indicators which some consider to be reliable when seen in adults. These indicators include a number of thought disturbances and perceptual disturbances. When present in clusters, these may be clinical predictors of past sexual abuse in adult survivors. Some day it may be found that these are predictive with children as well. Keep in mind that we are still not looking at just one indicator. Rather, significance in assessment increases as we look at clusters of these indicators. The research indicates that a combination of

> *seven or more* [italics mine] symptoms is predictive of a history of chronic sexual abuse in childhood. A combination of five, including at least one perceptual disturbance, is highly predictive, as are any two perceptual disturbances.... Thought disturbances can include recurring nightmares with violent themes, recurring and unsettling intrusive obsessions, recurring dissociations, and persistent phobias. (Bagley & King, 1990, pp. 113, 114).

Perceptual disturbances can include "illusions such as a feeling of evil in the person's home or body as well as auditory, visual, and tactile hallucination" (Bagley & King, p. 113). At the risk of stating the obvious, I would add that these indicators would be reliable only when accompanied by some memory of the abuse.

Caution continues to be the wisest route. You may be working with a client who has recurring nightmares with violent themes, or you yourself may have recurring nightmares with violent themes. This does not mean that there has been sexual abuse. All that it is safe to assume about people who have recurring nightmares with violent themes is that they have recurring nightmares with violent themes. Again, keep in mind that we are looking for a cluster of symptoms and indicators which paint a picture of trauma and abuse, combined with a memory and disclosure of abuse. Any one of these indicators in isolation tells us nothing with regard to abuse. Nor do they mean a whole lot if there is no memory of abuse.

With regard to the previous list of thought and perceptual disturbances, recurring and unsettling intrusive obsessions may include things like an impulse to harm a child, a loved one or oneself, or fear of a child, loved one or self being harmed. A common perceptual disturbance is an auditory hallucination of a child crying in the periphery or behind the person. I have never in practise heard it reported that people thought they heard a child crying in front of them in the frontal 120 degrees of perception. It is always metaphorically as if they are turning to their own lost childhood behind them. I believe this perceptual disturbance really is a metaphor for the lost childhood. Individuals are turning to the past behind them, so to speak. Another auditory hallucination may be an intruder in the home. This same kind of illusion goes for visual hallucinations. Tactile hallucinations include sensations such as the feeling that one is being tapped from behind and, upon turning, there is no one there.

Even if any of these indicators does have some accuracy, there is still a great risk of misuse. They can be used very destructively by therapists who have problems of their own. I will give an example of how this could occur. A couple of years ago there was a major storm where I live. It was a long weekend and my kids were having a sleepover, so there was lots of fun and excitement in the house as the storm hit. There was a sudden change in mood. Something felt (physically/environmentally) very weird and I opened the front door and looked outside to see the sky gone green and winds intensifying rapidly. I yelled at the kids to "get in the basement now!" Everyone ran to the basement and there was a great roar, then a crash in the back of the house. Our favourite maple tree had been pulled from the ground and was lying across the power lines, which had ignited, and the hydro pole was on fire. We still had one active phone line after the lines had gone down so I was able to call the fire department. They arrived and took care of the situation until everything was both safe and secure. The hydro company also arrived and took care of the live power lines that were down on the ground.

At that point, with no power, no air conditioning and a lot of stress in the evening, I decided that the best thing for everyone was to "camp out" in the living room. We all got to sleep eventually. Somewhere around 2 in morning I was awakened by a crash in the basement, or what I thought was a crash. I was a bit shaken and lay there wondering what I had heard. I eventually convinced myself I had imagined or dreamed it. So there I lay, wide awake, having trouble getting back to sleep due to the stress of the night combined with the high heat and humidity. Suddenly, there was a very clear crash in the basement. This time I knew I heard it and did not wonder if I had been dreaming. Quite concerned about an intruder, I gently woke up all the kids and said "I think there's someone in the basement. We're all going next door to call the police."

Why anyone would break into our house with us home on the long weekend when neighbours were away and don't bother to lock their doors did not occur to me. The police arrived, searched the house top to bottom and found absolutely nothing. Now back in the house, I lay there trying to figure out why I had been "hearing things." Had I been vulnerable on account of a painful past and a screwed up therapist who urged me to reexamine my past for abuse that causes present problems, I could have easily been led to believe that the situation I described above resulted from abuse in my past, even if I had no memory of it.

To sum up this story, later in the day, in order to save our frozen food, we decided to move food from our freezer to a neighbour's across the street who still had power. When I opened the freezer lid, a big chunk of ice fell and made the crashing sound I had heard in the night. Our "intruder" was actually ice melting in the freezer due to the power failure.

Please keep in mind that behaviours, thoughts, and perceptions that I am calling "indicators" of abuse are in no way conclusive of sexual abuse in and of themselves. A child having experienced another kind of unresolved crisis, stress or trauma may also exhibit similar behaviours. Or, as seen in the above example, there may be a very straightforward explanation.

The bottom line is something most mental health professionals do not want to hear: there will always and often be situations where we will never know exactly what happened or whether a child has truly been abused. This raises the unpleasant possibility of perpetrators going free. Such a situation is a reality with which we must live. Rather than looking for some pat answers and cute checklists that will allow us to determine if this or that child has been abused or whether this or that person is an abuser—such quick and scientifically validated checklists will likely never truly exist—we should be devoting our attention to political issues and social issues that will help create a better and safer world in which children can grow up. The alternative is a world where we use cute "projective techniques" and checklists and pretend we can know exactly what went on and easily identify and then prosecute perpetrators.

We can pretend to have this information, we can use simple-minded checklists and narrow ideas and put people in jail as child abusers, regardless of whether or not they actually are, and still end up with the real perpetrators living free. This is exactly what has happened over the past two decades in the hysteria which has developed around sexual abuse. Many trials have occurred, many incompetent and/or zealous social workers and child protection workers testified and applied their simple (and totally erroneous) theories to determine what exactly happened, many innocent people went to jail, many of these innocent people were, fortunately, later acquitted—many with ruined finances and careers, and the real perpetrators (in cases where there really were perpetrators) have remained free. The child advocates have done at least as much harm as the perpetrators they were attempting to find.

To leave this section on child abuse, I turn to the superb work of Debbie Nathan (1991, 1995). She has extensively examined the problems of false allegations, justice for victims, a frequent lack of evidence combined with many child victims being too young or

> compromised by family ties to testify convincingly. The only real answer to these dilemmas is to cease thinking obsessively about what to do after sexual abuse has occurred, and take real steps to prevent it in the first place. Here we are not talking about current good-touch/bad-touchprograms, which are little more than laundry lists of taboo body parts and warnings about accepting candy bars from sex killers. Such presentations are one-shot affairs that do very little to help children define their psychological and sexual integrity or be able to react effectively when it is being threatened or denied. These abilities do not come from occasional didactic sessions. Children develop them by being given the chance to live in egalitarian families, to study in schools that value their intellectual, moral, and creative capabilities, and to live in a society where they are encouraged to engage in meaningful decision making, with peers and with adults. Prevention lessons do not address these needs. Neither do they help make nurturers of fathers, encourage economic parity between parents, or otherwise change family relations so that if abuse happens, or is about to, a mother – or children themselves – can muster the economic and emotional independence to stop the mistreatment, or leave home if need be. In the long run, nothing short of these changes will make much of a dent in the frequency of incest, the most common type of sexual abuse (Nathan & Snedeker, 1995, p. 251-252).

Obviously, what is needed are not more techniques for dealing with sexual abuse, but political action and social change. All the social workers, psychiatrists, child protection workers and psychologists in the world will not make an ounce of difference if they fail to address these issues.

MEDICAL PROBLEMS – THE HOSPITALIZED CHILD

Children entering the hospital deserve much caregiver support. Whenever there is an awareness that children will need to enter a hospital for some reason, a pre-admission visit is advisable for them to have a tour of the facility beforehand. If this is not possible, perhaps some time could be arranged with their own physicians about what will be happening and allowing children some time for any questions.

With children under the age of about 10 or 11, a puppet can

be a useful guide through the experience. Some of the best material around on the therapeutic use of puppets in a hospital setting is available from Nancy Cole, who works as Puppetry and Visual Arts Specialist at the Hugh MacMillan Rehabilitation Centre in Toronto, Canada. Her material is published as *Lend Them A Hand: Therapeutic Puppetry* (1993). Another excellent resource on a number of general activities for hospitalized children is the manual, *Therapeutic Play Activities for Hospitalized Children* (Hart, Mather, Slack & Powell, 1992).

It is a wise hospital which creates an environment where a caregiver can sleep with or beside children in the same room and which allows a caregiver to be present at all times during medical procedures. This is especially true in "pre-op" and in the recovery room. It is most beneficial for children to see their caregiver's face as the last vision prior to the aesthetic taking effect and the first vision upon coming out of anaesthetic in the recovery room. There is no reason to keep well-prepped (and the being well-prepped is a key to this working) caregivers away from the child. The caregivers should certainly be present up to the moment of entering and the moment of leaving surgery.

Upon discharge from a hospital or residential care setting, children may experience a phase of considerable sadness. This may seem like a contradiction, since their stressful medical treatment is over and recovery has begun. However, emotionally there is a letdown in two areas. First, while in a hospital setting children are constantly monitored and, thereby, given attention. There is lots going on—sounds, staff involvement, visitors. Upon returning home, they are no longer the centre of attention. They are not surrounded by hustle and bustle and interesting new things. The other issue is a natural grief. Children can become very attached to all of these people who are caring for them. These skilled and caring medical professionals care about children and the children know this. They feel the concern and love that all of the paediatric specialists have for them. When the time comes to end this relationship and separate from the staff, it is a natural response for children to feel deeply sad. Children should be allowed a significant goodbye while in the hospital. Perhaps they could take some pictures of staff or have an autograph book that staff and friends can sign and write notes in. Upon returning home, some extra cuddles and hugs, more than the usual amount of storytime together, and a general sensitivity to children's sadness is called for. This does not mean that they should be given any special privileges or have lowered expectations for discipline, manners, etc. It is important that they are grounded in the reality of their home. Children could easily become tyrants and rule the roost if they are rewarded for or receive sympathy for being "sick."

Animals can be quite important and helpful to physically handicapped or medically ill children.

> When children are hospitalized, the things they love the most are taken away; these are the very things that could contribute to their recovery and happiness. Chronically ill children have personalities that are developing (George, 1988, p. 403).

The very presence of a pet can promote a normal development and counteract any emotionally negative effects from their physical illness or disability. Children who are disfigured or physically "different" in any way often benefit immensely from a pet. There may come a time when young children with any kind of physical disability are, or feel, rejected by their peer groups. This is a moment when the pet is there, accepting, caring not an ounce about the physical challenges or difficulties of the child. What the pet gives the child is love, love, and more love.

Footnotes

[1] The research actually refers to "symptoms." However, I cannot accept this word. Diseases have symptoms. Children under stress have reactions and responses, not symptoms. Use of the word "symptom" is typical mental health professionals' mystified medical model terminology.

[2] The *DSM IV* is not accepted with open arms by everyone. It is a classification system that can be both exclusive and rigid. There are many who believe that classifying people into predetermined moulds does not, in any way, help them. I remember a wonderful professor, Maurice Moreau, in graduate school. On the wall of his office was a fabulous

poster that read: "Label jars, not people." As well, if you take the *DSM* to its logical (or illogical) extreme, every one of us could be labelled as mentally disturbed.

[3] This description sounds too simplistic: "I was sad and felt really bad so held this ceremony and then everything was better." That is certainly not the impression I intend to convey here. Many months after witnessing this dead teen, I was still having flashbacks of the bleeding corpse at the scene, still having difficulty sleeping and continued to experience intense distress. It is not an easy moment or vision from which to recover.

[4] The actual title, Magic Bottle, is derived from a treatment method created by Bridget Revell (Barnes & Revell, 1995, pp. 50-53). The method described here is quite different.

CHAPTER 15

Methods

MAIL BOX
FEELINGS GAMES
HAVE A PUPPET DO THE WORK/DRAW
LETTERS
DREAMCATCHER/WEBS
LETTER/PHONE CALL TO DEAL WITH UNFINISHED BUSINESS
IF YOU WERE...
YOUR FAVOURITE STORY/BOOK/MOVIE

Over the course of this book, I have presented a number of methods and techniques which can be used with children. There are many others which I have not yet mentioned. I will highlight some of my favourites in this chapter.[1]

MAIL BOX

This started out as a method for use in groups to help allow issues to arise which may be scary for children to raise directly themselves. The mail box involves having a nicely decorated box outside the group room and a pen and paper beside the box. The box has a slit in the top to put notes in. If there is some issue that a child does not want to raise in group but would really like it to be discussed, he or she puts a note or question in the box. Then, at the beginning of each children's group, the box is always checked by the group leaders and the notes are read aloud.

This method worked so well over the years that I started to use it all the time in group and individual sessions. Anything which the person in therapy wants to discuss but doesn't know how to bring it up can be written on a note and placed in the box. Before every session, the therapist can check the box and begin a session by reviewing items in the box.

Since my professional work these days involves training professionals who work with children and working with large corporations and human resources teams, one day I decided to use this same method in my training sessions. It seemed quite appropriate, since not all participants are extroverted or want to put their hands up to ask questions or raise issues. This method allows everyone to have specific issues dealt with. It may not need stating, but this has worked extremely well in our training programs.

What is interesting in children's groups is that a large proportion of the time, after the note is read aloud by a group leader, the child who put the note in claims it as his or her own. This should not be too surprising, though, since it is less stressful to own it after it has been raised than it is to actually raise the concern.

FEELINGS GAMES

There are many variations on games which can be played with children to deal with their emotions. Like most techniques, these games can be played in group or with a child individually.

Feelings Bag/Feelings Box/Feelings Treasure Chest

Most therapists who work with children use one or more variations of this method. A number of feelings can be written on recipe cards and placed in a nicely decorated bag, box, or "treasure chest." In group, the children take turns. Each child, when it is his or her turn, pulls out a card and talks about the feeling on the card. There are any number of questions which can be used. For example:

"When was the last time you felt that way?"

Children may say they don't remember. You can ask them if

they can remember anytime they felt that way, or when they think they might feel that way.

"What do you do when you feel that way?"

Here we are exploring how their behaviour relates to the feeling.

"What do you need when you feel that way?"

"Who can you talk to or ask for help when you feel that way?"

If there is violence in the child's life and home situation, it is important to build in the idea of choice. For example, perhaps the child's father has a tendency toward violent outbursts. It is important when processing these kinds of questions to be asking questions like "What does dad *choose* to do when he feels sad, angry, frustrated, etc.?"

The child may simply have trouble identifying with the feeling. In situations like this you can use some substitute: a puppet, a best friend, some admired person. For example, "what do you think Winnie (a big bunny) would do if she felt sad?"

Targets

Many of the feelings games that we use are very passive. You can add action by some simple modifications. The following is one I learned from Bridget Revell. It can draw in a child who is otherwise not attracted at all by feelings games. As originally designed, this method involved a chalk board with a target made up of different colours. Children get to throw a wet nerf ball at the target. The colour that is hit and splashed is the colour dealt with. For example, if children splat the colour red, then they reach down to the floor and pick up a corresponding piece of red construction paper. They turn it over and, on the other side, is a feeling. This feeling is then processed just like any other feelings game from this point.

HAVE A PUPPET DO THE WORK/DRAW

For people who feel they have absolutely no art skills—and even if they do—it can be quite a relief and release to have puppets hold the crayon and have puppets do the drawing. I tried this a number of times over the years and it worked so well that I started to build it into my work as a very valuable exercise. It also acts as a safety valve. After all, I don't have to deal with this directly, it's not me, it's the puppet who has the feeling.

LETTERS

The use of letters allows a child to discuss feelings that may have been difficult to confront directly. For example, after a parental separation, children can write a letter to either or both of their parents asking them something they've been scared to ask directly or telling them something they've really wanted to let them know.

Letter to Other Kids in the Same Situation

In some children's groups or in work with individual children I have made up letters based on a number of children's questions and concerns. Since, on some level, children are their own best experts, I would ask the children in the group to help me answer the letter. This builds in two processes. First, it normalizes things for kids in the group. They see that others have the same feelings and concerns. Second, it helps kids start to access resources and build some coping skills. The following is an example:

> Dear Mark and Cindy,
> Our cousin Brendan told us you help kids who have operations. I heard you even have groups for kids just like me. I am scared. I am going into the hospital in two weeks to have a heart transplant. I don't know what is going to happen. Can you help me? Brendan said you folks know a lot about kids and hospitals. What should I do?
> Yours truly,
> Wendy (9 years old)

This is a very simple yet powerful exercise. The issues can be changed in this letter. It could be about being HIV positive or having a family member with AIDS. Perhaps you are running a bereavement group. Then the issue could become how to deal with feelings about someone dying. The important points in the letter are the sentences "I don't know what's going to happen" and "What should I do?" The first allows you to incorporate a sense of the normal. When what's going to happen is discussed, by hearing others talk about the issues, it makes children feel included. The question of "What should I do?" allows resources to be discussed.

By discussing such a letter with children in group or in an individual session, their own responses help to normalize the feelings that surround the actual issues. As well, the children's suggestions and recommendations for what Wendy should do become resources they themselves can use. The therapist's role here is to encourage participation in the exercise and to edit (gently) any negative suggestions. For example, if little Billy says "when you are upset you can kick the cat," the therapist could respond with "Hey Billy, that might get you in trouble and will certainly hurt the cat. I've often heard you come up with really great ideas in the group. How about giving me a suggestion that won't get you in trouble and won't hurt anyone!"

Letter to Kids Entering Therapy

I have often used this when near the end of my work with a child or a group of children. I would ask each child to write a letter to other kids about to enter therapy or about to come into group. They are to tell other kids what to expect, what they liked and disliked about our time together. They write about what they learned in group or in individual counselling and how this helped them.

This method has indirectly served as a self esteem booster as well. Many kids do not have a sense of importance. Nor do they have a sense of their place in an intergenerational history. They simply do not feel that they have roots. The past is not seen as connected to the present or future. By creating this letter to other kids entering therapy, they are giving something to others, making a contribution to the future. This method was initially meant as a simple little goodbye tool. Kids were often beaming with joy after doing this, and

I realized that they were proud of what they had to offer and what they could give to others. It was a fine example of a positive secondary effect not built into the original rationale for the design.

DREAMCATCHER/WEBS

A dreamcatcher is a creation that looks like a spider's web. It is meant to be hung in one's window or over the bed, although these days there are even beautiful dreamcatcher earrings. The dreamcatcher catches bad dreams and lets only good ones through. It is a protective tool for children's rooms with its origins in Native culture.

This exercise, which I adapted from Bharat Cornell (1989, pp. 185-186), can be done in a children's group with six kids or in an adult training group with two hundred. The largest group I have done it with involved over two hundred and fifty people. The exercise was very touching when that many people all combined to form the dreamcatcher. This is an activity that deeply impresses participants. Through visually being in touch with what we are doing in the exercise there is great personal impact. I have done this exercise in many training programs and find it has just as much impact with adults as it does with children. All you need for the exercise is a very long roll of string, rope or twine. If you are using string, get as coarse a roll as possible. String that is too fine tends to tangle easily, and you can't wind it up after to reuse it. If your group is not too large (less than 40 or 50 people[2]), you can use different colours of drapery cord available at many fabric shops.

In conducting this exercise I like to use very comforting music such as that created by Enya or Maire Brennan. It is also useful to have at least two people leading the exercise so one person is not running all over the room.

> I would start by asking all those interested in participating to stand in a large circle. With the tone for this exercise already set by the choice of music, there is a flowing sense felt in the room. I tell people that we are doing an exercise on the interconnectedness of all men and women with the natural world. I would then ask if anyone in the room felt like any animal or plant. Whoever called out what they felt

like would be handed a piece of the rope...next, anybody feel like the wind—someone on the other side of the room is the wind, so rope is taken across to them...the sun...a wolf, a butterfly, a tree, a rock, waves on the ocean, water in the river...anyone feel like the autumn breeze or the scent of flowers on a spring morning.... I keep rhyming off different aspects of nature.... I ask what I've missed and let people call out what they are.... Finally, I ask anyone not already joined in the web to hold onto the nearest piece of rope as it is taken around the entire circle.

Next, I ask who was the butterfly or some other fragile insect.... I go to that person and tell them that someone has recently sprayed their front yard to rid it of broadleaf plants like plantain and dandelions. Unfortunately, it also kills the butterfly—you can use any example of destruction here: the cutting of a forest for logging purposes, the dumping of sewage in the lake or ocean, the smog created by automobiles. The point here is that there is some destruction of our natural world. I ask the person playing the butterfly to fall down onto the ground and sit there or lie there. Anyone who feels any physical pressure from this (through the tugging on their rope) is asked to respond. Very quickly a number of people have fallen onto the ground. I do not let this negative imagery proceed very far. I want to build in hope, not pessimism. As soon as the message is clear I tell the group that I am planting a new tree. As I do this I lift up the person who was playing the butterfly and again ask people to respond to any pressure they feel through the pull on the rope. Soon, all the circle is standing again. I end with two messages. The first is that we are all very connected to each other and to the natural world. The second message is about healing—ourselves and our planet. Reports have focused on the negative impact of humans. There is a much more important point to make. All individuals can have intense positive impact on the world around them. There really is nothing else that needs to be said after such an exercise. For that reason we usually use this exercise as an ending to training programs.

If you were using this exercise in an ongoing program I would allow a little time after the exercise to process how individuals can offer to the natural world around them and what they can offer to fellow human beings. In future weeks you can follow through on the exercise and build in a commitment to ideals.

LETTER/PHONE CALL TO DEAL WITH UNFINISHED BUSINESS

Much in life remains unspoken. There are many things in relationships that we wish we had said, and sometimes things we wish we hadn't said. Perhaps a child's parents have divorced. The child may have all kinds of hidden and unexpressed feelings or questions. He or she can pretend to be talking on the phone with mum or dad or someone else, asking their questions or expressing the things he or she would like to express. A letter could also be written dealing with the same issues. The letter is not actually sent. It is an exercise, to help the child express things. However, some children, after completing the exercise, do wish to give the letter to the intended recipient and may ask the therapist to help with this.

There is a caution needed with this exercise. If the issue involved is the death of a significant person in the child's life, an exercise like this can be used. However, I would not recommend the exercise be used to "communicate" with the deceased person at first. This is taking the process very deep, and it should not be rushed. I would make sure a child had excellent emotional support at home prior to an exercise that directly deals with the deceased person. First express something to or ask something of a living caregiver about the death or about the person who died. Later, the expression of feelings and questions for the actual person who has died could be dealt with.

IF YOU WERE....

Many therapists use variations on exercises like those that follow. Each of the exercises in this section can be quite revealing about the participant. Most of these can be used with any age child and will tell you a great deal about the child and the world around them.

A Musical Instrument...what would you be? You can also choose to ask the child to pick a parent or parents. In other words: "If your mum/dad/parents were musical instruments what would they be?" Is this musical instrument loud and boisterous, or soft and quiet? Does it play by itself or in orchestras with other instruments?

A Tree...what would you be? Does this tree need lots of space or just a little? How much sunshine does it need? If there was no one around to take care of it, how long would it survive? Does it give shade to others, have big branches for kids to climb on, have shallow roots or deep roots? Are there any animals that like to live in this tree?

A Toy...what would it be? Whose toy would you be? Who would you live with? Where would you be kept and spend most of your time during the day, at night, when your child was away? How would you be played with? How often would someone play with you? Would they take good care of you or just leave you lying around?

A Plant...what would you be? Again, a great deal of information about being nurtured can be gained from this little exercise.

A Garden...what kinds of plants and animals would live in you? Who would take care of the garden? What kind of care would the garden need? What happens to the garden if it is ignored?

An Animal...what would it be? When children pick an animal that they would be, they are sharing much about themselves if we choose to follow their choices. For example, the child who picks a cat could be asked questions like: "How do you know what a cat is feeling?" "How do you know what a cat needs?" "What happens if the cat doesn't get what it needs?"

A Rock...what would it be? Where does it exist? What colours is this rock made up of? Would this rock like to be hidden away somewhere or would it like to be on display? Where? What could this rock be used for?

YOUR FAVOURITE STORY/BOOK/MOVIE

You could also choose a favourite television show. However, I try and stay away from this, as I like to do little or nothing to encourage children to spend time in front of a television. They spend far too much time there to start with, without me in any way seeming to encourage it.

In this exercise, children are initially simply asked what their favourite stories are. Then these stories are explored with them. It is quite possible that the stories emphasize themes from their own lives. What do they like and dislike about the stories? Where do the stories take place? Are there safe places, sanctuaries or symbolic healing sites in the stories? With whom do they identify? What are the heroes like in the stories? What powers and strengths do they have? How would they like to be like the hero? Is there anyone in their lives like that?

This is a projective exercise but, like all projective exercises, its usefulness does not come from going in with a preconceived checklist of what different aspects of the stories or symbols mean. The value in projective tests is exploring stories with children or adults and finding out what aspects of the stories mean for them.

Footnotes

[1] Some of these methods, like *The Mail Box*, *Feelings Bag*, *Letters*, and *If You Were...* are adaptations of methods learned during brief training in 1985 with Families in Transition in Toronto, Canada.

[2] When I say 40 to 50 people, I am referring to training groups I have run. I would never run a children's group with more than 8 to 10 children in it.

CHAPTER 16

The Professional Play Therapist

Training, Supervision, Referral

INTERNATIONAL STANDARDS FOR CERTIFICATION
SUPERVISION, CONSULTATION, BURNOUT PREVENTION
STRESS AND BURNOUT PREVENTION
EVALUATING A CHILD'S THERAPIST

Working with children is fascinating and enchanting. I am often approached by people who would like to be involved in the field and who would like to become play therapists. The standards of the International Board of Examiners of Certified Play Therapists for Certification (IBECPT) as a Child Psychotherapist and Play Therapist are described here. The Canadian Association for Child and Play Therapy was the first organization in the world to establish standards for those working in the field. The international standards were based on those used in Canada and are the highest standards in the world for those wishing a career in play therapy.

INTERNATIONAL STANDARDS FOR CERTIFICATION

The international standards for certification as a child psychotherapist and play therapist are:

Education

a) A minimum of a Masters or medical degree in an appropriate profession. Such professions include, but are not limited to, psychology, paediatrics, psychiatry, education, recreation therapy, child life, creative arts, occupational therapy, speech/language therapy, and social work. Regardless of the degree certain core academic areas must have been completed. These are described in the following section "b."

b) The areas of study and knowledge must include:

1) Child and Human Development including psychosocial, sexual and physiological development through the life cycle. One full university year course (two semester courses).
2) Childhood and adolescent behavioral disorders and psychopathology. One full university year course.
3) Theories of personality. One half-course or one semester.
4) Marital and family issues. Two full university year courses (four semesters).
5) Principles of the Therapeutic Process. One full university year course.
6) Ethics (including legal issues of child protection and family law).
7) Research and Evaluation Methods. A thorough knowledge of: i) statistics; ii) empirical research methods; and iii) up-to-date research in developmental psychology and child therapy. A minimum of two full university year courses (a thesis or dissertation completion may count as one of these full course requirements).
8) Child psychotherapy and play therapy. A minimum of two full university year courses (or 200 hours in IBECPT accredited or pre-approved conference/ training program attendance). This requirement means courses in child play therapy. Up to 25% of this course work may include work in play therapy/creative arts modalities with adolescents and adults. The term “child psychotherapy” is used to differentiate this work from adult psychotherapy.

Clinical Experience

a) A minimum of 2500 hours of direct clinical practise (face to face therapeutic client contact) in the area of child psychology and play therapy in both individual and group process. Of these 2500 hours, 500 may include therapeutic work other than child play therapy. It is highly recommended that it involve work with caregivers/families.

b) A minimum of 200 hours of direct clinical supervision of the applicant's practice of child psychotherapy and play therapy. A minimum of 100 of these hours must be in individual supervision. Supervision must be with a Certified Supervisor/Professor or by a Supervisor/Professor pre-approved by IBECPT. Supervision must include either a "live" component using a one-way mirror system or extensive use of videotapes.

Professional Behaviour

a) Demonstrated professional and personal readiness for the independent practise of child psychotherapy and play therapy. The professional association will request whatever information which may be necessary to secure satisfactory evidence of this, including letters of reference, contact with supervisors of the applicant, and so on.

b) All Certified Child Psychotherapists and Play Therapists are required to comply with the ethical standards of the profession.

Interview/Examination/Evaluation Process

a) Attendance, participation and successful completion of a certification interview.

b) Candidates are required to submit a minimum of three unedited videotapes of their therapeutic work. These are to be submitted prior to the certification interview and are returned to the candidate.

c) Candidates may be required to complete a written examination in any of the areas of study and knowledge where there appears to be a background which could be considered inadequate.

Continuing Education

Certified Child Psychotherapists and Play Therapists must complete 48 hours of IBECPT accredited or approved continuing education specifically in the area of child psychotherapy and play therapy every 3 years in order to maintain their Certification status. Of these 48 hours, 30 must be in the play therapy. The remaining 18 may be in related therapeutic areas.

SUPERVISION, CONSULTATION, BURNOUT PREVENTION

Despite the vital importance of supervision, there is little research on it in the mental health fields. Fortunately, there is considerable data available from organizational psychology concerning the effectiveness of different supervisors and leadership styles.

Some things that have been found from this research indicate that neither the authoritative nor *laissez-faire* supervisor make a particularly good supervisor.

Although there has not been much empirical research in the mental health field regarding effective supervision, there has been an abundance of empirical studies by organizational psychologists in industry. It is clear from this research that there are certain things to look for in an effective supervisor. In studies on front line supervisors, it was found that "effective supervisors were found to be more competent, caring and committed to their work and to their subordinates. They emphasized quality, provided clear directions, and gave timely feedback to their workers. Effective supervisors described themselves more as coaches than directors. They freely shared with subordinates information about organizational policies and procedures and the reasons for their own decisions" (Klein & Posey, 1986).

From further research within the field of organizational psychology (Schultz & Schultz, 1994) we know that the most effective supervisors in any kind of setting are person-centred. They focus on consideration rather than quotas, deadlines, and costs. It is interesting that this even applies in an industrial setting where measured productivity is of significant importance. It has been shown that in settings where supervisors focus on output and productivity, that very productivity is actually lower than when the supervisor is person oriented.

Effective supervisors are supportive of their employees and helpful to them. They will defend their direct employees against criticism from higher management. They are loyal both to the organization and to their employees. It has been found that supervisors who give their main loyalty to the company are less effective. Keep in mind that this effectiveness has been measured in industrial settings in terms of productive output by employees.

The supervisor who is effective will be both democratic and flexible. There will be frequent, meaningful meetings soliciting the views of employees and encouraging participation. The effective supervisor will also have the flexibility to

> allow employees to accomplish their goals in their own way whenever possible. Less effective supervisors dictate how a job is to be performed and permit no deviation (Schultz & Schultz, 1994, p. 237).

It has been argued that "supervisors have more difficult jobs than executives do, yet they receive less formal training in how to manage other people. Supervisors may receive no training at all, and they are not selected as carefully as people who enter higher-level management positions. Often, the most competent workers are selected to be supervisors, and there is little assessment of their leadership potential" (Schultz & Schultz, 1994, p. 240). One of the difficulties for front-line supervisors is the fact that they are relating to the needs and expectations of both the front-line workers and to management. These needs and expectations can be very much in conflict and the front-line supervisor may often feel that they are walking on a tight-rope in a circus.

Keep in mind here that I am talking about front-line supervisors, not managers and executive directors. It is a very dangerous situation if the front-line clinical supervisor is also a manager or executive director. This is a time bomb waiting to explode. At higher levels of management and organization, the manager may need to be more work-oriented and less people-oriented. However, in studying the characteristics of effective managers it has been shown that

> they were tolerant of change, had clear goals, and were thorough, persistent, and persuasive. They shared rewards and recognition

> with their subordinates and exercised a democratic style of leadership (Kanter, 1982).

On the other hand, a study of failed executives found that they

> lacked consideration behaviours. Insensitive, arrogant, and aloof, they displayed an abrasive and domineering leadership style and were overly ambitious to attain personal rather than organizational goals (McCall & Lombardo, 1983).

Even at the management and executive levels, a high level of people skills are still required.

These kinds of studies have far ranging implications for the supervisor in the mental health, educational and social service fields. It is clear that good clinical supervisors will feel like they are part of your team. A vulnerable person and insecure professional will make a very poor supervisor. You should feel that what you say and do matter and make a difference and similarly for what your supervisor says and does. Over my years in practise I have heard of and seen far too many situations in the social services where supervision and the supervisor are resented and even hated by employees. Supervision then becomes known as "stupidvision," "snoopervision," or "superbitchin." It is probably a severe case of supercollusion. This reflects a situation where the worker is burnt out, the supervisor is burnt out, or both. It is highly negative, undesirable and unnecessary. There is absolutely no need for such situations to develop.

Good and effective supervisors will be those who can provide direction, know policy and procedures but don't cling to them obsessively, and can provide feedback on your work. They are caring and emphasize quality of work rather than the number of appointments you have and clients that have been seen in a week.

Good supervisors have a solid knowledge base, but do not cling to it like the dogma of a religion. They are competent in their own practises and have abilities to communicate ideas and concepts and to teach others individually and in groups.

They should be providing direction rather than always asking you "what do you think?" Over time there will need to be a shift from direct teaching and direction to increasing flexibility in allowing you to try out new methods, some of which may never have been used by the supervisor. With time and your own growth, you will increasingly hear things like "explain your rationale for that decision or approach" or "what do you think?" But these kinds of statements come later in the supervisory relationship rather than when you are working with your first client and craving direction.

They are able to accept differences of opinion and are not threatened by differing views of students. In backing up their opinions in honest disagreement, they can defend their approaches and access relevant empirical studies to support their views. They should expect you to do the same. Supervisors who base their decisions and recommendations and confrontations based on "my years of experience" (their years of experience could be the basis for well ingrained superstitious beliefs) are not scientists. Clinical decisions need to be made based on scientific knowledge and empirical studies, not belief systems.

Beware the supervisors who are always giving you homework and not answering your questions early in the supervisory process. They may be doing this because they don't know, rather than to help you learn.

Good supervisors will sometimes say to you "I don't know," or "I've never heard of that." They will be honest when they don't know something and work as partners with you to find the doors to open which will enable you both to find the answers.

> Nobody has all the answers. Knowing that you do not know everything is far wiser than thinking you know a lot when you really don't.... It is a relief to be able to say: "I don't know" (Heider, 1988, p. 141).

Supervisors who can help students learn will be those who are willing to take risks. For example, a student whom we'll call Bob presents a situation where he is working with a child or a family and he believes it will provide a significant amount of information and allow the family to feel listened to if a home visit is made, yet your agency does not provide home visits. Nor does your agency have any policy on this matter. Bob has read the literature and found that seeing this kind of family and child with which he is working at home could be beneficial. A good supervisor would support Bob in this, rather than tell him it's not done with an explanation involving all kinds of psychobabble.

It is important for supervisors to confront, support, critique and to have understanding and compassion. Perhaps the day after the intern's dog died is not the time to raise key issues of concern about the intern's work. (In fact, I would give the professional three to five days off—as well as the offer of a shoulder to listen—after the death of a pet to allow some immediate grieving space.) Timing is crucial to effective supervision. The phase of development of the supervisee needs to be taken into account. I have met some supervisors who treat all supervisees as if they are at the same stage. Early in one's career there may be very legitimate feelings of inadequacy and the need for the supervisor's wisdom, intuitive sense and knowledge. Later, the supervisee may need to be trying out his or her own wings with new methods and a new approach the supervisor has never tried. There is no such thing as non-directive supervision or supervisee centred supervision.

One of my strongest recommendations and directives with regard to supervision is the need for videotapes. You can dance all around issues with words and paint all kinds of wonderful descriptive pictures of your work when it is not actually seen. Videotapes (or live supervision using a one way mirror) allow a supervisor immediate and first-hand access to your work. There can be no greater aid to the supervisory process than videotapes of your work, even though the use of videotapes can make you feel very vulnerable and insecure at times. In the long run, your skills will develop at an optimum pace when you are able to videotape your work.

An area of concern that I have had over the years is when I hear of supervisors who are also the supervisee's therapists. Your supervisor should not be your therapist. These are very different roles with clearly different boundaries. Supervisors help you with professional development. This hopefully has a resultant personal development, but personal development is neither the goal nor focus. A variation on this theme would be supervisors who are more concerned with your personal life and problems than your work skills. This only meets the voyeuristic needs of supervisors to share in the intimate lives of supervisees. If your personal life and personal issues seem to be interfering with your work, then supervisors need to confront this. That still does not make them your therapist, nor should it make them privy to what the issues are. Such situations as these only seem to develop within certain theoretically oriented training situations and this caution may seem like stating the rather obvious. However, since I have seen it, it exists and should be cautioned against.

When you are receiving effective and competent supervision you know it. You may disagree with your supervisors, but you respect them and they respect you. If you aren't sure if you are getting the supervision you need, either you aren't, or you are in the wrong field. Effective supervisors should be excited and energized by the process of supervision. They can discuss what they know based on experience, theory and research. They are not threatened by being asked to explain their work. Above all, they are open to learning themselves and to gaining knowledge of new things. This will mean they are comfortable with having their old beliefs challenged and possibly changed.

STRESS AND BURNOUT PREVENTION

One of the most important tasks of supervisors is to help staff deal with stress. This is of such vital importance in a field where the issues with which we are dealing can be so emotionally painful—child abuse, suicide, divorce, death. Each of these and many more issues may be right in front of us in any given week. So, supervisors need to help you deal with stress and empower your professional growth. It doesn't take long for stress to begin to lead to burnout if we do not build support and renewal into our work. Yet, it is so easy to prevent burnout with proper supports and personal outlets.

As discussed earlier in this text with regard to self-care for the healer, we need to build lifestyles as professional healers that involve regeneration and rebirth; otherwise, our life force will become drained and we will start to feel helpless. It is only a short step from that point to becoming resentful of our work and burnt out.

A burnt out professional may not always be easy to identify initially. There may simply be a case of the "Monday morning blues," a general lack of enthusiasm for work, a tired and drained feeling at the thought of going to work. However, I would maintain that these "Monday morning blues" are, almost always, an early symptom of burnout. We should be excited about our work and overjoyed at being able to be at work on Monday mornings. Our work should be rewarding and exciting, and we should find passion in being able to be part of it. If not, you may be suffering early signs of burnout. Alternately, you may be in the wrong job or the wrong career. If this is the case, and you do not quickly change the situation, you will then be on the burnout path.

Once full burnout sets in, professionals become "grouchy" about their work or the field. They are openly resentful of their employers, the mental health field, the "system" and, most unfortunately, their clients. Professionals who are burnt out eventually stop taking any responsibility for their professional position. They sink into a victim role of helplessness, hopelessness and powerlessness. Everything they see wrong relates to "the system." It is a vicious spiral cycle. The more anyone looks outside themselves for the cause of their problems, the more they feel helpless and blame the outside for everything that is wrong in the world. When they take a passive view that some outside impersonal system factor is making them ineffective, the deeper the burnout becomes.

Supervisors need to point out when they are seeing early signs of burnout and help you build in burnout prevention to your work. This necessary self care still remains your responsibility, not your supervisors'. It is simply their job to help you identify professional issues and needs.

One reason for burnout is something I have seen far too many times: a professional sinks into a "swamp" as a result of being a professional full-time, all the time. They talk shop constantly, their friends are all professionals, and work is always nagging at them. They start losing sleep and are stressed out by work issues even at home and at play, if they even play anymore.

There are some key burnout prevention tools. In the demanding human service fields, all supervisors should include a focus on burnout prevention in their supervision strategies. It is important for you to have many outside interests beyond the work of your professional expertise. Work can only be expected to meet some of your needs. If your major energy and focus are all oriented to work, you will be left drained at some point in your career. Although this still relates to your specific career orientation, it is important to become involved in a professional organization relating to your work. This may be a professional association, a board relating to an agency in the mental health field, or political canvassing for a party which supports the values of your profession.

However, it is crucial that you also become involved in your community in some manner not related to your work. Perhaps you are a psychologist. Volunteer some time outside the field of psychology doing direct work at a local humane society, public speaking for a wildlife conservation group or delivering meals for Meals on Wheels. It needs to be completely different from your day to day work.

You need to also take care of yourself. In the early pages of this text I discussed the needs of children. Apply these needs to yourself. Take care of yourself—as a professional or as a parent. Physically take care of yourself through relaxation, beneficial nutrition, an exercise program and lots of rest and sleep. Allow for your own development in spiritual and cultural areas. Explore the background of your family's culture. Perhaps plan a trip to the place where you were born or the home town of your family of origin in their country of origin. Set aside time to be in touch with the Divine: five minutes between counselling sessions to sit quietly and say a prayer; an hour at the end of the day to be alone in your own home, or by the beach or in the park; a significant time each week to be in touch with your spiritual life at church, talking with your Divine Creator in the garden. Something in this realm is important to your own personal and professional development.

Continued Growth

Professionals in all fields need to keep up-to-date on current knowledge in the field, treatment issues and skills, research, and effective methods. I recommend that every professional spend at least a full day every month in an up-to-date reference library reviewing current literature, research and relevant texts in the field in order to maintain a current knowledge base. I also recommend professionals explore views that contradict their own. This encourages self-critiquing and helps prevent us from taking too narrow an approach. This learning process should be a part of every professional's life, but only a *part* of your life. We all need to learn in a holistic manner. We need to grow, to fly (metaphorically), to explore our wonderful world. If you've always wanted to learn to fly, or to dance or to grow herbs, go for it. There is nothing stopping you except that tiny voice inside that says things like "you're broke right now or you don't have the time, you can't possibly take that workshop on organic gardening or herbs." Perhaps there is some legitimacy for the reasons for such hesitation, but, even if there is, that doesn't mean you can't check some books out of the local library on growing herbs and, then, in one small pot in your tiny apartment, start your very first herb garden. Imagine the joy of having some friends over some evening for a dinner you've prepared yourself and saying to them, "I grew the herbs myself." Truly a divine moment. I remember having dinner with a friend some time ago. She was an Irish model and lived "on the road" a great deal between Canada, Ireland, New York and England. I had dinner with her in a small apartment she kept in Toronto (a large city with a population of over two million, so not exactly "close to nature"). She had made some fancy dish, and I don't remember what it was called. But the glow in her eyes when she said: "I grew me own herbs on the windowsill and made the pasta meself." There was such pride and she clearly was so proud of her work and it was deeeeliscious. This was a woman who died all too young of a congenital heart condition. Yet, while alive, she lived every moment to the fullest and never came anywhere close to burnout in her very demanding and stressful career.

It is never too late to learn something completely new. I am always amazed at the wonderful new things my friends get into. Cultivate your old hobbies or develop new ones. You know, three of the most loving and encouraging words in the English language are "go for it!"

I think we also need to be our own monitors and supervisors and always keep the following statement in our minds: "As a professional in this healing field I need to...." You fill in the rest and keep on taking care....

EVALUATING A CHILD'S THERAPIST

Should you find that your own child or a child with whom you are working is in need of some outside support that you are not able to give, there are a number of issues to consider in searching for an appropriate source of support. An important safety precaution is to always interview anyone to whom you wish to refer clients or whom you wish to hire as a therapist. Feel free to ask any professional about his or her training and professional work. There are a number of questions you may wish to ask before referring a child to a therapist. Any qualified and skilled therapist will be quite open to any questions you may have. This is the first thing to look for in a therapist. You need to be referring to or working with someone who is open to a working relationship. Such a person will be only too happy to answer any questions you have and deal with any legitimate concerns.

It may be important for you to know where therapists trained, with whom they trained and how long they trained in each setting. What are their credentials? These don't necessarily make for a better therapist, but they do give you an idea of personal commitment to professional development. Are they recognized by a legitimate licensing body and licensed in their specialty? Find out what professional journals and texts this therapist reads—this will give you a glimpse of how up-to-date he or she is in an awareness of research into clinical effectiveness of different methods. His or her awareness of present research is crucial, for it means that he or she is more likely to be familiar with methods that have been shown to be effective.

If a child is being referred for play therapy, make sure the therapist is a Certified Child Psychotherapist and Play Therapist with the International Board of Examiners of Certified Play Therapists or, in Canada, by The Canadian Association for Child and Play Therapy. The standards set by these organizations are the highest in the world. If the therapist is not Certified, is he or she supervised by a Certified Play Therapist?

You should know what the working model(s) are that the therapist uses. If he or she says eclectic, ask what models they draw from. A holistic approach that draws from an eclectic framework is in any individual's best interest, since it means the therapist is not restricted to one viewpoint. However, too many times I have heard the word eclectic uttered by someone who uses it to cover the fact that he or she has no thorough understanding of any particular model and basically grasps in a chaotic way here and there to see what works.

How many children with similar issues has the therapist to whom you are referring dealt with? And don't turn away just because the therapist may say "I've never actually dealt with this specific issue before." You are looking for a therapist who is generally competent in the field and who is open to new ideas and consultation. This is the next area to explore: where does the therapist currently turn for consultation or supervision? What kind of continuing education is undertaken over a year? You may be seeing a recent graduate of a graduate program in child studies. Your child may be the very first referral. The research clearly indicates that the there is no better therapeutic outcome for clients of professionally trained therapists than there is for paraprofessionals.

Each of these areas provides relevant decision making material for you to determine if this is the right professional with whom you should work.

This begs the question whether or not you really need a highly credentialed, seasoned and highly paid therapist. The answer is: not really. But it really depends on the issue involved. We know that success in therapy is highly influenced by the personal qualities of a therapist rather than the type or amount of professional training or the theoretical model used. "Nevertheless, a well-trained and experienced professional psychologist or similar professional may better understand what people—particularly distressed ones—are like, why particular individuals act and feel as they do, and how to diagnose individual problems, however much of a hodgepodge the resulting classification system may be. If so, then the professionalization of the mental health field, the fees, its status, and its public acceptance may all be justified" (Dawes, 1995, pp. 75-76).

Ideally, you will find a therapist who is willing to work with the child as needed and who is willing to work with the caregiver. The goal is reintegration in a positive way with the caregiver, not a severing of the family bonds.

CHAPTER 17

Commonly Asked Questions

The following are a number of questions that have arisen during the course of training programs I have presented throughout North America and the Pacific. Actual questions from participants have been used. They have been chosen based on their representation of general questions which seem to be on a number of professional's minds in the mental health field.

Q. What would be some advice for parents who want to see their children's art work, feelings packets, or papers that they are completing in sessions? (or ask what their children are saying in session?)
A. This is a very important question and one that arises frequently. Parents tend to be naturally concerned about their children. This carries over into curiosity about the work the therapist is doing with their children. The parents have a right to be concerned, they have a right to know what is going on and they have a right to have final say. I cannot overemphasize that point. Every parent does, in fact, have the full right to know exactly what is going on in any session involving their children. However, children also need privacy. Children need to not be intruded upon. For that reason, it is crucial to work with the parents, not to fill them in on every detail of sessions, but to help them understand the therapeutic process, the needs of children for their own space and time and privacy. I would discuss it with

parents from the perspective of their own needs as much as possible. I would, first, let the parents know that yes, they very much do have the right to see their children's art work, know what is being said in session and have full access to the child's world. Then I would ask them, in the best interest of the child, not to exercise that right. I would ask them how they would feel and how much they would share with a therapist if they knew that everything they were doing in a session was going to be shared with a supervisor or boss who had power over them or with a romantic partner. I would let them know my view that children need some space to work on their issues and they can ask me anything about me and how I work but please—even though they have the right—don't ask me about the details of sessions. Parents need to hear from me that if I have concerns or if there is something with which they can help, they will hear from me immediately.

Q. With regard to sandplay, do you encourage the child to disassemble their sand tray, or do you do it after they leave the session? I have been told that it is dangerous to "erase" the scene in front of the child.
A. I think it is important to clean up with kids. To me, the process of therapy is a joint process and I tend to perceive cleanup time as a joint process as well. I have heard some sandplay therapists maintain that you should not ever clean up children's sandbox scenes in front of them since it will symbolize the destruction of the ego and so on. Give me a giant break. This is reality. If they are that fragile, they probably need to be in the hospital, not in the sandbox. I get rather tired of such professional gobbledeegook. Cleanup should be a fun, playful, quieting time together. These types of statements by professional therapists lead me to wonder about their stability. Maybe it's the therapist who can't handle the end of the session. If this is the case, they should get some help, and it would probably be in everyone's best interest if they got out of the field.

Q. How do you channel a child's aggressive behaviour or anger without reinforcing negative behaviour?
A. I think it is important to realize that angry children have energy in their systems that has to be dealt with prior to peacefully and calmly dealing with the anger. They have an adrenalin flow activated, and

this has to be channelled. However, that is different from channelling aggressive behaviour. I always try to philosophically take the approach which reflects the attitude, "Lord, make me an instrument of your peace." I would highly recommend any physical activity that "shakes off" energy. For example, running, jumping, splashing, or throwing a ball against a wall and catching it. I strongly advise against the use of such methods as hitting "bobo" dolls or anything else used to represent a person or other living thing. Use of such "toys" is simply self indulgent participation in an aggressive approach to dealing with issues and should be abandoned. The approach of hitting some inanimate object that looks like a person or living being only serves to model striking someone as a legitimate way of dealing with anger. It is but a short step from a bobo doll to another child at the playground: "Gee, I'm feeling angry, guess I'll hit someone to get it out of my system." Children need guidance in learning that there are other ways of dealing with anger than hitting or striking someone. Children may need some physical release, but they don't have to pretend they are hitting someone as part of that release. They can scream in a pillow, even flail at a pillow, splash in a pool or bathtub, or splash their hands into a tub full of water. They can run around a track or around the block, they can chop wood or rake leaves or jump in leaves or jump on egg cartons (empty egg cartons preferably!). Part of their activity never involves directions to pretend the egg carton is the sister at whom they are angry. This, again, is far too close to modelling aggression. They would simply be given instructions similar to: "Billy, I know you are very angry and it looks like you'd like to hit someone you are so angry. I won't let you hit anyone or do anything like that. I will let you stomp on that pile of egg cartons and let all your anger out as you are stomping. Let all that angry energy go back to the earth as you are stomping. After you do that, we can talk about all the things you are angry about."

Q. Can you discuss working with children who seem non-responsive or who are quite non-verbal in a session?
A. Please keep in mind, in reality there is no such thing as non-responsive children. We may not be able to see what is going on inside of them, but they are not non-responsive. With these kind of children, always keep in mind the metaphor of following them along a path. Go at their pace and never attempt to change their direction

along the path. Watch them, face them, and try to see what their eyes are doing. You may make a comment like "I see your head facing down and I am wondering what your eyes see." This allows them to answer if they want, or to remain silent. When you simply comment that "I wonder," you have not asked them to reply. If you do see them look around, you could comment "I see you looking around. I wonder what you see" or "I saw your eyes move, I wonder what they were looking at." You could ask a direct question: "I saw your eyes look over there, what did you see? Is there something over there you would like to play with?" You need to be prepared for the possibility that you may get no answer. At some point, you could start playing yourself. Perhaps you could start to colour on a piece of paper to see if you can capture their attention. In my career, I have rarely, if ever, seen a child who remained non-responsive for a long period of time. Showing them respect, going at their pace, and truly being there with them and for them prompts children to open up to you when they feel safe and ready. Patience is the key here.

Q. How are your children's groups physically structured? Where are the children in relation to each other, to you in the room—young groups as well as older?
A. I like to be where most kids are, on the floor. Children's groups we have run have always been on the floor in a circle, with everyone facing each other. With some adolescent and adult groups we have used big comfy chairs or couches, but still all facing each other. Many adolescent and adult groups have been run on the floor as well.

Q. I've heard that unless you are a Certified Play Therapist, you shouldn't try to use the sand box, etc., because you'll bring up issues without realizing or addressing them. You could do more harm than good. Could you please address this issue?
A. This is professional gobbledeegook and typical of mystification within and by the mental health field. This kind of nonsense is most often heard with regard to Jungian sandplay and some art therapy approaches where therapists too often consider themselves to be some omnipotent guru. I refer you to the fascinating text *The Jung Cult* by Richard Noll, who describes Jung as the founder of a "new religion", for an examination of how "professionals" can take themselves so seriously they function as a "cult". If you are following

at a child's pace and not imposing, then no harm will be done. As noted more than once in this text, the view expressed in this question is not consistent with known facts. Research clearly shows that level of experience, credentials and level of training are in no way related to outcome.

Q. Is there any indication that children of same sex parents have more or different issues when their parents separate than do children of heterosexual parents?
A. Separation issues are separation issues and that is what you will see following any separation. However, there may be many other issues for children of same sex parents, but these would not be issues related to the separation.

Q. I work in a mental health clinic with a requirement of a certain number of "billable hours" per month. This means back-to-back appointments all day. How many hours of direct work do you recommend scheduling per day, and how do you recommend arranging "down time" to avoid exhaustion by day's end?
A. I am hesitant to answer this kind of question, but will usually take a shot at it. The level and amount of work at which any individual is going to function most effectively is always going to be unique to each individual. However, I do not want to avoid this kind of question either. Personally, I would never want to see a professional therapist doing more than twenty-five hours of clinical work in a week, nor would I allow any staff I was supervising to do more than that. Somewhere between fifteen and twenty-five hours should allow a professional to function effectively for very long periods of time and work for many years without fear of burnout. This allows time for a walk between some sessions, time for a glass of juice and a sprawl in your favourite chair with your feet up, time for recording and for chats with colleagues, for supervision, for training, for phone calls and all the other administrative duties with which a clinician is faced. It also means therapists are allowing themselves a full outside life with time available for many other interests. Without this, you will be facing physical, emotional, psychological, and spiritual burnout.

Q. Can you please comment on the extent that the play therapist should become involved in the play activity? I have a child who loves to play competitive games using a nerf ball. My role, for him, is to play basketball, soccer, etc. I am often uncertain about the amount of participation I should initiate. Another child wants me to be the student, her the teacher.

A. I never allow myself to be put in a degraded or degrading position with a child. Some children wish to play out degrading situations. They wish to verbally, sometimes even physically, abuse me in role play or, quite often, they want me to be the abusive partner in play. I had one little girl replaying what she had heard many times. She wanted me to be a bad daddy and say things to her that were degrading and simply awful. I told her that, even in pretend play, I would not say such things to her. She could play her story with toys, but I was not willing to say such things to her and at her. I do not want to ever put myself in the position of having this child attach such words to an image of an adult who cares about her and is working with her in therapy. That is far too potent a combination with great negative impact. Aside from this concern, I always let the kids decide on my role and position in play. Keep the children's issues as a focus always. For example, when children tell me to play the teacher, I won't directly go into teacher role and start playing with them. I would ask them to tell me what kind of teacher to play, what kinds of things to say. I would get their own images of the role and then simply act out their own directions. They maintain responsibility for the entire production involved in the play.

Q. I have been through a training program where I was made to feel unprofessional and foolish because I actually got on the ground, "down and dirty," so to speak, and played with children. I was told that I would lose all objectivity by doing this and I would influence the child's play and that I should, at all times, maintain a professional stance. I was literally told that I was "overinvolved," yet all I thought I was doing was playing with the child at her own level and in her own space. Does play therapy really mean "don't play with children?" Was it really that wrong for me to be on the floor playing with kids?

A. Unfortunately, there are professionals in the field of play therapy who believe that adults should not play with children in their professional work. They think the professional should sit and watch children play, comment on their play, and reflect on what they interpret the play to mean. They actually believe themselves to be very professional and caring people by taking this approach. This just shows what a powerful negative influence people like John Watson, Sigmund Freud, and Luther Emmett Holt have had on the mental health field. Watson and Holt advocated adult distance from children (refer to pages 53-58 of this text). Beware of professional play therapists who advocate not playing with children, keeping your distance, and interpreting children's play. What you should maintain is a playful perspective. Keep in mind that children and their play are not neat and tidy. My guess is that whoever told you what you described in your question was probably a therapist who was told too many times by his or her own parents "Don't get dirty," or "Don't you make a mess. Go outside if you are going to play." Remember that many therapists are in the mental health field because of their own problems or neglectful pasts. As for your question, keep playing on the floor with kids.

Q. You have talked about the need for confidentiality in play therapy. As a school counsellor who needs to work with teachers, foster parents, social workers and others, what can I reveal about what is going on in the play sessions without violating the child's right to confidentiality?
A. It is important to realize that, if you are working as a team, this should be clear up front from the start of your work with a child. That way, there is no betrayal later if others do have access to a child's file. On the other hand, if you are not part of a team but are working with other colleagues in the community, I would never share something without a child's permission unless there were issues of safety or protection of the child involved. I could let colleagues know the general kinds of issues we are working on at the moment, but would never share specific details of the content of a child's session. Neither do you want to alienate colleagues by putting up a dogmatic wall and refusing to ever share anything with them about a child for reasons of confidentiality.

Q. Is play therapy always an individual process, or can there be more than one child in the play room at a time? Perhaps siblings?
A. Play therapy can certainly be done in group format, and, many times, this is preferred. For example, in dealing with separation and divorce issues, group is an ideal approach. With regard to siblings,

this may be possible when working with a goal of building family relationships. But there are times when each of these siblings will need time on his or her own in session, too, to work on issues that could possibly involve the other sibling.

Q. Can you please comment about the child who has had few limits in the family and comes to school with much acting out, is rebellious to authority figures, often lies or steals? Is play therapy the most effective technique? How could it best be utilized?
A. I think play therapy can be a very effective technique with this kind of child. By being involved in play therapy, children have an opportunity to act out symbolically all their fears and issues. A child with few limits is a very insecure child who is not protected. The rebellious child needs a safe place to deal with that rebellion. A non-directive play therapy process would be most beneficial with this child.

Q. Could you speak a bit about interpretation (vs. analysis) and how to draw out important information for the child to work with again and again? Also, the importance of interpretation of the child's creative process in individual therapy?
A. I do not draw out important information for the child. Neither do I interpret the child's creative process in therapy. The first involves leading the child rather than following, and my work as a clinician has always meant following, whenever realistically possible. The second involves a degradation, and I will not do this to a child, or anyone else.

Q. Are there children with whom you would not use play therapy?
A. In general, I think that play therapy can be useful with most any child. However, there are some limitations. If I am working with attention deficit children, I would have to alter the physical arrangement and general structure of session, or they will be overwhelmed by too many choices. Rather than having everything available for them to play with, I would have very few items out from which they could choose. If I am working with children when impulse control is the main issue, then a very structured and behavioral approach is the best route to take. Rather than exploring their inner worlds, they need assistance in dealing with the concrete outer world.

One important caution involves work with abused children, especially children of domestic violence. If my working with those children in any way makes them more vulnerable to abuse at home, despite my desire to help them and work with them on painful issues, it may be in the children's best interest to not be involved in therapy while still in jeopardy at home. Obviously, child protection agencies must be involved, but that is not always a useful alternative in terms of making children safe while therapy proceeds. Finally, cultural issues must be considered in determining whether play therapy is an appropriate approach. Refer to pages 268-288 of this text for a discussion of cultural considerations.

Q. What would be some responses for a therapist to group members that continually state that group activity is stupid, they are bored or they consistently do not wish to participate?
A. I might play their own advocate and ask the members to help me understand what it is that is stupid or boring. Keep in mind that what they are saying may be true and maybe you do need to consider that what you have planned is stupid or boring or not relevant or appropriate to this particular group. It can be rather unpleasant if children (perhaps young adolescents) are sitting there saying, "you are such an asshole, why do I have to come here every week?" A couple of things to keep in mind—the children don't know the real you, so they cannot possibly really know if you are truly an asshole in your day to day life. This is therapy, not a personal attack. Don't take it as such. On the other hand, I may simply play devil's advocate and say, "that really upsets me. I don't want to be an asshole. Can you help me see how I am being an asshole? That is something I would really like to change about myself." With regard to this specific question, I would wonder why children who do not wish to participate are present. Unless children are somehow endangering themselves or others, therapy should be a voluntary process.

Q. Could you recommend specific titles of tapes or CDs (instrumental or sounds of nature) for progressive relaxation or guided imagery and other resources to use with children in the hospital dealing with pain?
A. This question has come up so many times in my public presentations that I have added a section at the end of this book with specific recommendations.

Q. What is the minimum number of sessions you can see a child and still be effective?
A. I am often asked this question and I think the minimum number of sessions would be one. There is much that can be done in one session. In being with children over an hour and respecting them, listening to them and caring about them, they may feel something they have never felt before or not felt very often. Such a new and positive picture can really stick with them and the things I say and do can have a high level of impact. In one session, I need to be a catalyst and help children learn ways to access other resources over the future. Perhaps I can give them some little tool to help them out in the world—for example, some little technique like *The Emotional First Aid Kit* described earlier in this book. I want them to gain the message that they are worthwhile people and that there are places for them to turn to where adults will help them.

Q. I work with sexually abused kids and for reasons of insurance or funding, we are often given just six sessions with each child. How can I meet my goals in six sessions?
A. If you only have six sessions, then your goals will have to be quite low compared to a situation where you had unlimited time. In the area of sexual abuse, it can take six months just for trust to develop, so do not plan on dealing with all or any big issues in only six sessions. In six sessions you can give children an image of an adult who can care for children and you can help them with some general coping and some day to day survival skills. Do not open deep emotional doors if you cannot see them through. If you only have six sessions it is not fair to children to delve into deep, painful issues only to end soon after.

Q. How do you establish therapy sessions in terms of frequency and in telling parents how long to expect the child will be there?
A. I think it is important to work cyclically so that there is a consistent and predictable time for the child to see a professional. For example, if you have weekly sessions, children know that every week on Tuesday at four o'clock they are going to see you. In general, if working in an outpatient setting, weekly is usually appropriate. If you are in an inpatient setting, try and keep the same time of day that you see a child. As far as telling parents how long to expect the child will

be there, I advise letting the parents know that you would like six sessions over six weeks with a child and will then offer a general opinion on issues, needs and how long you think the child will need to be with you. If you think the child needs indefinite, long-term work, be very clear on your reasons and review the situation every two to three months with the caregivers. It is important to be involving the caregivers in the process of decision making as much as possible. They are your partners and allies and spend much more time with the child than you do. That is very important to remember.

Q. How do you tell the difference between a joyful kid and a kid in denial?
A. I talked earlier in this book and often mention in my training programs how important it is to deal with the children's issues, not our own. Sometimes, we think we have to constantly deal with problems in the therapeutic process, and we lose our focus on the child. Perhaps the child comes in some week joyful and we feel the need to bring them down to our agenda of problem issues rather than dealing with the fact that the child has come in "up" and joyful some particular week. So how do you tell the joyful kid from a kid in denial? The body language and directness of contact should give it all away. Joy involves an opening up, denial a closing down. Joy brings eye contact, exuberance, spontaneity, even a certain silliness at times. Denial is an avoidance response. This avoidance will show itself through a lack of eye contact or a lack of ability to sit deeply with any issue or topic.

Q. What happens, what do you do if the child steps over a limit that has been set?
A. It is important to restate the limit once and this should include the spelling out of the consequences of stepping over the limit. It is possible that in the heat of the moment a child truly has forgotten the limit. You should know the consequences and be ready to fulfil those consequences when the limit is stepped beyond again. What I have found over the years is that therapists who are secure in themselves and are comfortable with setting limits (which might mean there will be times that the child does not like you) and dealing with consequences do not have to fulfil consequences nearly as often as those who are wishy-washy or unclear about limits or consequences.

Q. What do you do when a child throws toys?
A. First, duck. Then, basic limit setting. They would be told which toys are not for throwing. Refer to the previous question on limits.

Q. Could you share some of your ideas and techniques on helping children learn coping skills? I work with many children of chronically mentally ill, substance abuse and abusive parents.
A. Children in these kind of places need as much outside support as possible. They need the outside resources to meet the needs the family is not meeting and to help them survive their painful families. Big Brothers or Big Sisters can be very helpful here in allowing the child to lead a normal life at times. Kids in this position also need skills in relaxation training and inner world building. Exercises in this text like *Your Sacred Space* (pp. 191-192), *Nature's Healing Arms* (pp. 201-204), and others like those can be most valuable when these children are very stressed out. The greatest gift for children growing up in such stressful environments is to build in external resources wherever possible and to help them access inner resources. One little fellow with whom I was working was in the unfortunate position of having two parents who were divorced and who had not dealt with their own issues very effectively and who were each getting remarried the same week. They seemed to be saying to each other "if you can do it, I can do it." So this little guy had to cope with the craziness of attending each of his parent's weddings the same week. To help him cope, in session we designed an emotional first aid kit. This consisted of ideas that he came up with for things that could make him feel better. It included some excellent ideas like curling up in a duvet or asking gramma for a hug. He carried this list with him to the weddings so, when he was stressed out and feeling out of control, he still had the resources to turn to this list. It was his own self-generated list of resources and by carrying this list he was able to tap these resources during times of need.

Q. As a therapist, how do you introduce the family to the concept of play therapy and/or activities in family therapy?
A. Ideally, family therapy involves a great deal of play. Family therapy needs to work at the level of the lowest common denominator (usually the youngest member). There are a number of good starting points with a family: you could ask the family members to take turns

playing in the sandbox and creating a story to express what each is feeling. You could also ask them to create a story together, perhaps to express their family history; you could use a creative art technique. They could together, or individually, draw a picture of their family as animals; you may want to give them a feel for some of the "games" used with children in play therapy. The family could take turns with the feelings bag; with storytelling they could work together to create a tale—for example, the method beginning with "Once upon a time there was a seed...." It is important for families to play together too. Perhaps there is no "purpose" to the exercise other than having fun. They could spend part of a session playing charades. This one is usually good for laughing and giggling together. When they are fully able to be spontaneous and playful together, it is unlikely they will need therapy as a group any longer.

Q. When children are playing with sand, dollhouses or whatever, what do you do yourself? I have no trouble playing with them, but what do you do when they are playing alone? Also, do you ever record notes or leave the room during a session?
A. First, I do not generally record notes in a session. I would never leave children alone in the room during the session. I have left the room with the child during sessions. Perhaps we have taken a break and gone for a run outside, or maybe it is appropriate some week to take a walk down to the lake to collect some stones together or play with the water on the shore. To answer the first part of the question, I try to take a zen-like approach of just being there and doing nothing other than being. Symbolically, I am probably somewhere on the floor close to them, but not smothering. It says "I am with you here. You are not alone or abandoned." But if the child is saying nothing, I am likely only watching and saying nothing as well. If there is a lot of intensity or activity in the play, I may raise a question like "what's happening over there between those people in the house?"

Q. How do you pace therapy (including group therapy) with sexually abused kids? How do you balance the therapist's directive need to address issues with a non-directive approach? Is it intrusive even to say: "This is a group for kids who have been sexually abused."?
A. I don't pace therapy with sexually abused kids, or any other children. They set the pace. I follow them. They lead at their pace

and raise their issues. If therapists have a need to address issues, then they should be doing something to deal with this need. A major problem in a great deal of work with sexually abused children is the therapist's own issues get in the way. Children get forgotten. In clinical work with children, therapists should not be—but often are—going in there with preconceived ideas on what the issues should be for children. To answer the specific question about saying "This is a group for kids who have been sexually abused," that is not leading. If all the kids have been sexually abused and that is why they have been referred, then you are just stating the obvious and letting the kids know what you know and the reality of why you are all in the room together.

Q. Can you comment on the use of videotaping children for the purpose of clinical supervision. If you do it, how do you talk to the child about it?

A. I have mentioned in this book how important I think it is to use videotapes in supervision. These tapes give a very clear glimpse into the work of the therapist. However, the child's needs must come first. Children must have the right to veto the use of a video recorder during their sessions. It is also important to explain to children why the video recorder is in the room and how it will be used in work with them. Most children will be quite content to be taped if you tell them something along the lines of "I like to tape our sessions. That way I don't have to take any notes. The things you are doing in here are important and I don't want to miss anything. Sometimes my supervisor watches these tapes. I let her do that because I want to do as good a job as I can when I work with children. When my supervisor watches them, she can see what I'm doing and tell me if there is anything I can do to do a better job in my work with children. So by having the video recorder on, it helps me do a better job with you and with many other children. I am always learning and always trying to do my best. That is why I like to have the tape on. But it is also important that you know that there may be something or many things that are so important to you to keep very private here that you do not want the tape machine on. I need to know two things from you. One is whether I have your permission to tape these sessions. The other is, if I do have your permission to tape, tell me at any time if you want the tape machine turned off for something you want to talk about without it being recorded. In fact, I will show you how to turn the machine on and off so you can do it yourself if you would like to when you need to."

Q. I work for an agency where investigative work and therapeutic work are expected from the same individual with the same child. Could you address the issues that may arise as a result of doing work on both sides of the coin?
A. I would be a false idealist if I simply said "Don't put yourself in the position of doing the investigative work and therapeutic work with the same child." You may be the only person available and be in the position of having to do both. Unfortunately, the fact is that once you are doing the investigative work, you are now working for the system, not the child. You are no longer proceeding at the child's pace, and, thus, you are no longer doing therapeutic work with children. In other words, you cannot do the investigative work and therapeutic work with the same child at the same time. You can switch roles, but you cannot do both at once. When you begin the investigative role, you will have to let the therapeutic work coast on neutral for a while. It may take some time to get back the full trust of children, which develops from the respect gained by proceeding at their pace, but it doesn't mean it is gone forever. The systemic investigative work is important. We need to get perpetrators off the streets for the sake of all children. Just keep it clear in your mind which role you are in and you will be able to do a good job in each of these roles consecutively.

Q. What are your thoughts about hugging children, for instance if they ask you for a hug or reach over to hug?
A. I have discussed in this book the importance of touch for children. I see no reason to avoid hugging children in session, especially if they are asking for a hug. If a child is particularly needy, I would try and make sure that his or her needs could start being met outside the session. In session, if the entire focus became the hugs, perhaps you could set aside hug time during each session when you could ask the child if he or she needs a hug during our time together. Perhaps some time at the beginning, a couple of minutes in the middle and some more time at the end. However, if the child is that needy, I do not really see a reason to limit the physical nurturing he or she is craving. Build in a cuddle and story time for each session. I know some people

are very uncomfortable about hugging children in session. Perhaps these people should choose another career.

Q. What is your opinion of parents sleeping with their children?
A. I think it is the ideal for emotionally stable caregivers and their children. For too long, professionals have frowned on this practice. The ridiculous reasons for this development are well documented in Jackson (1989), Montague, (1986), Liedloff (1985) and Davis (1991). This situation is briefly discussed in this book in *Chapter 2, What Do Children Need?*

Q. Do you personally give children treats or snacks during sessions? I had a prof who was opposed to giving children treats due to not wanting to lure kids to therapy. So if they were hungry, they would have good-for-you snacks—carrots, celery, etc.
A. The only time I have given children treats is in situations of community forming. For example, in some group work with children, it can be a pleasant touch to snack at the end of group. It is a time for the kids to socialize and act as their own little community. We have no task other than the snack time at that point. If you are going to have snack, do it at the end, not the beginning. Otherwise, you have no group. The snack becomes the issue. As for the quality of the food, yes, we like to have some kind of good-for-you food like carrots and celery, healthy juices, maybe some cheese and crackers. But this is reality, and kids do like to have fun and be kids, so we usually also have potato chips, soft drinks and other such snacks. I am not sure what it means not wanting to lure kids into therapy. Hey, I will do whatever I can to make it an experience that they will want to return for more.

Musical Resources

Maire Brennan

Maire (Atlantic CD 82421)
Misty Eyed Adventures (Atlantic CD 82701)

The Clancy Brothers and Tommy Makem

Brian Eno

Ambient 1: Music For Airports. Very calm and relaxing music.

Enya

Celts
Watermark (WEA CD 43875)
Book of Days (WEA LC 4281)
Shepherd Moon (WEA CD 75572)
Christmas CD
In Memory of Trees (WEA CD 12879)

All of Enya's work is inspirational. Some of the songs in this collection are soothing and calming, some energizing. All of the songs are enchanting.

The Rankin Family

Scott Fitzgerald and Richard Hooper

Mother Earth Lullabies (Planet Me! CDK22)

Arlo Guthrie

Woody Guthrie

Both Woody Guthrie and his son Arlo have written and recorded some fine children's songs. Make sure you preview your material first. Each of these artists has also written much material that would not be appropriate for children.

Tommy Makem

Much of the work of Tommy Makem is appropriate for use with children. Especially recommended fun songs are *Waltzing with Bears* and *The Garden Song.*

Bob Marley

Martina McBride

My Baby Loves Me (the song—from the CD *The Way That I AM* (RCA 66288-2))

Loreena McKennit

A Canadian Harpist. Celtic and Moroccan inspiration. A wide range of styles and moods through her music.

Elemental (Quinlan/Wea CD101)
To Drive the Cold Winter Away (Quinlan/WEA CD 76310)
Parallel Dreams (Quinlan/WEA CD76309)
The Visit (WEA CD 75151)
The Mask and the Mirror (WEA CD 95296)
A Winter Garden (WEA CD 12290)

Parents

The Lullaby Album (Angel CD 64897)
The Playtime Album (Angel CD 64898)

Tom Paxton

Songs for Children

Kim Robertson

A Celtic Harpist. Anything by Kim Robertson is highly recommended. Very soothing and enchanting music.

Angels in Disguise

Kim Robertson with Singh Kaur, *The Crimson Collection*

Volume 1, *Guru Ram Dass*
Volume 2, *Mool Mantra*
Volume 4, *Har Har Mukande*
Volume 5, *Mender of Hearts*

Buffy Sainte-Marie

Up Where We Belong (EMI CD835059)

Pete Seeger

One of the greatest versions of "The Lion Sleeps Tonight" (entitled Wimoweh) ever recorded is by Pete Seeger. He has recorded and written many good children's songs. Again, preview your material. Pete Seeger is a highly aware and active political songwriter. Much of his material is geared to the mature adult. It's still great, but not for children.

Tchaikovsky

The Nutcracker. Magical music for children. Not necessarily relaxing, though. Some of it is enchanting, some quite energetic.

Vision

The Music of Hildegard von Bingen (Angel CDC 724355524621)

Sources for Play Supplies

Model train stores. In model train stores or hobby shops, you will find very realistic looking scenery, vegetation, trees, fences, hydro poles, people, buildings, town construction materials (traffic lights, street signs and so on), vehicles and so on.

Cake decorating supply stores. The joy of teaching and training. We all can learn much from our interns and students. Thanks to Mary McIntyre, who was doing her graduate internship with me, I discovered this treasure chest of "toys". Mary showed up for work one Monday morning several years ago and was thrilled with the little figurines she had found on the weekend at a cake decorating supply store. This source has been a real treat for me over the years. I have found the most realistic people of many sizes, ages and races in cake decorating supply stores. I have also found quite a wide variety of other figures like boats, cars, teepees and imaginary characters.

Yard sales. These allow you to save a great amount of financial resources and you also help the planet through recycling.

Zoo and museum shops. The gift shops of both zoos and museums have provided some wonderful surprises of toys in general and figurines for the sandbox in particular. Where else can you find an Egyptian mummy?

Disney stores. Here is the place for pixies and magic carpets. Keep your eyes on the ever changing displays in places like Disney Stores for unique little figurines. I actually found a tiny toy magic carpet in a Disney store. I now include it in my sandbox collection.

Independent toy stores. This is where some of the nicest "finds" occur.

Teachers supplies stores. All kinds of goodies and creative arts supplies.

Christmas stores. Lots of angels and sparkly things here.

Other Resources

Play Therapy International (PTI)

Many locations and affiliates throughout the world.
North American contact:
11E - 900 Greenbank Road, Suite 527
Nepean (Ottawa), Ontario,
Canada K2J 4P6
Telephone: (613) 634-3125.

This is the international organization for professional child psychotherapists and play therapists. The mandate of Play Therapy International includes: the maintenance of an internationally representative professional association for child psychotherapists and play therapists; the provision of a professional body offering Certification as a Child Psychotherapist and Play Therapist on an international basis; the provision of training for child psychotherapists and play therapists, and; the promotion and advancement of discussion, education and research in child psychotherapy and play therapy. Hosts and Co-hosts international conferences on play therapy.

The International Board of Examiners of Certified Play Therapists (IBECPT)

11E - 900 Greenbank Road, Suite 527
Nepean (Ottawa), Ontario,
Canada K2J 4P6
Telephone: (613) 634-3125.

The International Board of Examiners of Certified Play Therapists (IBECPT) is the professional body governing play therapy Certification on an international basis and is accountable to Play Therapy International. Certification is a rigorous process with stringent requirements. These requirements are outlined in *Chapter 16, The Professional Play Therapist.*

The Canadian Association for Child and Play Therapy (CACPT)

2 Bloor St West, Suite 100
Toronto, Ontario,
Canada M4W 3E2
1-800-361-3951 (800 phone line is active in Canada only)

The Canadian Association for Child and Play Therapy (CACPT) is the Canadian professional organization governing play therapy Certification in Canada. They are a registered non-profit, charitable organization and, as such, hold an annual general meeting open to all members each year where decisions are made concerning the Association's activities. As well, they provide travelling training programs where practical techniques for working with children are shared with Association members and members of the public. The Association's newsletter, *Playground*, is provided to members.

The Canadian Play Therapy Institute (CPTI)

P.O. Box 2153
Kingston, Ontario,
Canada K7L 5J9
Phone: (613) 384-2795
Fax: (613) 634-0866
email: cplayti@limestone.kosone.com
Internet Web Site: www.playtherapy.org/

The Canadian Play Therapy Institute provides hundreds of training programs with a variety of presenters throughout the world. These programs are often open to the public, including parents and students. They offer an annual five day Summer Play Therapy Institute in Canada. A complete calendar of presentation topics and locations is available by contacting their office directly. Supervision as well as programs of independent study in play therapy are available through the Canadian Play Therapy Institute.

CPTI is a fully accredited training institute with the International Board of Examiners of Certified Play Therapists/Play Therapy International and the Canadian

Association for Child and Play Therapy (CACPT) for play therapy training credit and continuing education credit. Many state/provincial boards of social work, marriage and family therapy and mental health counselling have approved the Institute for status as a Continuing Education Provider and they are approved by the American Psychological Association (APA) to offer continuing education for psychologists.

The Canadian Play Therapy Institute was the first play therapy organization in the world to go on the Internet with its own web site. At this site there is a listing of resources, training opportunities, accredited professionals in child psychology and play therapy, bibliographies, music and other resources, and, of great interest to many, **a discussion group** where you can participate with professionals from throughout the world in discussion of relevant issues, cases and concerns in play therapy and child psychology. Do make sure to visit and cyberplay!

Viktoria, Fermoyle and Berrigan Publishing House

P.O. Box 698
Kingston, Ontario, Canada
K7L 4X1
email: vfbpubl@limestone.kosone.com

VFB publishes children's books and material specifically related to children, parenting, child psychology and play therapy concerns. Submissions by authors are accepted and must include self-addressed and stamped return envelopes.

Mandala Therapeutic Services

P.O .Box 1654
Kingston, Ontario,
Canada K7L 5C8

Mandala Therapeutic Services provides play therapy training supplies including puppets, stuffed toys, CDs, tapes, and books.

References and Bibliography

Please note that, while some of these references are highly recommended, some are included only for historical understanding of the development of the field and treatment methods suggested in them may not be useful or appropriate. Others have been negatively critiqued and methods in them are considered irrelevant or inappropriate. Approach all material with a critiquing mind.

Achenbach, T. (1978). Psychopathology of childhood: Research problems and issues. *Journal of Consulting and Clinical Psychology, 46*, 759-77.

Adams, C.P. & Fay, J. (1981). *No More Secrets: Protecting Your Child From Sexual Assault*. San Luis Obispo, CA: Impact Publishers. This book is quite useful for parents and professionals in helping children learn to say "no" to sexually assaultive and manipulative acquaintances and how to get help that is needed.

Adler, M. (1986). *Drawing Down the Moon*. Boston: Beacon Press. A fascinating and honest look at the religious experiences of those who call themselves neopagans.

Aikman, L. (1977). *Nature's Healing Arts: From Folk Medicine To Modern Drugs*. Washington DC: National Geographic Society.

Ainsworth, M.D.S., Blehar, M.C., Waters, E., & Wall, S. (1978). *Patterns of Attachment: A Psychological Study of the Strange Situation*. Hillsdale, NJ: Lawrence Erlbaum.

Aldridge, A., Sung, C., & Knop, C. (1945). The crying of newly born babies. *Journal of Pediatrics, 27*, 95.

Allen, F. (1942). *Psychotherapy With Children*. New York: Norton.

American Broadcasting Corporation. (1995, September 13). Who's rocking the cradle? *ABC News Primetime Live*.

American Psychiatric Association. (1994). *Diagnostic and Statistical Manual of Mental Disorders* (4th ed.). Washington, DC: Author.

American Psychological Association. (1982). *Report of the Task Force on the Evaluation of Education, Training, and Service in Psychology*. Washington, DC: Author.

Ammann, R. (1991). *Healing Transformation in Sandplay: Creative Processes Become Visible*. Trans. W.P. Rainer. La Salle, IL: Open Court Publishing. (Original work published in German as *Heilende Bilder der Seele*.)

Anderson, R.S. (Ed.). (1975). *Pet Animals and Society*. Baltimore: Williams & Wilkins.

Anderson, R.S. & Gantt, W.H. (1966). The effect of person on cardiac and motor responsivity to shock in dogs. *Conditioned Reflex, 1*, 181-189.

Areheart-Treichel, J. (1982). Pets: The health benefits. *Science News, 121*, 220-223.

Armstrong, T. (1985). *The Radiant Child*. Wheaton, IL: Theosophical Publishing House.

Associated Press. (1995, July 14). Hugh Grant not ready for analyst's couch yet. *The Whig Standard*. Kingston, Ontario, 19.

Axline, V. (1947). *Play Therapy*. Boston: Houghton-Mifflin. One of the classics in the field of child therapy. The text is full of love for children.

Bagley, C. & King, K. (1990). *Child Sexual Abuse: The Search for Healing.* London: Tavistock/Routledge. An interesting study combining up to date research findings with healing methods.

Barnes, M. (1981, June). The art of sensuous healing. *Bodywork*, 3-10.

Barnes, M. (1982, August). Healing the senses. *Bodywork*, 12-13.

Barnes, M. (1983, July). Holistic approach. *Newsmagazine*, 8-11.

Barnes, M. (1991, Winter). Endings. *Playground*, 8.

Barnes, M. (in press). A conversation with Dr. Thomas Szasz. *The World of Play.* This is a fascinating, intense and intimate conversation with Dr. Thomas Szasz in his living room. This was a wonderful and relaxed discussion with one of my mentors who has never failed to keep me on my toes and keep me thinking. The transcript of this videotaped conversation is very challenging to the mental health field in general and specifically to the specialty of child psychotherapy.

Barnes, M. (in press). Evaluation in and of the field of play therapy. *The World of Play.*

Barnes, M. & Revell, B. (1994). *Exploring the Play Therapy Journey.* Unpublished manuscript. Presented at their conference presentation of the same title, Toronto, Canada.

Barnes, M. & Revell, B. (1995). *Self Discovery Through Inner Play: A Manual of Guidelines for Going Inward with Creative Imagery Exercises and Experiential World Exploration.* Ottawa, Canada: Viktoria, Fermoyle and Berrigan Publishing House.

Barnett, L. (1984). Research note: Young children's resolution of distress through play. *Journal of Child Psychology and Psychiatry*, *25*, 477-483.

Barrett, C., Hampe, T.E. & Miller, L. (1978). Research on child psychotherapy. In S. Garfield, & A. Bergin (Eds.). *Handbook of Psychotherapy and Behavior Change* (2nd ed.). New York: Wiley.

Barton, M. & Williams, M. (1993). Infant day care. In C.H. Zeanah (Ed.). *Handbook of Infant Mental Health*, pp. 445-461. New York: Guilford Press.

Behjati-Sabet, A. (1990). The Iranians. In N. Waxler-Morrison, J. Anderson, & E. Richardson (Eds.). *Cross Cultural Caring: A Handbook for Health Professionals*, pp. 91-115. Vancouver: UBC Press.

Bennett, S.J. & Bennett, R. (1994). *Kick the TV Habit: A Simple Program for Changing Your Family's Television Viewing and Video Game Habits.* Toronto: Penguin.

Bentov, I. (1988). *Stalking the Wild Pendulum: On the Mechanics of Consciousness.* Rochester VT: Destiny Books.

Bergler, R. (1988). *Man and Dog: The Psychology of a Relationship.* Palo Alto: Blackwell Scientific Publicatios.

Berman, J.S. & Norton, N.C. (1985). Does professional training make a therapist more effective? *Psychological Bulletin*, *98*, 401-407.

Berne, E. (1970). *Sex In Human Loving.* New York: Simon and Schuster. A fun, actually hilarious, text on sex and the part it plays in relationships.

Bernstein, S.C. (1991). *A Family That Fights.* Morton Grove, Illinois: Albert Whitman & Co. A helpful little book for use with children involved in family violence situations.

Bettleheim, B. (1977). *The Uses of Enchantment: The Meaning and Importance of Fairy Tales*. New York: Vintage Books.

Bharat Cornell, J. (1989). How to be an effective nature guide (a few suggestions for good teaching). In A. Carson (Ed.). *Spiritual Parenting in the New Age*, pp. 181-187. Freedom CA: The Crossing Press.

Bills, R.E. (1950a). Non-directed play therapy with retarded readers. *Journal of Consulting Psychology, 14*, 140-149.

Bills, R.E. (1950b). Play therapy with well-adjusted readers. *Journal of Consulting Psychology, 14*, 246-249.

Bixler, R. (1949). Limits are therapy. *Journal of Consulting Psychology, 13*, 1-11.

Bonwick, J. (1986). *Irish Druids and Old Irish Religions*. New York: Dorset Press. (Originally Published 1894.)

Bowlby, J. (1969). *Attachment and Loss*. Vol. 1, *Attachment*. New York: Basic Books.

Bowlby, J. (1980). *Attachment and Loss Loss*. Vol. 3, *Sadness and Depression*. New York: Basic Books.

Bowyer, R. (1970). *Lowenfeld World Techniques*. New York: Pergamon Press.

Bradway, K., Signell, K.A., Spare, G.H., Stewart, C.T., Steward, L.H., & Thompson, C. (1981). *Sandplay Studies: Origins, Theory and Practice*. San Fransisco: C.G. Jung Institute. Republished (1990) Boston: Sigo Press.

Brant, C.B. (1990). Native ethics and rules of behaviour. *Canadian Journal of Psychiatry, 35*, 534-539.

Briggs, D. C. (1975). *Your Child's Self Esteem*. Garden City, NY: Doubleday. Good material for mental health professionals, teachers and parents. Practical and down-to-earth reading that conveys methods, rather than just theory, for helping children of all ages create feelings of self-worth.

Brown, L. K. & Brown, M. (1986). *Dinosaurs Divorce*. Boston: Atlantic Monthly Press. This is one of the best available books to help children understand the divorce process. It gently tells the story of how a dinosaur family deals with divorce and all the feelings that result. It also presents many of the changes that can occur after parents divorce and offers positive suggestions for helping children to get on with their lives.

Bruner, J.S., Jolly, A., & Sylva, K. (1976). *Play—It's Role in Development and Evolution*. Middlesex: Penguin.

Cabot, L. & Cowan, T. (1989). *Power of the Witch: The Earth, the Moon, and the Magical Path to Enlightenment*. New York: Delacourte Press.

Caduto, M.J. & Bruchac, J. (1989). *Keepers of the Earth: Native American Stories and Environmental Activities for Children*. Golden CO: Fulcrum.

Carlsson-Paige, N. & Levin, D.E. (1990). *Who's Calling the Shots: How to Respond Effectively to Children's Fascination with War Play and War Toys*. Gabriola Island BC: New Society Publishers.

Carson, A. (Ed.). (1989). *Spiritual Parenting in the New Age*. Freedom, CA: The Crossing Press. A superb book on the importance of spirituality for children. Examines a number of different issues for children of different ages. Carson includes a number of different religious perspectives.

Carson, R. (1965). *The Sense of Wonder*. New York, NY: Harper & Row.

Casey, R.J. & Berman, J.S. (1985). The outcome of psychotherapy with children. *Psychological Bulletin, 98*, 388-400.

Cassell, S. (1965). Effect of brief puppet therapy upon the emotional responses of children undergoing cardiac catheterization. *Journal of Consulting Psychology*, *29*, 1-8.

Cautela, J.R. & Groden, J. (1978). *Relaxation: A Comprehensive Manual for Adults, Children & Adolescents With Special Needs.* Champaign IL: Research Press.

Chess, S. (1978). The plasticity of human development. *Journal of the American Academy of Child Psychiatry*, *17*, 80-91.

Chess, S. (1979). Development theory revisited. *Canadian Journal of Psychiatry*, *24*, 101-112.

Chess, S. & Thomas, A. (1982). Infant bonding: Mystique and reality. *American Journal of Orthopsychiatry*, *52*, 213-222.

Chess, S., Thomas, A. & Birch, H. (1959). Characteristics of the individual child's behavioral responses to the environment. *American Journal of Orthopsychiatry*, *29*, 791-802.

Chilton, D. (1989). *The Wealthy Barber: The Common Sense Guide to Successful Financial Planning*. Toronto: Stoddart.

Chisholm, P. (1996, January 8). Coping with stress: Canadians look for new ways to reduce pressures that threaten their careers, families and even health. *Macleans, 109*, 32-36.

Chopra, D. (1990). *Quantum Healing: Exploring the Frontiers of Mind/Body Medicine.* Toronto: Bantam.

Clason, G.S. (1955). *The Richest Man In Babylon*. New York: Hawthorn/Dutton.

Cole, N.A. (1993). *Lend Them A Hand: Therapeutic Puppetry*. Available through Box 45, RR #2, Milford, Ontario, Canada, K0K 2P0.

Columbia Broadcasting System. (1996, February 21). Who will watch the kids when Mom and Dad cannot? *CBS This Morning.*

Condren, M. (1989). *The Serpent and the Goddesss: Women, Religion, and Power in Celtic Ireland*. Toronto: Harper & Row. Simply one of the best studies on Irish history, and the suppression, repression and oppression of Irish and Celtic culture and spirituality ever written.

Conway, D.J. (1990). *Celtic Magic*. St. Paul MN: Llewellyn.

Conway, D.J. (1995). *By Oak, Ash, & Thorn: Modern Celtic Shamanism*. St. Paul MN: Llewellyn.

Cooper, G. (1981). *One Unicorn*. New York: E.P. Dutton. Although quite a recent story, the author (who is also a psychiatrist) manages to weave a tale rich in the fairy-tale tradition.

Coren, S. (1994). *The Intelligence of Dogs: Canine Consciousness and Capabilities.* Toronto: Macmillan.

Covitz, J. (1986). *Emotional Child Abuse – The Family Curse*. Boston: Sigo Press. A fascinating study on the effects of parenting on children. Refreshing philosophical approach typified by a line from the book "Just because a pattern has been set up doesn't mean that it has to be followed. I've always done it that way is not a valid reason for continuing destructive behavior."

Cowan, T. (1993). *Fire in the Head: Shamanism and the Celtic Spirit*. San Francisco: Harper Collins.

Cox, F. (1953). Sociometric status before and after play therapy. *Journal of Abnormal and Social Psychology, 48*, 354-356.

Crockenberg, S., Lyons-Ruth, K., & Dickstein, S. (1993). The family context of infant mental health: Infant development in multiple family relationships. In C.H. Zeanah (Ed.). *Handbook of Infant Mental Health*, pp. 38-55. New York: Guilford Press.

Culbertson, J. (1993). Clinical child psychology in the 1990s: Broadening our scope. *Journal of Clinical Child Psychology*, *22*, 116-122.

Cunningham, S. & Harrington, D. (1988). *The Magical Household*. St. Paul MN: Llewellyn.

Danaher, K. (1981). Irish folk tradition and the Celtic calendar. In R. O'Driscoll (Ed.) *The Celtic Consciousness*, pp. 217-242. Toronto: McClelland and Stewart.

Davis, P.K. (1991). *The Power of Touch*. Carson, CA: Hay House.

Dawes, R.M. (1994). *House of Cards: Psychology and Psychotherapy Built on Myth*. New York: The Free Press.

DeAngelis, T. (1993). Chaos, chaos everywhere is what the theorists think. *The APA Monitor*, *24(1)*, 1, 41.

Diaz, A. (1992). *Freeing the Creative Spirit*. San Fransisco: Harper.

Dobson, J.C. (1992). *The New Dare to Discipline*. Wheaton IL: Tyndale House Publishers.

Dorfman, E (1951). Play therapy. In C. Rogers, *Client-centered Therapy*. Boston: Houghton Mifflin.

Dorfman, E. (1958). Personality outcomes of client-centered child therapy. *Psychological Monographs, 72* (3).

Dossey, L. (1982). *Space, Time & Medicine*. Boston: Shambhala.

Dossey, L. (1993). *Healing Words: The Power of Prayer and Medicine*. New York: HarperCollins.

Drell, M.J., Siegel, C.H., & Gaensbauer, T.J. (1993). Post-traumatic stress disorder. In C.H. Zeanah (Ed.). *Handbook of Infant Mental Health*, pp. 291-304. New York: Guilford Press.

Drescher, J. (1988). *Seven Things Children Need*. Scottdale, Pennsylvania: Herald Press. This is one of those rare gems and unfortunately a rather obscure book that is truly one of the best references available for parents and families or for people who want to do healing work in the processes of family life. The author provides insight into how to meet these needs. This little book may be hard to find, but is well worth the search.

Dubos, R. (1971). A Theology of Earth. In R.T. Harney, R. Disch (Eds.). *The Dying Generations: Perspectives on the Environmental Crisis*, pp. 402-415. New York: Dell Publishing.

Dubos, R. (1972). *A God Within*. New York: Charles Scribner's Sons.

Dundas, E. (1978). *Symbols Come Alive in the Sand*. Aptos CA: Aptos Press.

Dunham, C., Myers, F., Barnden, N., McDougall, A., Kelly, T.L, & Aria, B. (1991). *Mamatoto: A Celebration of Earth*. London: Virago Press.

Ehrlich, A. (Ed.). (1985). *The Random House Book of Fairy Tales*. New York: Random House. A fine addition to a family's or professional's library. Excellent bedtime reading.

Evans-Wentz, W.Y. (1966). *The Fairy Faith In Celtic Countries*. Don Mills, Ontario: Musson Book Company. (First Published 1911.)

Everett, F., Protcor, N., & Cartmell, B. (1983). Providing psychological services to American Indian children and families. *Professional Psychology: Research and Practice, 14*, 588-603.

Eysenck, H. (1985). *Decline and Fall of the Freudian Empire*. New York: Viking Penguin.

Fagot, B.I. & Kavanagh, K. (1991). Play as a diagnostic tool with physically abusive parents and their children. In C.E. Schaefer, K. Gitlin, & A. Sandgrund, (Eds.). *Play Diagnosis and Assessment*, pp. 203-218. New York: John Wiley & Sons.

Felson, R.B. (1984). The effects of self-appraisal ability on academic performance. *Journal of Personality and Social Psychology, 47*, 944-952.

Field, T., Schanberg, S., Scarfidi, F., Bauer, C., Vega-Lahr, N., Garcia, R., Nystrom, J., & Kuhn, C. (1986). Tactile/kinesthetic stimulation effects of preterm neonates. *Pediatrics, 77*, 654.

Fish, M.C. (1988). Relaxation Training for Childhood Disorders. In C.E. Schaefer (Ed.). *Innovative Interventions in Child and Adolescent Therapy*, pp. 160-192. Toronto, ON: Wiley-Interscience.

Fischer, J. (1976). *The Effectiveness of Social Casework*. Springfield IL: Charles C. Thomas Publisher.

Fischer, K.F. (1980). A theory of cognitive development: The control and construction of hierarchies of skills. *Psychological Review, 87*, 477-531.

Fleming, L. & Snyder, W. (1947). Social and personal changes following non-directive group play therapy. *American Journal of Orthopsychiatry, 17*, 101-116.

Ford, C. & Beach, F. (1951). *Patterns of Sexual Behavior*. New York: Harper & Row. A fascinating look by a psychologist and anthropologist at cross cultural and cross species sexual behaviours. Sexual behavior in cultural and evolutionary terms is described in a well integrated and unopinionated fashion.

Frank, J.D. (1973). *Persuasion and Healing* (2nd ed.). Baltimore: Johns Hopkins University Press.

Frankl, V. (1985). *The Unconscious God.* New York, NY: Washington Square Books. Frankl argues that not only is there an instinctual unconscious but a spiritual unconscious as well. Frankl shows that unconscious religious belief is not only a universal reality, but a vital element of the human condition.

Freeman, R. (1985). Separation & divorce: What about the children? *Toronto Parent, 2(2)*, 4-6.

Freud, S. (1914). *Pscyhopathology of Everyday Life*. London: Unwin.

Freud, S. (1932) [1909]. The analysis of a phobia in a five-year-old boy. *The Standard Edition of the Complete Works of Sigmund Freud*, Vol. 10. London: Hogarth Press.

Freud, S. (1949). *Three Essays on the Theory of Sexuality*. London: Hogarth Press.

Fung, Y. (1973). *A History of Chinese Philosophy*. Trans. D. Bodde, Princeton, NJ: Princeton University Press.

Funk, J.B. (1980). Management of sexual molestation in preschoolers. *Clinical Pediatrics, 19*, 686-688.

Gabel, S., Oster, G., & Pfeffer, C.R. (1988). *Difficult Moments in Child Psychotherapy.* New York: Plenum Publishing.

Garb, H.N. (1989). Clinical judgment, clinical training, and professional experience. *Psychological Bulletin, 105*, 387-392.

Garbarino, J. (1995). *Raising Children in a Socially Toxic Environment*. San Francisco: Jossey-Bass.

Garcia Coll, C.T., & Meyer, E.C. (1993). The sociocultural context of infant development. In C.H. Zeanah (Ed.). *Handbook of Infant Mental Health*, pp. 56-69. New York: Guilford Press.

Gardner, R. (1970). *The Boys and Girls Book About Divorce*. Toronto: Bantam. This is a good reference book for kids whose parents are separating, separated or divorced. Many kids keep it beside their beds and refer to it out of interest or in times of confusion and difficulty. An excellent gift from group leaders to children at the end of a separation and divorce group.

Gardner, R. (1971). *Therapeutic Communication With Children: The Mutual Storytelling Technique*. New York: Jason Aronson.

Gardner, R. (1977). *The Parents Book About Divorce*. Toronto: Bantam. A parent's companion volume to *The Boys and Girls Book About Divorce*.

Garfield, P. (1984). *Your Child's Dreams*. New York: Ballantine. An excellent resource on children's dreams and nightmares.

Garfield, S.L., & Bergin, A.E. (1986). *Handbook of Psychotherapy and Behavior Change* (3rd ed.). New York: John Wiley.

George, H. (1988). Child therapy and animals: A new way for an old relationship. In C.E. Schaefer (Ed.), *Innovative Interventions in Child and Adolescent Therapy*, pp. 400-418. Toronto: Wiley-Interscience. Excellent material on this often ignored important topic. What better way to integrate nature, creativity and everday experience than through the use of domestic animals.

Gil, E. (1991). *The Healing Power of Play: Working With Abused Children*. New York: Guilford Press.

Ginott, H. (1959). The theory and practice of therapeutic intervention in child treatment. *Journal of Consulting Psychology, 23*, 160-166.

Glasgow, J.H. & Adaskin, E.J. (1990). The West Indians. In N. Waxler-Morrison, J. Anderson, & E. Richardson (Eds.). *Cross Cultural Caring: A Handbook for Health Professionals*, pp. 214-244. Vancouver: UBC Press.

Greven, P. (1992). *Spare the Child: The Religious Roots of Punishment and the Psychological Impact of Physical Abuse*. New York: Vintage Books. This is best described as "one of those rare works of scholarship that have the power to change our lives."

Griffin, S. (1981). *Pornography and Silence: Culture's Revenge Against Nature*. New York: Harper & Row. The title says it all. Very astute examination of the processes functioning behind the phenomenon of pornography. Excellent examination of the psychodynamics of projection and the shadow concept.

Grof, S. (1985). *Beyond the Brain: Birth, Death and Transcendence in Psychotherapy*. Syracuse, NY: State University of New York Press.

Grof, S. & Grof, C. (Eds.). (1989). *Spiritual Emergency: When Personal Transformation Becomes a Crisis*. New York: Putnam.

Guerney, L.F. (1983). Client-centered (Nondirective) Play Therapy. In C.E. Schaefer & K.J. O'Connor (Eds.). *The Handbook of Play Therapy*, pp. 21-64. New York: John Wiley & Sons.

Hacking, I. (1995). *Rewriting the Soul: Multiple Personality and the Sciences of Memory.* Princeton NJ: Princeton University Press.

Haller, I. (1987). *How Children Play.* Edinburgh Scotland: Flovis Books. (Originally published in German as *Das Spielende Kind* by Verlag Freies Geistesleben, Stuttgart, 1987).

Hambridge, G. (1955). Structured play therapy. *American Journal of Orthopsychiatry, 25,* 601-617.

Hammerschlag, C.A. (1988). *The Dancing Healers: A Doctor's Journey of Healing with Native Americans.* San Fransisco: Harper & Row.

Hart, R., Mather, P.L., Slack, J.F., & Powell, M.A. (1992). *Therapeutic Play Activities for Hospitalized Children.* St. Louis MO: Mosby-Year Book.

Harter, S. (1980). Children's understanding of multiple emotions: A cognitive developmental approach. *Proceedings of Jean Piaget Society.* Hillsdale NJ: Lawrence Erlbaum.

Harter, S. (1982). A cognitive-developmental approach to children's use of affect and trait labels. In F.C. Serafica (Ed.). *Social Cognition in Context.* New York: Guildord Press.

Harter, S. (1983). Cognitive-developmental considerations in the conduct of play therapy. In C.E. Schaefer & K.J. O'Connor (Eds.). *Handbook of Play Therapy* pp. 95-127. Toronto: John Wiley & Sons

Heaton, J.A. & Wilson, N.L. (1995). *Tuning in Trouble: Talk TV's Destructive Impact on Mental Health.* San Francisco: Jossey-Bass.

Heider, J. (1988). *The Tao of Leadership.* Toronto: Bantam.

Heinicke, C. & Goldman, A. (1960). Research on psychotherapy with children: A review and suggestions for further study. *American Journal of Orthopsychiatry, 30,* 483-494.

Heinicke, C. & Strassman, L. (1975). Toward more effective research on child psychotherapy. *Journal of Child Psychiatry, 14,* 561-588.

Hellendoorn, J., van der Kooij, R. & Sutton-Smith, B. (Eds.). (1994). *Play and Intervention.* Albany: State University of New York Press.

Henley, N.M. (1973). The politics of touch. In Phil Brown (Ed.). *Radical Psychology,* pp. 420-433. New York: Colophon Books.

Hicks, R.D. (1991). *In Pursuit of Satan.* Buffalo: Prometheus.

Hindman, J. (1985). *A Very Touching Book.* Ontario OR: AlexAndria Associates. Very good book for ideas to use with children to help them learn about different kinds of touch, sexual abuse, prevention. Highly recommended for all parents and professionals. One word of caution: this little book has certain pictures which can give odd messages to children who have been traumatized and may tend toward certain distortions of reality. For that reason, I tend to use some of the ideas and words from the book rather than the actual book with children.

Hindman, J. (1989). *Just Before Dawn.* Ontario OR: AlexAndria Associates. Myth shattering material concerning abuse, trauma and assessment and treatment methods.

Hindman, J. (1991). *The Mourning Breaks.* Ontario OR: AlexAndria Associates. Another welcome addition to the field. Specific guidelines and treatment strategies and numerous exercises and techniques for working with victims of sexual abuse.

Hoffman, E. (1981). *Huna: A Beginner's Guide*. West Chester PA: Whitford Press.

Holt, L. (1894). *The Care and Feeding of Children*. East Norwalk CT: Appleton-Century. This text, first published in 1894, went on through 15 editions.

Hood-Williams, J. (1960). The results of psychotherapy with children. *Journal of Consulting Psychologist*, *24*, 84-88.

Hug-Hellmuth, H. (1921). On the technique of child-analysis. *International Journal of of Psycho-Analysis*, *2*, 287-305. This is definitely one of those "don't try this at home" efforts. Hug-Helmuth was murdered by a nephew who was actually an adopted son. Hug-Helmuth was treating him with psychoanalytic methods. I guess he didn't believe in the Oedipus complex.

Irwin, E.C. (1991). The use of a puppet interview to understand children. In C.E. Schaefer, K. Gitlin, and A. Sandgrund (Eds.), *Play Diagnosis and Assessment*, pp. 617-635. Toronto, ON: Wiley-Interscience.

Jackson, D. (1989). *Three In A Bed: Why You Should Sleep with Your Baby*. London: Bloomsbury.

James, B. (1989). *Treating Traumatized Children: New Insights and Creative Interventions.* Toronto: Lexington Books.

James, B. (1994). *Handbook for Treatment of Attachment-Trauma Problems in Children.* Don Mills, Ontario: Maxwell Macmillan. Highly recommended material on this complex issue.

Jernberg, A.M. (1979). *Theraplay—A New Treatment Using Structured Play for Problem Children and Their Families.* San Fransico CA: Jossey-Bass.

Johnson, R. (1986). *Inner Work*. San Fransisco: Harper & Row. Dreamwork and Jungian therapy demystified and made accessible.

Jones, M.C. (1974). A laboratory study of fear: The case of Peter. *Pedagogical Seminary, 31*(*2*), 308-315.

Jourard, S.M. (1966). An exploratory study of body accessibility. *British Journal of Social and Clinical Psychology*, *5*, 221-231.

Jourard, S.M. & Rubin, J.E. (1968). Self-disclosure and touching: A study of two modes of interpersonal encounter and their interaction. *Journal of Humanistic Psychology*, *8*, 39-48.

Jourard, S. (1971). *The Transparent Self*. New York: Van Nostrand Reinhold.

Jung, C.G. (1972). *Mandala Symbolism*. Priceton NJ: Princeton University Press. (Originally published in 1959.)

Jung, C.G. (1981). *The Development of Personality*. Princeton NJ: Princeton University Press. (Originally published in 1954.)

Kagan, J. (1984). *The Nature of the Child*. New York: Basic Books.

Kalat, J.W. (1995). *Biological Psychology*. Toronto: Brooks/Cole Publishing Company.

Kalff, D. (1980). *Sandplay: A Psychotherapeutic Approach to the Psyche*. Trans. W. Ackerman. Santa Monica: Sigo Press. (Originally published (1966) in German as *Sandspiel*. Zurich: Rascher.) (First published (1971) in English as *Sandplay: Mirror of a Child's Psyche*. Trans. H. Kirsch. San Francisco: Browser Press.)

Kanter, R. (1982). The middle manager as innovator. *Harvard Business Review, 60*(*4*), 95-105. Cited in D.P. Schultz, & S.E. Schultz (1994). *Psychology and Work Today: An Introduction to Industrial and Organizational Psychology*. New York: Macmillan.

Kaplan-Williams, S. (1985). *The Jungian-Senoi Dreamwork Manual.* Berkeley CA: Journey Press.

Kaplan-Williams, S. (1992). *Dreamworking.* San Fransisco CA: Journey Press. The work of Kaplan-Williams tends to be very respectful of the client and does not impose external meaning on symbols for individuals.

Katchadourian, H. (1972). *Fundamentals of Human Sexuality.* New York: Holt, Rinehart and Winston. An excellent all round resource in the field of human sexuality. This text does justice to all areas covered: biology of human sexuality; sexual behaviour, sexual development, variations and deviations; sex and culture. The text continues to be updated and reissued in new editions. The 1972 edition has some of the best material on history and culture.

Kazdin, A.E. (1988). *Child Psychotherapy: Developing and Identifying Effective Treatments.* New York: Pergamon Press.

Keleman, S. (1979). *Somatic Reality.* Berkeley, CA: Center Press.

Keller, K. (1991). Legal requirements for the use of phytopharmaceutical drugs in the Federal Republic of Germany. *Journal Ethnopharamacol, 32,* 225-229.

Kilcommons, B. & Wilson, S. (1995). *Good Owners, Great Cats.* New York: Warner Books.

Kissel, S. (1990). *Play Therapy: A Strategic Approach.* Springfield IL: Charles C. Thomas.

Klein, J.A. & Posey, P.A. (1986). Good supervisors are good supervisors—anywhere. *Harvard Business Review, 64(6),* 125-128 cited in Schultz, D.P. & Schultz, S.E. (1994). *Psychology and Work Today: An Introduction to Industrial and Organizational Psychology.* New York: Macmillan.

Kline, S. (1993). *Out of the Garden: Toys and Children's Culture in the Age of TV Marketing.* Toronto: Garamond Press.

Knell, S. (1993). *Cognitive-Behavioral Play Therapy.* Northvale NJ: Aronson.

Koocher, G. & Broskowski, A. (1977). Issues in the evaluation of mental health services for children. *Professional Psychology, 8,* 583-592.

Koocher, G. & D'Angelo, E.J. (1992). Evolution of practice in child psychotherapy. In D.K. Freedheim (Ed.). *History of Psychotherapy.* Washington DC: American Psychological Association.

Kramer, E. (1971). *Art As Therapy With Children.* New York: Schocher Books.

Krauss, D.A., & Fryrear, J. (1983). *Phototherapy in Mental Health.* Springfield IL: Charles C. Thomas. Interesting approach to access inner material through the use of photographs.

Laing, R.D. (1967). *The Politics of Experience and The Bird of Paradise.* Middlesex, England: Penguin.

Laing, R.D. (1969). *The Politics of the Family.* Toronto: Canadian Broadcasting Corporation Publications.

Laing, R.D. (1970). *Knots.* Middlesex, England: Penguin.

Laing, R.D. (1982). *The Voice of Experience: Experience, Science and Psychiatry.* Middlesex, England: Penguin.

Lamb, M. (1990). *2 Minutes a Day for a Greener Planet.* Toronto: Harper Collins.

Landman, J.T. & Dawes, R.M. (1982). Psychotherapy outcome: Smith and Glass' conclusions stand up to scrutiny. *American Psychologist, 37,* 504-516.

Langs, R. (1988). *Decoding Your Dreams.* New York: Ballantine.

Lanning, K.V. (1989, October). Satanic, occult, ritualistic crime: A law enforcement perspective. *Police Chief*, National Center for the Analysis of Violent Crime—FBI Academy.

Laudenslager, M.L. & Reite, M.L. (1984). Losses and separations: Immunological consequences an health implications. In P. Shaver (Ed.). *Review of Personality an Social Psychology: Emotions, Relationships, and Health*, pp. 285-312. Beverly Hills: Sage Publications.

Laughingbird, G. (1978). The healing sounds of Patricia Sun. In E. Bauman, A.I, Brint, L. Piper, & P.A. Wright (Eds.) *The Holistic Health Handbook*, pp. 274-280. Berkeley CA: And/Or Press.

Lazarus, A.A. (1990). If this be research. *American Psychologist*, *37*, 504-516.

Leach, P. (1994). *Children First: What Our Society Must Do—and Is Not Doing—For Our Children Today*. New York: Alfred A. Knopf.

Lebo, D. (1952). The present status of research on nondirective play therapy. *Journal of Consulting Psychology*, *17*, 177-183.

Leboyer, F. (1976). *Loving Hands—The Traditional Indian Art of Baby Massage.* New York: Alfred A. Knopf.

Lenett, R. & Crane, B. (1985). *It's O.K. To Say No!* New York: Tom Doherty Associates. A fun yet very serious book for parents and children. The book's subtitle says it well: "A parent/child manual for the protection of children." A number of stories and scenarios are presented for discussion that will help children learn to be street safe.

Lenett, R. & Barthelme, D. with Crane, B. (1986). *Sometimes It's O.K. To Tell Secrets.* New York: Tom Doherty Associates. A companion book to *It's O.K. To Say No!*, this is another excellent selection of stories and scenarios for discussion that will help children learn the dangers of sexual abuse without frightening them into a shell.

Lester, P.F. (1995). *Aviation Weather*. Englewood CO: Jeppesen Sanderson.

Levinson, B. (1969). *Pet-Oriented Child Psychotherapy.* Springfield IL: Charles C. Thomas. Levinson is the pioneer in the field of "pet therapy." This is one of the earliest, or the earliest legitimate, work on the subject ever published.

Levinson, B. (1972). *Pets and Human Development*. Springfield IL: Charles C. Thomas.

Levitt, E.E. (1957). The results of psychotherapy with children: An evaluation. *Journal of Consulting Psychology*, *21*, 189-196.

Levitt, E.E. (1963). Psychotherapy with children: A further evaluation. *Behavior Research and Therapy*, *1*, 45-51.

Levy, D. (1938). Release therapy in young children. *Psychiatry*, *1*, 387-389.

Levy, S.J, & Rutter, E. (1992). *Children of Drug Abusers*. Toronto: Lexington Books.

Liedloff, Jean (1985). *The Continuum Concept.* Don Mills, ON: Addison-Wesley. The author offers a new understanding of how we have lost much of our natural well-being and shows us practical ways to regain it for our children and ourselves. In Liedoff's own words: "Once we fully recognize the consequences of our treatment of babies, children, one another, and ourselves, and learn to respect the real character of our species, we cannot fail to discover a great deal more of our potential for joy." Most highly recommended.

Lowenfeld, M. (1935). *Play In Childhood*. London: Victor Gollancz. Reprinted (1976) New York: John Wiley & Sons.

Lowenfeld, M. (1993). *Understanding Children's Sandplay: Lowenfeld's World Technique.* Cambridge: Margaret Lowenfeld Trust.

Lubimiv, G.P. (1994). *Wings for Our Children: Essentials of Becoming a Play Therapist.* Burnstown, Ontario: General Store Publishing House. This brief little text has some wonderful material in it dealing with termination, techniques and interactive stances.

Lynch, J.J., Fregin, G.F., Mackie, J.B., & Monroe, R.R. (1974). The effect of human contact on the heart activity of the horse. *Psychology, 11*, 472-478.

Lynch, J.J. & McCarthy, J.F. (1969). Social responding in dogs: Heart rate changes to person. *Psychology, 5*, 389-393.

Lynch, J.J. & McCarthy, J.F. (1977). The effect of petting on a classically conditioned emotional response. *Behavioral Research and Therapy, 5*, 55-62.

Lyons-Ruth, K. & Zeanah, C.H. (1993). The familiy context of infant mental health: Affective development in the primary caregiving relationship. In C.H. Zeanah (Ed.). *Handbook of Infant Mental Health*, pp. 14-37. New York: Guilford Press.

Maguire, J. (1985). *Creative Storytelling.* New York: McGraw-Hill.

Mails, T. E. (1988). *Secret Native American Pathways: A Guide to Inner Peace.* Tulsa, OK: Council Oak Books. Wonderful material from a Lutheran pastor who approaches another culture and religious orientation with a great deal of respect and a non-threatened, non-threatening attitude. Highly recommended.

Martel, S. (Ed.). (1981). *Direct Work With Children.* London: Bedford Square Press.

Masheder, M. (1994). Play and creativity. In J. Thomson (Ed.). *Natural Childhood*, pp. 126-213. Toronto: Simon & Schuster.

Masson, J.M. (1988). *Against Therapy: Emotional Tyranny and the Myth of Psychological Healing.* New York: Athenium.

Matthews, C. (1989). *The Elements of The Celtic Tradition.* Worcester, Great Britain: Element Books.

May, R. (1981). *Freedom and Destiny.* New York: W.W. Norton & Company. This text, although not related specifically to the field of child psychology or child therapy, is a highly recommended study on freedom, responsibility, limits, and boundaries. It has definite implications for our understanding of children and their own needs for protection, limits, choices, and responsbilties.

McCall, M.W., Jr., & Lombardo, M.M. (1983, February). What makes a top executive? *Psychology Today*, 26-31. Cited in D.P. Schultz, & S.E. Schultz (1994). *Psychology and Work Today: An Introduction to Industrial and Organizational Psychology.* New York: Macmillan.

McIntyre, M. (1988). *Sandplay: A Tool of Therapy.* Unpublished master's thesis. University of Waterloo, Waterloo ON, Canada.

McVicar, J. (1994). *Herbs for the Home: A Definitive Sourcebook to Growing and Using Herbs.* Toronto: Penguin.

Mead, M. (1935). *Sex and Temperament in Three Primitive Societies.* New York: William Morrow.

Mead, M. (1949). *Male and Female: A Study of the Sexes in a Changing World.* New York: William Morrow. A classic study on human sexual behavior, sex role stereotyping, cross cultural behaviours and modern sex roles.

Meehl, P.E. (1973). Why I do not attend case conferences. *Psychodiagnosis: Selected Papers*. New York: Norton.

Meighan, R. (1994). Education and schooling. In Thomson, J. (Ed.). *Natural Childhood*, pp. 290-335. Toronto: Simon and Schuster.

Mendell, A.E. (1983). Play therapy with children of divorced parents. In C.E. Schaefer & K.J. O'Connor (Eds.). *Handbook of Play Therapy*, pp. 320-354. John Wiley & Sons.

Meyer, K. (1913). *Ancient Irish Poetry*. London: Constable and Company. Republished by Constable and Company, 1994.

Mills, A. (1995, September 9). School Issues: The Kingston Area's four "generals" of education know there is a lot riding on any decisions that will affect the students in their charge. *The Kingston Whig Standard*, p 3. Kingston, Ontario.

Mills, J.C. & Crowley, R.J. (1986). *Therapeutic Metaphors for Children and the Child Within*. New York: Brunner/Mazel.

Mitchell, R.R. & Friedman, H.S. (1994). *Sandplay: Past, Present & Future*. New York: Routledge. A thorough and broad overview of the treatment method known as sandplay.

Monks of New Skete. (1991). *The Art of Raising a Puppy*. Toronto: Little, Brown & Company.

Montague, A. (1986). *Touching: The Human Significance of Skin* (3rd ed.). New York: Harper & Row.

Montour, S. (1992). *Eagle Child*. Ohsweken ON: Ganohkwa Sra Publications. *Eagle Child* is available from Ganohkwa Sra, Family Assault Support Services, P.O. Box 257, Ohsweken, Ontario, Canada, N0A 1M0, phone (519) 445-4324, fax (519) 445-4825.

Montour, S. (1993). *Eagle Child Book 2*. Ohsweken ON: Ganohkwa Sra Publications.

Moore, R. (1991). *Awakening the Hidden Storyteller: How To Build a Storytelling Tradition in Your Family*. Boston MA: Shambhala.

Morris, R.J. & Kratochwill, T.R. (1985). Behavioral treatment of children's fears and phobias: A review. *School Psychology Review*, *14*, 84-93.

Moss, D.C. (1988, December). "Real" dolls too suggestive. *American Bar Association Journal*, 24-26.

Moustakas, C. (1959). *Psychotherapy With Children*. New York: Harper & Row.

Mrazek, P.J. (1993). Maltreatment and infant development. In C.H. Zeanah (Ed.). *Handbook of Infant Mental Health*, pp. 159-170. New York: Guilford Press.

Nathan, D. (1991). *Women and Other Aliens*. El Paso: Cinco Puntos Press.

Nathan, D. (1995). *Satan's Silence: Ritual Abuse and the Making of a Modern American Witch Hunt*. New York: BasicBooks.

National Museum of Science and Technology. (1991). *The Amazing Potato: History and Culture*. Ottawa, Canada: Government of Canada.

Nelson, R.E. & Galas, J.C. (1994). *The Power to Prevent Suicide: A Guide for Teens Helping Teens*. Minneapolis: Free Spirit Publishing. This is a highly recommended text, not just for "teens helping teens," but for anyone involved in the helping professions. It is clear, concise, full of highly recommended suggestions, and completely free of mystified jargon behind which mental health professionals sometimes hide.

Newhouse, S. & Amodeo, J. (1978). Native American healing. In E. Bauman, A.I. Brint, L. Piper, & P.A. Wright (Eds.) *The Holistic Health Handbook*, pp. 64-70. Berkeley CA: And/Or Press.

Nieberg, H.A., & Fischer, A. (1996). *Pet Loss: A Thoughtful Guide for Adults and Children*. New York: HarperCollins.

Nilsson, L. (1977). *A Child is Born*. New York: Delacourte Press.

Noll, R. (1994). *The Jung Cult: Origins of a Charismatic Movement*. Princeton NJ: Princeton University Press.

Oaklander, V. (1978). *Windows To Our Children*. Highland NY: Gestalt Journal Press. Violet Oaklander, a psychologist, has put together a wonderful "toolchest" of methods that is most beneficial to both the beginning practitioner and seasoned professional. She thoroughly deals with the therapeutic process without getting bogged down in professional jargon, mystified theory or degrading arrogance so rampant in the mental health field.

O'Connell Higgins, G. (1995). *Resilient Adults: Overcoming a Cruel Past*. Scarborough, Ontario: Prentice-Hall.

O'Connor, K.J. (1991). *The Play Therapy Primer*. New York: John Wiley & Sons.

Odent, M. (1986). *Primal Health: A Blueprint for Survival*. New York: Century Hutchinson.

O'Driscoll, R. (Ed.) (1981). *The Celtic Consciousness*. Toronto: McClelland and Stewart.

Ofshe, R. & Watters, E. (1994). *Making Monsters: False Memories, Psychotherapy, and Sexual Hysteria*. Toronto: Charles Scribner's Sons.

O hOgain, D. (1991). *Myth, Legend & Romance: An Encyclopaedia of the Irish Folk Tradition*. New York: Prentice-Hall.

Okabe, T., Takahashi, K., & Richardson, E. (1990). The Japanese. In N. Waxler Morrison, J. Anderson, & E. Richardson (Eds.). *Cross Cultural Caring: A Handbook for Professionals*, pp.116-140. Vancouver: UBC Press.

Oldfield, L. (1994). The unfolding world. In J. Thomson (Ed.). *The Natural Child*, pp. 214-265. Toronto: Simon & Schuster.

O'Toole, P. (1990, March 17). You don't have to be Irish: The symbolism of St. Patrick's Day. *The Kingston Whig-Standard*, 8. Kingston, Ontario.

Payne, H. (1988). The use of dance movement therapy with troubled youth. In C.E. Schaefer (Ed.). *Innovative Interventions in Child and Adolescent Therapy*, pp. 68-97. New York: John Wiley & Sons.

Pearce, J.C. (1977). *Magical Child*. New York: Penguin.

Pearce, S. (1991). The bond: Understanding pet power. *Dogs Annual In Canada*, *82*, 18-23.

Phillips, F.B. (1990). NTU psychotherapy: An Afrocentric approach. *Journal of Black Psychology*, *17*, 1, 55-74.

Phillips, R. (1985). Whistling in the dark?: A review of play therapy research. *Psychotherapy*, *22*, 752-760.

Piaget, J. (1952). *The Origins of Intelligence in Children*. New York: International Universities Press.

Piaget, J. (1962). *Play, Dreams and Imitation in Childhood*. New York: International Universities Press.

Piaget, J. & Inhelder, B. (1969). *The Psychology of the Child*. New York: Basic Books.

Pinkson, T.J. (1978). Native American consciousness: A modern survival paradigm. In Bauman, E., Brint, A.I., Piper, L., Wright, P.A. (Eds.). *The Holistic Health Handbook*, pp. 71-76. Berkeley CA: And/Or Press.

Poznanski, E.O. (1982). The clinical phenomenology of childhood depression. *The American Journal of Orthopsychiatry, 52*(*2*), 308-313.

Prescott, J.H. (1971). Early somatosensory deprivation as an ontogenetic process in the abnormal development of the brain and behavior. In E.I. Goldsmith and J. Moor-Jankowski (Eds.). *Medical Primatology*, pp. 1-20. New York: S. Karger.

Prescott, J.H. (1975, April). Body pleasure and the origins of violence. *The Futurist*, 64-74.

Prescott, J.W. & Wallace, D. (1976). Developmental sociobiology and the origins of aggressive behavior. Paper presented at the *XXIst International Congress of Psychology*, July 18-25, Paris.

Psychology Today Staff. (1995). How to build a dream: Dreams have no inherent meaning—but they do have lots of emotion. *Psychology Today*, *28*(*6*), 47-54, 62.

Rabinowitz, D. (1990, May). From the mouths of babes to a jail cell. *Harper's Magazine*, 52-63. A very challenging article for mental health professionals.

Rae, W., Worchel, F., Uupchurch, J., Sanner, J., & Daniel, C. (1989). The psychosocial impact of play on hospitalized children. *Journal of Pediatric Psychology*, *14*, 617-627.

Rainbow-Wind, S. (1978). T'ai Chi Ch'uan as a healing art. In Bauman, E., Brint, A.I., Piper, L., & Wright, P.A. (Eds). *The Holistic Health Handbook*, pp. 359-361. Berkely CA: And/Or Press.

Rank, O. (1936). *Will Therapy*. New York: Knopf.

Reams, R. & Friedrich, W. (1994). The efficacy of time-limited play therapy with maltreated preschoolers. *Journal of Clinical Psychology, 50*(*6*), 889-899.

Reed, J.P. (1975). *Sand Magic Experience in Miniatures: A Non-Verbal Therapy for Children* (2nd ed.). New York: Lexington Books.

Reich, C.A. (1971). *The Greening of America*. New York: Bantam.

Reichard, G. (1977). *Navajo Medicine Man Sandpaintings*. New York: Dover.

Reichert, E. (1994). Play and animal-assisted therapy: A group-treatment model for sexually abused girls ages 9-13. *Family Therapy*, *21*(*1*), 55-62.

Reisman, J.M. & Ribordy, S. (1993). *Principles of Psychotherapy with Children* (2nd ed.). New York: Lexington Books.

Rienow, R. & Train Rienow, L. (1967). *Moment in the Sun: A Report on the Deteriorating Quality of the American Environment*. New York: Ballantine Books.

Robins, D. (1988). *The Secret Language of Stone*. London: Rider. A fascinating look at the mysteries of stone, the search for the mechanism behind "power" contained in stone and how stone has been used in different cultures. A highly respected solid state chemist and archeologist, Dr. Robins is internationally recognized for his development of the technique of electron spin resonance as an archaeological analytic tool and has more recently been involved in energy anomaly research. This text takes some of the beliefs behind the use of stones in ancient and modern healing ceremonies out of the new age parapsychology field and into modern scientific examination.

Robson, K.S. (Ed.) (1994). *Manual of Clinical Child and Adolescent Psychiatry* (Rev. ed.). Washington DC: American Psychiatric Press.

Rogers, F. (1988). *When A Pet Dies*. New York: Putnam.

Rogers, L., TenHouten, W., Kaplan, C., & Gardner, M. (1977). Hemispheric specialization in language: An EEG study of bi-lingual Hopi Indian children. *International Journal of Neuroscience*, *8*, 1-6.

Rosen, C., Faust, J. & Burns, W.J. (1994). The evaluation of process and outcome in individual child psychotherapy. *International Journal of Play Therapy*, *2*, 33-43.

Ross, P. (1991). The family puppet technique: For assessing parent-child and family interaction patterns. In C.E. Schaefer, K. Gitlin, & A. Sandgrund (Eds.). *Play Diagnosis and Assessment*, pp. 609-616. Toronto: Wiley-Interscience.

Rozman, D. (1976). *Meditation for Children*. Boulder Creek CA: University of the Tree Press.

Rubin, J. (1984). *The Art of Art Therapy*. New York: Brunner/Mazel.

Russ, S.W. (1995). Play psychotherapy research. In T.H. Ollendick & R.J. Prinz (Eds.). *Advances in Clinical Child Psychology, Volume 17*, pp. 365-391. New York: Plenum Press.

Sadeh, A. & Anders, T.F. (1993). Sleep disorders. In C.H. Zeanah (Ed.). *Handbook of Infant Mental Health*, pp. 305-316. New York: Guilford Press.

Saltz, E., Dixon, D. & Johnson, J. (1977). Training disadvantaged preschoolers on various fantasy activities: Effects on cognitive functioning and impulse control. *Child Development*, *48*, 367-380.

Sapolsky, R.M. (1994). *Why Zebras Don't Get Ulcers: A Guide to Stress, Stress-related Diseases, and Coping*. New York: W. H. Freeman.

Sattler, J.M. (1992). *Assessment of Children* (3rd Ed.). San Diego: Jerome M. Sattler Publisher.

Schaefer, C.E. & O'Connor, K.J. (Eds.). (1983). *Handbook of Play Therapy*. New York: John Wiley & Sons.

Schaefer, D. & Lyons, C. (1993). *How Do We Tell The Children: A Step-By-Step Guide for Helping Children Two to Ten Cope When Someone Dies*. New York: Newmarket Press.

Schmidtchen, S., & Hobrucker, B. (1978). The efficiency of client-centered play therapy. *Praxis Der Kinderpsychologie and Kinderpsychiatric, 27(4)*, 117-125.

Schultz, D.P. & Schultz, S.E. (1992). *A History of Modern Psychology* (5th Ed.). Fort Worth: Harcourt Brace Jovanovich.

Schultz, D.P. & Schultz, S.E. (1994). *Psychology and Work Today: An Introduction to Industrial and Organizational Psychology*. New York: Macmillan.

Scott, S. & Richards, M. (1981). Nursing low-birthweight babies on lambswool. *The Lancet*, *12*, 1028.

Seeman, J., Barry, E., & Ellinwood, C. (1964). Interpersonal assessment of play therapy outcome. *Psychotherapy: Theory, Research, and Practice, 1*(2), 64-66.

Seligman, M.E.P. (1995). *The Optimistic Child*. New York: Houghton Mifflin.

Selman, R. (1980). *Interpersonal Understanding*. New York: Academic Press.

Selye, H. (1974). *Stress Without Distress*. New York: Lippincott.

Sgroi, S. (1982). *Handbook of Clinical Intervention in Child Sexual Abuse*. Toronto: Lexington Books.

Shamoo, T.K. & Patros, P.G. (1990). *Helping Your Child Cope with Depression and Suicidal Thoughts*. Toronto: Lexington Books.

Sharkey, J. (1979). *Celtic Mysteries: The Ancient Religion*. New York: Thames and Hudson.

Sinclair, M. (1992). *Massage for Healthier Children*. Oakland CA: Wingbows Press.

Sisson, E. (1982). *Nature with Children of All Ages*. New York: Prentice Hall.

Skolimowski, H. (1993). *A Sacred Place To Dwell: Living With Reverence Upon The Earth*. Rockport MA: Element Books.

Sloan, J., Rivera, F., Reay, D., Ferris, J., & Kellerman, A. (1990). Firearm regulations and rates of suicide: A comparison of two metropolitan areas. *New England Journal of Medicine*, *322*, 369-373.

Smilansky, S. (1986). *The Effects of Sociodramatic Play on Disadvantaged Preschool Children*. New York: Wiley.

Smith, B. & Sechrest, L. (1991). The treatment of aptitude x treatment interactions. *Journal of Consulting and Clinical Psychology*, *59*, 233-244.

Smith, M.L. & Glass, G.V. (1977). Meta-analysis of psychotherapy outcome studies. *American Psychologist*, *32*, 752-760.

Smith, M.L., Glass, G.V. & Miller, T.I. (1980). *The Benefits of Psychotherapy*. Baltimore: Johns Hopkins University Press.

Soloman, J. (1938). Active play therapy. *American Journal of Orthopsychiatry*, *8*, 479-498.

Starhawk (1979). *The Spiral Dance*. San Francisco, Harper & Row.

Stein, D.M., & Lambert, M.J. (1984). On the relationship between therapist experience and psychotherapy outcome. *Clinical Psychology Review*, *4*, 127-142.

Stein, S. (1993). *Noah's Garden: Restoring the Ecology of Our Own Back Yards*. Boston: Houghton Mifflin.

Stern, D.N. (1985). *The Interpersonal World of the Infant: A View from Psychoanalysis and Developmental Psychology*. New York: Basic Books.

Stillerman, E. (1992). *Mother Massage: A Handbook for Relieving the Discomforts of Pregnancy*. New York: Delta.

Strauss, M.B. (1994). *Violence in the Lives of Adolescents*. New York: W.W. Norton.

Strupp, H.H. & Hadley, S.W. (1979). Specific versus nonspecific factors in psychotherapy. *Archives of General Psychiatry*, *36*, 1125-1136.

Szasz, T.S. (1980). *Sex By Prescription*. Garden City NY: Anchor Press/Doubleday. An outstanding and, as often is the case with Dr. Szasz's work, controversial book which serves as a focus of reality in the face of the questionable (yet largely unquestioned) and at times ludicrous field of sex therapy. There is interesting and challenging material here in a chapter concerning sex education for children.

Szasz, T.S. (1987). *Insanity: The Idea and Its Consequences*. Toronto: John Wiley & Sons. A must for anyone having anything to do with the field of mental health. An excellent critique of our typical ways of perceiving and doing things in this field.

Szasz, T.S. (1988). *The Myth of Psychotherapy*. Syracuse NY: Syracuse University Press.

Szasz, T.S. (1989). *Law, Liberty, and Psychiatry*. Syracuse NY: Syracuse University Press.

Szasz, T.S. (1990). *The Untamed Tongue: A Dissenting Dictionary*. La Salle IL: Open Court Publishing.

Szasz, T.S. (1994). *Cruel Compassion: Psychiatric Control of Society's Unwanted.* New York: John Wiley & Sons.

Taft, J. (1933). *The Dynamics of Therapy in a Controlled Relationship.* New York: Macmillan.

Takacs, V.R. (1993). Talking with rocks. *Playground, Spring,* 5-6. A most useful play therapy technique created by the author. Helpful in allowing children to be in touch with themselves and with nature.

Takacs, V.R. (1995). For an expecting mother. In M. Barnes & B. Revell, *Self Discovery Through Inner Play,* pp. 87-88. Ottawa, Canada: Viktoria, Fermoyle & Berrigan Publishing House.

Terr, L. (1983). Play therapy and psychic trauma: A preliminary report. In C.E. Schaefer & K.J. O'Connor (Eds.). *Handbook of Play Therapy,* pp. 308-319. New York: Wiley.

Terr, L. (1988). What happens to memories of early trauma? A study of twenty children under age five at the time of documented traumatic events. *Journal of the American Academy of Child and Adolescent Psychiatry, 27,* 96-104.

Terr, L. (1990). *Too Scared to Cry.* New York: Harper & Row.

Terr, L. (1991). Childhood traumas: An outline and overview. *American Journal of Psychiatry, 148,* 10-20.

Thevenin, T. (1987). *The Family Bed: An Age-Old Concept in Child-Rearing.* Minneapolis: Avery.

Thomas, A. & Chess, S. (1980). *The Dynamics of Psychological Development.* New York: Brunner/Mazel.

Thomson, J. (Ed.). (1994). *Natural Childhood.* Toronto: Simon & Schuster.

Trungpa, C. (1984). *Shambhala: The Sacred Path of the Warrior.* Boulder CO: Shambala Publications.

Verny, T. (1981). *The Secret Life of the Unborn Child.* New York: Delta. Very interesting reading for expectant parents or for those who work in obstetrics. Well documented material in the new and, at times, controversial, field of prenatal and perinatal psychology.

Verny, T.R. & Weintraub, P. (1991). *Nurturing the Unborn Child: A Nine-Month Program for Soothing, Stimulating, and Communicating With Your Baby.* New York: Delacorte.

Von Franz, M.L. (1970). *Interpretation of Fairy Tales.* Dallas: Spring.

Wadeson, H. (1980). *Art Psychotherapy.* New York: Wiley-Interscience. A good reference in the field of art therapy. However, a great deal of mumbo jumbo gets read into the work of others so this must be included in the category of "interesting, but take it with a grain of salt."

Walker, B.G. (1983). *The Woman's Encyclopedia of Myths and Secrets.* San Francisco: Harper & Row.

Walker, B.G. (1988). *The Woman's Dictionary of Symbols and Sacred Objects.* San Francisco: Harper & Row.

Walker, B.G. (1989). *The Book of Sacred Stones.* San Fransisco: Harper & Row. Debunks new age beliefs and tall tales surrounding crystal mysticism and brings things into workable perspective. The author looks upon stones and crystals for what they are – wonderful creations – and proceeds to completely debunk new age beliefs in the use of numerous stones and crystals.

Walker, L. (1988). *Handbook on Sexual Abuse of Children.* New York: Springer Publishing Company.

Walker, P. (1988). *The Book of Baby Massage.* New York: Simon & Schuster.

Wallace Budge, E.A. (Trans.). (1967). *The Egyptian Book of the Dead: The Papyrus of Ani.* New York: Dover. Originally published in 1895 by the Trustees of the British Museum.

Walsh, D.A. (1994). *Selling Out America's Children: How America Puts Profits Before Values—And What Parents Can Do.* Minneapolis: Fairview Press.

Wassil-Grimm, C. (1995). *Diagnosis for Disaster: The Devastating Truth About False Memory Syndrome and its Impact on Accusers and Families.* Woodstock NY: The Overlook Press.

Waxler-Morrison, N., Anderson, J., & Richardson, E. (Eds.). (1990). *Cross Cultural Caring: A Handbook for Health Professionals.* Vancouver: UBC Press.

Webster-Doyle, T. (1988). *Facing the Double Edged Sword.* Ojai CA: Atrium Publications. A book about children's inner and outer conflicts and how to resolve them in a non-violent manner. The philosophy stresses the importance of understanding one's inner feelings and the causes of violence and of developing the skills to resolve conflict non-violently. The book is easily understood by both adults and children. Included are chapters on roleplaying non-violent alternatives and one for parents and teachers on positive conflict resolution skills.

Weinrib, E. (1983). *Images of the Self: The Sandplay Therapy Process.* Boston: Sigo Press. Once again, although this is a very valuable resource book, at times an awful lot gets read into the scenes of clients where numerous alternate interpretations could be just as relevant. Despite this, the book is worth owning as one of the pioneering efforts in the sandplay technique.

Weisz, J.R. & Weiss, B. (1989). Assessing the effects of clinical-based psychotherapy with children and adolescents. *Journal of Consulting and Clinical Psychology, 57*, 741-746.

Weisz, J.R. & Weiss, B. (1993). *Effects of Psychotherapy with Children and Adolescents.* Newbury Park CA: Sage.

Weisz, J.R., Weiss, B., Alicke, M.D., & Klotz, M.L. (1987). Effectiveness of psychotherapy with children and adolescents: A meta-analysis for clinicians. *Journal of Consulting and Clinical Psychology, 55*, 542-549.

Wells, H.G. (1911). *Floor Games.* London: Palmer. Reprinted (1976) New York: Arno Press.

Wexler, R. (1990). *Wounded Innocents: The Real Victims of the War Against Child Abuse.* New York: Prometheus Books.

WGBH-PBS-TV (1980, December 9). A touch of sensitivity. *Nova.* Boston MA.

White, J. & Allers, C.T. (1994). Play therapy with abused children: A review of the literature. *Journal of Counseling & Development, 72(4)*, 390-394.

Wicks, B. (1995). *Born to Read.* Toronto: Ben Wicks.

Wilhelm, H. (1985). *I'll Always Love You.* New York: Crown Publishers. A beautiful little book about a young boy and the death of his dog. Excellent material for children grieving the loss of a pet.

Williams, M. (1984). *The Velveteen Rabbit*. New York: Holt, Rinehart and Winston. One of the great classics of children's literature. Life's hopes, hurts, and joys come alive in this beautifully illustrated edition of the story. The tale is about honesty, loyalty, being "REAL" and, above all, being loved.

Wilson, K., Kendrick, P., & Ryan, V. (1992). *Play Therapy: A Non-Directive Approach for Children and Adolescents*. London: Bailliere Tindall.

Winnicott, D.W. (1971). *Therapeutic Consultation in Child Psychiatry*. New York: Basic Books.

Winnicott, D.W. (1984). *The Child, The Family and the Outside World*. London: Norton.

Wolpe, J. (1958). *Psychotherapy By Reciprocal Inhibition*. Stanford CA: Stanford University Press.

Worwood, S.E. (1995). *Essential Aromatherapy: A Pocket Guide to Essential Oils & Aromatherapy*. San Rafael CA: New World Library.

Wright, M.S. (1987). *Behaving As If The God In All Life Mattered*. Warrenton VA: Perelandra.

Yavari, S. (1995). *A Study of Play Therapy Research, Methods and Assessment Tools*. Unpublished paper submitted in partial fulfilment of the requirements for an independent studies program in play therapy through the Canadian Play Therapy Institute, Kingston, Ontario, Canada.

Yeats, W.B. (1913). *The Celtic Twilight: Myth, Fantasy and Folklore*. Bridport, Great Britain: Prism Press. Republished, 1990.

Zeanah, C.H. (Ed.). (1993). *Handbook of Infant Mental Health*. New York: Guilford Press.

Index

About The Author

Mark Barnes is an internationally renowned lecturer and author in the field of child psychology and play therapy. He has travelled extensively presenting programs in play therapy, mental health and holistic issues throughout North America and the Pacific for numerous mental health organizations, educational institutions, churches, businesses and corporations. He was, with Cindy Taylor, the co-founder of the Canadian Association for Child and Play Therapy in 1985 and President of the Association from 1986-1990. He received the 1993 CACPT award for outstanding contribution to the field of play therapy, in 1995 was elected to the International Who's Who of Professionals, and in 1996 was awarded the PTI International Play Therapy Award for outstanding career contributions to child psychology and play therapy. He specializes in cross cultural healing processes. Beyond his undergraduate training in wildlife biology, psychology and geology, graduate degree in social work, and doctorate in psychology, he has also trained in Japanese shiatsu therapy, the Bach Flower Remedies and natural healing methods of the Irish Celts. He is a former director and faculty member of the Canadian Play Therapy Institute. Mark is a frequent speaker at international conferences and programs on child psychology, play therapy, and holistic issues and has been featured in many television, radio, newspaper and magazine interviews. His present practise is as an ecopsychologist studying humans in the natural world. His interests include many forms of music (playing and listening), flying (as a pilot), gardening, herbalism, wildlife, wolves, collecting natural healing artifacts, Celtic history and healing, rock collecting, anthropology, enjoying warm weather and Disney World.